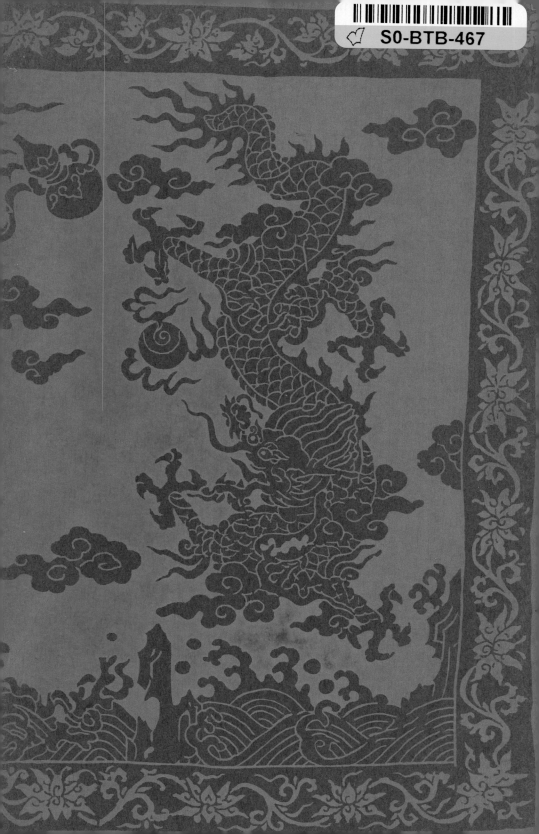

SHAMBHALA DRAGON EDITIONS

The dragon is an age-old symbol of the highest spiritual essence, embodying wisdom, strength, and the divine power of transformation. In this spirit, Shambhala Dragon Editions offers a treasury of readings in the sacred knowledge of Asia. In presenting the works of authors both ancient and modern, we seek to make these teachings accessible to lovers of wisdom everywhere.

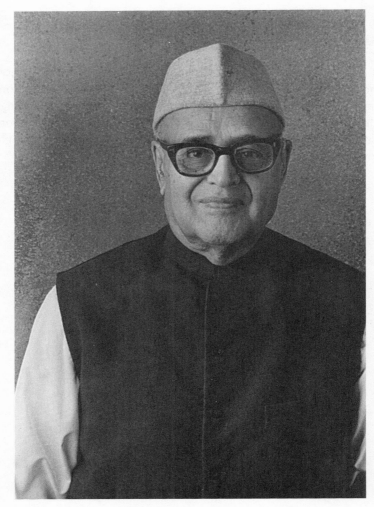

LIVING WITH KUNDALINI

The Autobiography of Gopi Krishna

EDITED BY LESLIE SHEPARD

SHAMBHALA
Boston & London
1993

Shambhala Publications, Inc.
Horticultural Hall
300 Massachusetts Avenue
Boston, Massachusetts 02115

9   8   7   6   5   4   3   2

Printed in the United States of America on acid free paper ⊚
Distributed in the United States by Random House, Inc.,
and in Canada by Random House of Canada Ltd

Library of Congress Cataloging-in-Publication Data

Gopi Krishna, 1903–
    Living with Kundalini: the autobiography of Gopi Krishna / edited
by Leslie Shepard.
        p.   cm.—(Shambhala dragon editions)
    ISBN 0-87773-947-1
    1. Gopi, Krishna, 1903–   .   2. Hindus—India—Biography.
3. Kuṇḍalinī.   I. Shepard, Leslie.   II. Title.
BL1175.G62A3   1993
294.5′092—dc20   93-21829
[B]   CIP

Contents

v

Editor's Foreword

THIS IS ONE of the most important books ever published.

This may seem like a sweeping claim when one considers the vast riches of literature—the revealed scriptures of various religions, the plays of Shakespeare, or the works of great novelists and religious geniuses. After all, this is the story of the life and philosophy of a very ordinary man, a minor Indian civil servant from Kashmir who failed in his college examinations. Yet this very ordinary man stumbled on the greatest secret of life, the key to that infinite ocean of consciousness from which all great geniuses and mystics draw inspiration. Throughout history, this secret has been known under many different names—*nirvana, samadhi, satori,* the Muslim concept of *hal,* mystic union, spiritual marriage, cosmic consciousness, God-realization.

It is one of the best-kept secrets, for the different paths to this supreme revelation have been obscured by the poetic metaphors and allegories of different faiths and philosophies, and many attempts to explain the ecstatic interpenetration of finite and infinite existence have failed, so that the experience itself has become legendary. Over centuries of material progress and scientific development, even the validity of the experience has been questioned or dismissed as a psychoneurotic phenomenon, half-believed in by the faiths of different religions whose very inception stemmed from the God-realization of inspired saints and sages. But that was all long ago and far away.

So for thousands of years, millions upon millions of men and women have struggled through life, richer or poorer, in sickness or health, without access to this great secret. They have known the joys and sorrows of life and sexual union, the rearing of children, suffered good and bad fortune, only to find at the end of their lives that everything in the material world—fame, fortune, wealth, possessions, and relationships—are all ephemeral and pass away at death. Even the consolations of religions have often dwindled to well-meaning platitudes or mere ritual and dogma, unable to cross the gap between life and death.

In modern times, under the banner of the New Age, there has been a new manifest hunger for something more meaningful in life than ambition, money, power or possessions. Hundreds of cults and revisionist religions have sprung up, claiming to offer transcendental meaning. Some, such as the Fundamentalist revivals in the Christian and Muslim worlds, have proved dangerous to world politics and peace, stirring up simplistic fanaticisms and racist empire building. Some of the New Age gurus have proven to be charlatans, enjoying the ego-satisfaction and adulation of thousands of devotees, misfit messiahs parroting the inspired teachings of the past but without any transcendental experience of their own. Other gurus have been dangerous messengers of death and destruction for their pathetically deluded followers, as with the cults of the Reverend Jim Jones, Charles Manson, or various neo-Satanist groups.

Another tragic blind alley was the Psychedelic Revolution, which promised cosmic consciousness in a capsule, but seduced millions of men, women and children into becoming dropouts, manipulated by an international cartel of Mafia-style crime barons and their empire of pushers.

Much of the New Age has been marked by trivial and banal novelties, with old and new gimmicks like astrology, tarot cards, the *I Ching*, crystals, and soothsayers, all enveloped in a stupefying heavy fog of incense and soporific music.

But the New Age and its mass media gurus at least revived the ancient Indian concept of kundalini, a latent energy in the universe and in the human body, the dynamic behind sexual expression and also, through meditation, the way to higher consciousness, with side effects of psychic phenomena. Although most of the time, the gurus were simply rehashing ancient teachings of the past as their own, without personal experience, the concept of kundalini is a true one. Only if you want to know about it, it is useless to follow teachers without real experience, who are only concerned with building their own reputations and cults. You will need to listen to someone with total experience of kundalini in both its negative and positive aspects, who knows its place in the evolution of the human race. This teacher is Pandit Gopi Krishna.

It is one of the ironies of fate that this supreme secret should have been revealed once more in modern times to an ordinary man, a gentle, modest individual without a cult, concerned only with sharing his transcendental knowledge with the rest of the world.

He founded no movement, demanded no money, refused to become the center of adoring crowds, and merely lived humbly in relative poverty, writing his inspired books about Kundalini and its place in human evolution.

The title "Pandit" is a traditional honorific bestowed on one who is recognized as an authority on a subject. Pandit Gopi Krishna is outstanding as an authority on Kundalini. There are few modern authorities on the subject who speak, as he does, from such detailed personal experience.

The beauty of the present work is that it describes in detail the stages of the awakening of the awesome power of kundalini in one individual, the years of struggle to balance and harmonize this force, the psychic gifts which it brought, and the validation of the subject in ancient treatises from India, China and other countries, and the mystery traditions of both East and West.

This autobiography opens with a prologue describing firsthand the incredible experience of the fabulous awakening of kundalini. The Pandit goes on to describe frankly the progress of this dynamic energy against the background of his daily life, the trials and agonies of taming the force, and harmonizing it, the paranormal side effects of prophecy and inspired verse, the obligation to live a socially productive life and share insights with the rest of humanity.

Much of this book is also a kind of protracted meditation on life

and the problems of our time. Inevitably there is some repetition of
thought or even occasional incoherence. His mind, or soul, if you
will, swamped by the total experience of higher consciousness often
struggles to express his insights through the limited apparatus of his
own simple education and background. If some of his perceptions
appear obvious or overstated, it is only because they are nonetheless
too important to overlook. At a time when atom bombs and global
pollution threaten the future of the human race and the planet itself,
it is proper to be reminded of those basic evolutionary laws that have
carried human beings from a primitive apelike existence to a high-
tech sophisticated modern society, and may yet, if properly observed,
carry us to an unimaginable splendid future, where individual
ambition is transformed into communal sharing, where knowledge
becomes wisdom, and a more profound and transcendental happiness replaces sensory satiation.

It has been an inspiring task for me to edit the Pandit's writings
into one autobiographical work. This book now contains all the
basic material formerly published in the earlier work *Kundalini: The
Evolutionary Energy in Man*, in a setting of later autobiographical
chapters written by the Pandit at different times of his busy life.

Editing this material has involved a few deletions and some minor
bridging phrases or sentences. Aside from routine editing of spelling
and punctuation, the only other changes to the original material
involve revision of hastily written passages and the use of outmoded
terms like *mankind*, where *human beings* or *humankind* are now
preferred usage.

In my own work as editor of the *Encyclopedia of Occultism and
Parapsychology* (3d ed., 2 vols., Detroit, 1991), I have studied the
stories of hundreds of mystics, psychics and other remarkable individuals. I can honestly affirm that I consider Pandit Gopi Krishna
one of the most important, since he belongs to the present time, and
his experiences provide guidance for the human race as a whole.
Moreover, I knew him personally and discussed with him many
issues of meaning and purpose in life. He remained an honest,

gentle, courteous, and modest man, anxious to avoid a cult following and desiring only to share his perceptions through his books.

Above all, he pleaded constantly for scientific validation of the kundalini phenomenon, claiming a biological basis for the changes in perception as evidence of an evolutionary development in human beings. It is unfortunate that while parapsychologists have spent much time and money testing and researching relatively trivial claimed phenomena of psychic gifts, no one was sufficiently interested to conduct research on the Pandit. Although much has been written on kundalini and transpersonal consciousness by cult leaders and by self-appointed authorities—all, in my opinion, equally lacking decisive experience of the subject—the opportunity of investigating a living subject has now been missed with the passing of Pandit Gopi Krishna.

Is this great secret to be lost to us again for more centuries? I think not. With books like the present one, as well as other important writings of the Pandit, we now know the way. He has charted in detail its disciplines, dangers, extraordinary physiology, and rewards in higher consciousness and ecstatically blissful experience. This book throws a flood of light on many enigmas of human existence, the true basis of great religions, and the possibilities of reconciliation between religion and science.

All that is needed now is study and practice.

Leslie Shepard

Acknowledgments

A GREAT DEAL OF SUSTAINED and complex hard work was necessary on the part of a group of friends of the late Pandit Gopi Krishna, in order to preserve and collate this autobiography. Special thanks are due to Michael Bradford, Margaret Kobelt, Philippe and Karen Minos, Dale and Paul Pond, Edie Siepi, and Janice St. Clair.

LIVING WITH KUNDALINI

INTRODUCTION

The Awakening of Kundalini

ONE MORNING DURING the Christmas of 1937 I sat cross-legged in a small room in a little house on the outskirts of the town of Jammu, the winter capital of the Jammu and Kashmir State in northern India. I was meditating with my face towards the window on the east through which the first gray streaks of the slowly brightening dawn fell into the room. Long practice had accustomed me to sit in the same posture for hours at a time without the least discomfort, and I sat breathing slowly and rhythmically, my attention drawn towards the crown of my head, contemplating an imaginary lotus in full bloom, radiating light.

I sat steadily, unmoving and erect, my thoughts uninterruptedly centered on the shining lotus, intent on keeping my attention from wandering and bringing it back again and again whenever it moved in any other direction. The intensity of concentration interrupted my breathing; gradually it slowed down to such an extent that at times it was barely perceptible. My whole being was so engrossed in the contemplation of the lotus that for several minutes at a time I lost touch with my body and surroundings. During such intervals I used to feel as if I were poised in midair, without any feeling of a body around me. The only object of which I was aware was a lotus of brilliant color, emitting rays of light. This experience has happened to many people who practice meditation in any form regularly for a sufficient length of time, but what followed on that fateful morning in my case, changing the whole course of my life and outlook, has happened to few.

During one such spell of intense concentration I suddenly felt a

1

strange sensation below the base of the spine, at the place touching the seat, while I sat cross-legged on a folded blanket spread on the floor. The sensation was so extraordinary and so pleasing that my attention was forcibly drawn towards it. The moment my attention was thus unexpectedly withdrawn from the point on which it was focused, the sensation ceased.

Thinking it to be a trick played by my imagination to relax the tension, I dismissed the matter from my mind and brought my attention back to the point from which it had wandered. Again I fixed it on the lotus, and as the image grew clear and distinct at the top of my head, again the sensation occurred. This time I tried to maintain the fixity of my attention and succeeded for a few seconds, but the sensation extending upwards grew so intense and was so extraordinary, as compared to anything I had experienced before, that in spite of myself my mind went towards it, and at that very moment it again disappeared. I was now convinced that something unusual had happened for which my daily practice of concentration was probably responsible.

I had read glowing accounts, written by learned men, of great benefits resulting from concentration, and of the miraculous powers acquired by yogis through such exercises. My heart began to beat wildly, and I found it difficult to bring my attention to the required degree of fixity. After a while I grew composed and was soon as deep in meditation as before. When completely immersed I again experienced the sensation, but this time, instead of allowing my mind to leave the point where I had fixed it, I maintained a rigidity of attention throughout. The sensation again extended upwards, growing in intensity, and I felt myself wavering; but with a great effort I kept my attention centered round the lotus.

Suddenly, with a roar like that of a waterfall, I felt a stream of liquid light entering my brain through the spinal cord.

Entirely unprepared for such a development, I was completely taken by surprise, but regaining self-control instantaneously, I remained sitting in the same posture, keeping my mind on the point of concentration. The illumination grew brighter and brighter, the roaring louder. I experienced a rocking sensation and then felt myself slipping out of my body, entirely enveloped in a halo of light.

It is impossible to describe the experience accurately. I felt the point of consciousness that was myself growing wider, surrounded by waves of light. It grew wider and wider, spreading outward while the body, normally the immediate object of its perception, appeared to have receded into the distance until I became entirely unconscious of it. I was now all consciousness, without any outline, without any idea of a corporeal appendage, without any feeling or sensation coming from the senses, immersed in a sea of light simultaneously conscious and aware of every point, spread out, as it were, in all directions without any barrier or material obstruction.

I was no longer myself, or to be more accurate, no longer as I knew myself to be, a small point of awareness confined in a body, but instead was a vast circle of consciousness in which the body was but a point, bathed in light and in a state of exaltation and happiness impossible to describe.

After some time, the duration of which I could not judge, the circle began to narrow down; I felt myself contracting, becoming smaller and smaller, until I again became dimly conscious of the outline of my body, then more clearly; and as I slipped back to my normal condition, I became suddenly aware of the noises in the street, felt again my arms and legs and head, and once more became my narrow self in touch with body and surroundings.

When I opened my eyes and looked about, I felt a little dazed and bewildered, as if coming back from a strange land completely foreign to me. The sun had risen and was shining full on my face, warm and soothing. I tried to lift my hands, which always rested in my lap, one upon the other, during meditation. My arms felt limp and lifeless. With an effort I raised them up and stretched them to enable the blood to flow freely. Then I tried to free my legs from the posture in which I was sitting and to place them in a more comfort-able position, but could not. They were heavy and stiff. With the help of my hands I freed them and stretched them out, then put my back against the wall, reclining in a position of ease and comfort.

What had happened to me? Was I the victim of a hallucination? Or had I by some strange vagary of fate succeeded where millions of others had failed? Was there, after all, really some truth in the oft-repeated claim of the sages and ascetics of India, made for thousands of years and verified and repeated generation after generation, that it was possible to apprehend transcendental reality in this life if one followed certain rules of conduct and practiced meditation in a certain way?

My thoughts were in a daze. I could hardly believe that I had experienced a vision of divinity. There had been an expansion of my own self, my own consciousness, and the transformation had been brought about by the vital current that had started from below the spine and found access to my brain through the backbone.

I recalled that I had read long ago in books on yoga of a certain vital mechanism called kundalini, connected with the lower end of the spine, which becomes active by means of certain exercises, and when once roused carries the limited human consciousness to transcendental heights, endowing the individual with incredible psychic and mental powers.

Had I been lucky enough to find the key to this wonderful mechanism, which was wrapped up in the legendary mist of ages, about which people talked and whispered without having once seen it in action in themselves or in others? I tried once again to repeat the experience, but was so weak and flabbergasted that I could not collect my thoughts sufficiently to induce a state of concentration.

My mind was in a ferment. I looked at the sun. Could it be that in my condition of extreme concentration I had mistaken it for the effulgent halo that had surrounded me in the superconscious state? I closed my eyes again, allowing the rays of the sun to play upon my face. No, the glow that I could perceive across my closed eyelids was quite different. It was external and had not that splendor. The light

I had experienced was internal, an integral part of enlarged consciousness, a part of my self.

I stood up. My legs felt weak and tottered under me. It seemed as if my vitality had been drained out. My arms were no better. I massaged my thighs and legs gently, and, feeling a little better, slowly walked downstairs. Saying nothing to my wife, I took my meal in silence and left for work. My appetite was not as keen as usual, my mouth appeared dry, and I could not put my thoughts into my work in the office. I was in a state of exhaustion and lassitude, disinclined to talk.

After a while, feeling suffocated and ill at ease, I left for a short walk in the street with the idea of finding diversion for my thoughts. My mind reverted again and again to the experience of the morning, trying to recreate in imagination the marvelous phenomenon I had witnessed, but without success. My body, especially the legs, still felt weak, and I could not walk for long. I took no interest in the people whom I met, and walked with a sense of detachment and indifference to my surroundings quite foreign to me. I returned to my desk sooner than I had intended and passed the remaining hours toying with my pen and papers, unable to compose my thoughts sufficiently to work.

When I returned home in the afternoon I felt no better. I could not bring myself to sit down and read, my usual habit in the evening. I ate supper in silence, without appetite or relish, and retired to bed. Usually I was asleep within minutes of putting my head to the pillow, but this night I felt strangely restless and disturbed. I could not reconcile the exaltation of the morning with the depression that sat heavily on me while I tossed from side to side on the bed. I had an unaccountable feeling of fear and uncertainty. At last in the midst of misgivings I fell asleep. I slept fitfully, dreaming strange dreams, and woke up after short intervals in sharp contrast to my usual deep, uninterrupted sleep.

After about 3:00 A.M. sleep refused to come. I sat up in bed for some time. Sleep had not refreshed me. I still felt fatigued and my thoughts lacked clarity. The usual time for my meditation was approaching. I decided to begin earlier so that I would not have the sun on my hands and face, and without disturbing my wife, went upstairs to my study. I spread the blanket, and sitting cross-legged as usual, began to meditate.

I could not concentrate with the same intensity as on the previous day, though I tried my best. My thoughts wandered, and instead of being in a state of happy expectancy I felt strangely nervous and uneasy. At last, after repeated efforts, I held my attention at the usual point for some time, waiting for results. Nothing happened and I began to feel doubts about the validity of my previous experience.

I tried again, this time with better success. Pulling myself together, I steadied my wandering thoughts and, fixing my attention on the crown, tried to visualize a lotus in full bloom as was my custom.

As soon as I arrived at the usual pitch of mental fixity, I again felt the current moving upward. I did not allow my attention to waver, and again with a rush and a roaring noise in my ears the stream of effulgent light entered my brain, filling me with power and vitality, and I felt myself expanding in all directions, spreading beyond the boundaries of flesh, entirely absorbed in the contemplation of a brilliant conscious glow, at one with it and yet not entirely merged in it. The condition lasted for a shorter duration than it had done the day before. The feeling of exaltation was not so strong. When I came back to normal, I felt my heart thumping wildly and there was a bitter taste in my mouth. It seemed as if a scorching blast of hot air had passed through my body. The feeling of exhaustion and weariness was more pronounced than it had been yesterday.

I rested for some time to recover my strength and poise. It was still dark. I had now no doubts that the experience was real and that the sun had nothing to do with the internal luster that I saw.

But, why did I feel uneasy and depressed? Instead of feeling exceedingly happy at my luck and blessing my stars, why had despondency overtaken me? I felt as if I were in imminent danger of something beyond my understanding and power, something intangible and mysterious, which I could neither grasp nor analyze. A heavy cloud of depression and gloom seemed to hang round me, rising from my own internal depths without relation to external circumstances. I did not feel I was the same man I had been but a few days before, and a condition of horror, on account of the inexplicable change, began to settle on me, from which, try as I might, I could not make myself free by any effort of my will.

Little did I realize that from that day onwards I was never to be my old normal self again, that I had unwittingly and without preparation or even adequate knowledge of it roused to activity the most wonderful and stern power in man, that I had stepped unknowingly upon the key to the most guarded secret of the ancients, and that thenceforth for a long time I had to live suspended by a thread, swinging between life on the one hand and death on the other, between sanity and insanity, between light and darkness, between heaven and earth.

ONE ======
Recollections of Childhood

I WAS BORN IN 1903 in the small village of Gairoo, about twenty miles from Srinagar, the capital of Kashmir. It was the parental home of my mother, and she went to stay there at the time of my birth to have the care and attention of her elder sister and brothers during her confinement. My father had constructed a small, two-storied hut of his own in their big compound. It was a humble structure, built of sun-dried bricks with a thatched roof and served as our residence for a long time: for the years of my childhood and afterwards at intervals, whenever, tired of the city, we returned for a breath of country air.

My first faint recollections of childhood circle round a medium-sized house in a quiet sector of the city of Srinagar. I can still recall a scene in which I was held tight in the arms of my oldest maternal uncle, who comforted me with soft, endearing words after a fit of prolonged weeping caused by the anger of my mother for having stayed out too long playing with the children. As I was the only son she never dressed me in fine clothes, to guard against the evil eye, nor allowed me long out of her sight for fear of mishaps.

Another indelible childhood memory is of a moonlit night with my mother and one of my maternal uncles, sleeping on an open-from-the-sides but roofed top of a small wooden cabin, used as a granary, a common structure in rural habitations in Kashmir. We had traveled all day on horseback on the way to the distant abode of a reputed hermit, but, failing to reach our destination at nightfall, had sought shelter in the house of a farmer, who accommodated us thus for the night.

I cannot recall the appearance of the saint, except that his long, matted hair fell on his shoulders as he sat cross-legged against one of the walls of his small room directly facing the door. I remember him taking me in his lap and stroking my hair, which my mother had allowed to grow long in conformity with a solemn vow she had taken not to apply scissors or razor to it except at the time of the sacred thread ceremony.*

Years later, when I had grown intelligent enough to understand her, my mother revealed to me the purpose of her visit to the saint. She said that years before he had appeared to her in a dream at a most anxious time. She had passed the preceding day in an extremely perturbed frame of mind caused by my inability to swallow anything owing to a swollen and badly inflamed throat. In the dream, the holy personage, of whose miraculous deeds she had heard astounding accounts from innumerable eyewitnesses, opened my mouth gently with his hand and touched its interior down to the throat softly with his finger. Then, making a sign to her to feed me, he had vanished from sight.

Awakening with a start, my mother pressed me close to her and to her immense relief felt me sucking and swallowing the milk without difficulty. Overjoyed at the sudden cure, which she attributed to the miraculous power of the saint, she then and there made a vow that she would go on a pilgrimage to his place of residence to thank him personally for the favor. Owing to household worries and other engagements she could not make the pilgrimage for some years and undertook it at a time when I was sufficiently grown up to retain a faint impression of the journey and the visit.

The more surprising part of the story is that, as my mother affirmed afterwards repeatedly, the hermit, at the very moment of our approach after entering the room, casually inquired whether I had been able to suck and swallow my milk after his visit to her in the dream. Wonderstruck, my mother had fallen prostrate at his feet, humbly invoking his blessings upon me.

---

*The *upanayana,* or investiture, with the sacred thread, is a Hindu religious ritual performed for a Brahmin youth in his eighth year. A loop of three strands of thread is placed over his head, supported on the left shoulder and hanging to the right hip, to the accompaniment of ritual prayers.

I cannot vouch for the miraculous part of the episode. All I can say is that my mother was veracious and critically observant in other things. I have related the episode merely as a faintly remembered incident of early childhood. Since then I have come across innumerable accounts of similar and even more incredible feats, narrated by trustworthy, highly intelligent eyewitnesses; but on closer investigation the bulk of the material was found to be too weakly supported to stand the force of rigid scientific inquiry. For a long time I lent no credence to such stories, and I can emphatically assert even today that a real yogi in touch with the other world, capable of producing genuine physical phenomena at will, is one of the rarest beings on earth.

Another remarkable event of my childhood at the age of eight, which I remember more vividly, occurred one day as I walked along a road in Srinagar in early spring on my way to the house of our religious preceptor. The sky was overcast and the road muddy, which made walking difficult.

All at once, with the speed of lightning, a sudden question, never thought of before, shot across my mind. I stood stock-still in the middle of the road confronted within to the depths of my being with the insistent inquiry, "What am I?", coupled with the pressing interrogation from every object without, "What does all this mean?" My whole being as well as the world around appeared to have assumed the aspect of an everlasting inquiry, an insistent, unanswerable interrogation, which struck me dumb and helpless, groping for a reply with all my strength until my head swam and the surrounding objects began to whirl and dance round me. I felt giddy and confused, hardly able to restrain myself from falling on the slimy road in a faint.

Steadying myself, I proceeded on my way, my childish mind in a ferment over the incident of which, at that age, I could not in the least understand the significance.

A few days later I had a remarkable dream in which I was given a glimpse of another existence, not as a child or as an adult but with a dream personality utterly unlike my usual one. I saw a heavenly spot, peopled by god-like, celestial beings, and myself bodiless, something quite different—diffused, ethereal—a stranger belonging to a different order and yet distinctly resembling and intimately close to me, my own self transfigured, in a gloriously bright and peaceful environment, the very opposite of the shabby, noisy surroundings in which I lived.

Because of its unique and extraordinarily vivid nature, the dream was so indelibly imprinted upon my memory that I can recall it distinctly even today. The recollection of the scene in later years was invariably accompanied by a feeling of wonder at, and a deep yearning for, the exotic, inexpressible happiness enjoyed for a brief interval. The dream was probably the answer to the overwhelming, unavoidable question that had arisen from my depths a few days before, the first irresistible call from the invisible other world which, as I came to know later, awaits our attention close at hand, always intimately near, yet, for those with their backs to it, farther away than the farthest star in the firmament.

In the year 1914 we migrated to Lahore, the capital of Punjab. In the same year I completed my primary education and had to seek admission to a high school. My father was receiving his pension from the government treasury in that town and he was required to present himself in person to receive it. Since his retirement from service we had been living in Kashmir and the treasury wished to satisfy itself that the pensioner was still alive as he had not been seen in person for a long time. When this formality was complied with, my father, for reasons of his own, refused to return immediately. This compelled my mother to stay on there, too.

From what my mother revealed to me about his active life in the service of the government, it was easy to see that my father was an extraordinary man, universally respected by all those who knew him. He was born in Amritsar, another important town of the Punjab, near Lahore. His ancestors were among the emigrants who fled from Kashmir to save themselves from the barbarous oppression which Kashmiri Hindus had to undergo for many centuries in their homeland. It was a terrible period. The atrocities committed on this historic community during this time rank among the most horrible in history. There was absolutely no protection for them from any outrage or indignity committed on them. Their houses could be plundered and their women outraged in broad daylight without let or hindrance. There was no court to hear their appeal and no police to heed the complaints.

In order to escape this terrible persecution, legions abjured the faith their ancestors had followed for thousands of years and submitted to conversion. Hundreds of families, disguising themselves, fled in terror, traversing the narrow tortuous mountain routes for weeks until they could draw a breath of relief outside the boundaries of the fear-ridden valley which was now a torture chamber and a slaughterhouse for them. Gruesome tales of the barbarities committed by the rulers on this defenseless population are still current in Kashmir.

The legend runs that only a small number of families of Kashmiri Hindus survived the massacre and all the present population of Kashmiri Pandits is descended from them. It was said that cartloads of sacred threads, which the Hindus wear, were collected and thrown into the Dal Lake from the decapitated bodies of the killed and tortured. Crowds of women committed suicide to escape the clutches of the ravishers. Women, it is said, carried lethal poisons in their pockets to be swallowed when no other way was left to save their honor.

My ancestors were among the refugees who settled in the Punjab. Others penetrated to more distant parts of India. They came friendless and penniless into their new surroundings, but with patient application and toil which adversity teaches and with their own native talent, soon adapted themselves to the changed conditions in the new places which they made their homes. The result was that not a few of them rose to eminent positions in the occupations or professions which they chose to adopt.

My father was born in 1855 and passed his childhood in Amritsar. He was an auditor in the service of the government when he came to Kashmir for the first time. There he joined the Public Works Department in Srinagar as an accountant, lent by the government of India to Kashmir. During that time the number of those with some knowledge of English and possessing administrative capabilities was very limited. Those who had the qualifications could easily obtain lucrative employment in the various departments of administration.

The first two marriages of my father proved unhappy. His first wife died soon after marriage and the second was mentally disoriented. The third was my mother. Born in 1877, she was sixteen years of age at the time of marriage in 1893 and my father was thirty-eight. The marriage proved very happy. In the whole course of my life I have seen few women as loyal and as devoted to their husbands as my mother remained to the end.

My father was brought up in a sophisticated, urban atmosphere and my mother in the simple, homely surroundings of a rustic village with a medieval mental climate and outlook. Every morning, when grown up, she went with other girls of the village to the nearby pasture, at the foot of the neighboring mountain to collect firewood and cow dung for the family. This daily hike of several miles, in the early hours of the morning, with a load on her head on her return journey, imparted to her body a symmetry of proportion, strength of muscle and ease of movement which lent an imposing form to her figure and continued to be a part of her personality to the last day of her life.

Born in a village, of a family of hardworking and God-fearing peasants, fate had destined her as a partner to a man considerably senior to her in age, hailing from Amritsar, at that time no less than six days journey by rail and cart from the place of her birth. The insecurity and lawlessness in the country had forced one of my forefathers to bid adieu to his cool native soil and to seek his fortune in the torrid plains of distant Punjab. There, changed in dress and speaking a different tongue, my grandfather and great-grandfather lived and prospered like other exiles of their kind, altered in all save their religious rites and customs and the unmistakable physiognomy of Kashmiri Brahmins.

My father, with a deep mystical vein in him, returned to the land of his ancestors when almost past his prime, to marry and settle there. Even during the most active period of his worldly life he was always on the lookout for yogis and ascetics reputed to possess occult powers, and never tired of serving them and sitting in their company to learn the secret of their marvelous gifts.

He was a firm believer in the traditional schools of religious discipline and yoga extant in India from the earliest times, which among all the numerous factors contributing to success allot the place of honor to renunciation, to the voluntary relinquishment of all worldly pursuits and possessions, to enable the mind, released from the heavy chains binding it to the earth, to plumb its own ethereal depths undisturbed by desire and passion.

The authority for such conduct emanates from the Vedas, nay, from the examples themselves set by the inspired authors of the Vedic hymns and the celebrated seers of the Upanishads, who, conforming to an established practice prevailing in the ancient society of Indo-Aryans, retired from the busy life of householders at the ripe age of fifty and above, sometimes accompanied by their consorts, to spend the rest of their lives in forest hermitages in uninterrupted meditation and preaching, the prelude to a grand and peaceful exit.

This unusual mode of passing the eve of life has exercised a deep fascination over countless spiritually inclined men and women in India and even now hundreds of accomplished and, from the worldly point of view, happily circumstanced family men of advanced age, bidding farewell to their otherwise comfortable homes and dutiful progeny, betake themselves to distant retreats to pass their remaining days peacefully in spiritual pursuits, away from the fret and fever of the world.

My father, an ardent admirer of this ancient ideal, which provides for many a refreshing contrast to the "dead-to-heaven and wed-to-earth" old age of today, chose for himself a recluse's life about twelve years after marriage, his gradually formed decision hastened by the tragic death of his firstborn son at the age of five. Retiring voluntarily from a lucrative government post before he was even fifty, he gave up all the pleasures and cares of life to shut himself in seclusion with his books, leaving the entire responsibility of managing the household on the inexperienced shoulders of his young wife.

She had suffered terribly. My father renounced the world when she was in her twenty-eighth year, the mother of three children, two daughters and a son. How she brought us up, with what devotion she attended to the simple needs of our austere father, who cut himself off completely from the world, never even exchanging a word with any of us, and by what ceaseless labor and colossal self-sacrifice she managed to maintain the good name and honor of the family would make fit themes for a great story of matchless heroism, unflinching regard to duty, chastity, and supreme self-abnegation.

I am convinced that it was this conjugation of a highly intelligent father with exceptional, noble traits of character, and a strong, able-bodied mother, with a deep religious bent, endowed with all the virtues of a simple unpretentious character, that helped me to brave, without succumbing, the psychic storm released in my body on the arousal of kundalini, the Serpent Fire. I honestly believe that the grace I have won I owe more to the mental and physical attributes that I inherited from my parents than to the efforts made by me. The law of karma does not work only in shaping one's own destiny but also in ordering the life of our progeny. The seeds of our actions live deep in the subliminal depths of our children and press their imprint on their thought and act.

The riddle of Life will prove to be the greatest mystery of creation. It may not be fathomed even in hundreds of thousands of years. The agnostical intellects of recent times only contrived to dig burrows of thought to shut themselves in, walling off their approach to Light. Whenever we speak of life it is wise to bear in mind that we are talking of a stupendous Intelligence, pervading every nook and corner of the universe, which at every moment of our lives reads our thoughts and knows precisely all about our actions even before we have formulated or performed them. We are merely the tiny droplets of an ocean which every moment supplies and controls the whole thinking of humankind.

My mother had never held a book in her hands nor could she read or write a word. Yet from what I can recall of her practical knowledge of life and the way in which she handled unexpected situations, I can say with confidence that perhaps even now with all my experience, I could not have handled things better than she did. There is a natural fount of wisdom in all of us which, alas, oversophistication, faulty education, crazy ideas imbibed from books and foolish indoctrination depletes or destroys. Some of the most enlightened spiritual teachers, some of the most successful and popular kings or rulers in history, were semiliterate or entirely unread. Why? We are still ill-skilled to handle the evolving human mind.

Integrity of character was perhaps the most prominent trait of my father. He was known not only in government circles but even in public for his high sense of honesty. In the Public Works Department of Kashmir, with the responsible post which he held, he had almost unlimited possibilities to make a fortune. My mother used to narrate many incidents when rich contractors came to the house, in the absence of my father, to press bags full of coins or costly presents on her. But my father already had her promise that she would never yield to a temptation of this kind. His honesty became almost proverbial.

At the same time he was very humane, generous, and kind. If he ever sent an attendant or subordinate in the office on a private errand of his own, during or after office hours, he invariably paid him from his pocket for the work done. He was also extremely kind to the domestic servants.

This is clear from an incident narrated to me. One day while cooking the meal, a servant felt the temptation to roast and eat a few pieces of meat he was about to prepare on the fire. The smell of the burning flesh was at once detected by my father sitting in his room in another floor of the building. He pointed this out to my mother and asked her to go down and investigate. She obeyed and came back with the admission of what had been done. The servant was called and in a momentary fit of anger my father, after pointing out his fault, gave him a slap on the face. The servant, conscious of his guilt, frightened and humiliated, went back to the kitchen.

After only a few minutes the mood of my father changed. He sat brooding over the incident for some time without speaking a word. My mother looked at him in silence, wondering what he was turning over in his mind. Suddenly he raised up his eyes to look at her and she found tears trembling on the lids.

"I have committed a sin," he said. "I must be as dear to him as his mother and he must have felt the same humiliation as I would have felt if treated in the same way. It is possible he might have been hungry and was tempted. I should have been more gentle with him." With these words tears began to stream down his cheeks. Wiping his eyes, he called the servant and made him sit beside him. Then, putting his hand into his pocket, he brought out a handful of coins and pressed them into the servant's hand saying he was sorry that he had been so harsh with him.

The servant, with folded hands, admitted his fault, saying that he had really done wrong and was sorry for it. He went down smiling to his work in the kitchen, having received a reward more than his wages for a month, as a gesture of atonement from my father.

I heard from my mother many stories of his generosity and compassion for the poor. What he received as his salary every month was a considerable sum, compared to the standard of prices during those days. But my mother never had the happiness of receiving the whole amount for the expenses of the family. My father's reputation for charity encouraged the poor and the needy who came to know of it to beseech his help. During the first days of the month when his pay was disbursed to him, they stood waiting on the road he took from his office to his residence. They related sorrowful tales of their misery to excite his pity. One had a grown-up daughter to marry and not a penny to defray the expenses, another had an illness or an incurable patient in the family with no money to pay for the treatment, the third was disabled without any resources to meet the cost of the food, and so on. My father would listen in silence and then put a handful of coins into the hands of the supplicant.

This happened at many places and by the time he arrived home a good part of his salary had vanished. The remainder went to my mother to meet the expenses of the household. She said to me that she almost always received only about one quarter of the amount which he drew as his pay. With even this depleted sum they could maintain a servant for the family and pay the charges for the boat that took him to the office. Even horse carriages were rare in Kashmir in those days.

He never cared to purchase property or even a residential house in Srinagar. Estates offered to him at throwaway prices were refused. He lived in a spirit of detachment, resigned to whatever he came across, kind and affectionate to everyone. By a strange vagrancy of fate this noble man was not allowed to experience a safe and blissful awakening of the Serpent Power. Ominous signs were evident from the very start in his passion for the uncanny and bizarre and his preference for eccentric and disoriented God-men and saints in whom also the power had gone astray.

Like attracts like in human association. The first symptom of a malfunctioning kundalini, even when slightly active, is an irrational and vagrant tendency of the mind towards the occult and the divine. All the monstrosities and horrors associated with religion are an outcome of this misdirection of thought. A skeptical mind which looks with suspicion at what is not demonstrable to reason is far more healthy than a credulous mind which accepts and acts on every supernatural story it encounters. Ascription of lawlessness to creation is the first sign of incipient chaos in the thoughts of an individual.

Every day some loaves of bread, a bottle of wine and a prescribed measure of roasted meat went from our house to a sadhu (Hindu holy man) known as Kakaji. My mother was asked to see to it that the offering was made every day. She obeyed without asking what good purpose it served to feed a person who, apparently, was of no use to the world and indulged his fancies without profit to anybody. But she never dared to express her feelings to her husband. Her sound intuition helped her to see clearly into the absurdity which, for my father, had the position of a religious duty which it was obligatory for him to fulfill.

The painful death of his son put an end to his association with sadhus and saints. The stark reality of the sudden blow made him realize he had been building his hopes on a base of shifting sand. He issued strict instructions that henceforth no sadhu should be allowed to enter the house. The tribute sent every day was discontinued and the deeds of charity brought to an end. There was also a lack of financial means, as he no longer attended the office. He became taciturn with friends and relatives and finally shut himself in his room, allowing no one to see him on any pretext whatsoever.

The crisis brought about by his isolation and rejection of vitally needed articles of diet, including milk, at last culminated in certain symptoms of abnormality which my mother had never noticed before. He would wake her up in the dead of night in a state of intense alarm, shouting that the house was shaking with an earthquake, and then rush down the stairs without waiting to see if she followed. Without stopping to reason, my mother, carrying some articles of bedding in her arms, would follow him to the graveyard adjacent to the house and sit by his side while he lay down breathing fast with the signs of fear still on his face. He was clearly passing through the upward and downward phases of a now active kundalini sending streams of impure prana (vital energy) into the brain. It was the impact of the stream that caused the hallucination of the earth-quake and the symptoms of fear.

It has to be understood that the awakening of kundalini does not mean merely the activation of a force which has been lying dormant at the base of the spine. It means much more than that. The bioenergy which runs the extremely complex mechanism of the human body and provides the fuel for thought is not split up into compartments or currents acting independently of each other. It is one homogeneous whole, performing all the functions of the body from the movement of a muscle to the highest flight of thought. It is a medium entirely beyond our conception, working in a hundred ways, with varied speeds, varied spectrums and varied material to perform the almost limitless functions of the body. But the energy is basically one, capable of assuming any pattern or any speed to suit every situation. This means, in other words, that prana assumes one form for digestive activity, another for the circulation of the blood, yet another for the movement of the muscles and so on. It is an incredible stuff which can manipulate atoms and molecules in any conceivable way, compound any organic substance and use every possible expedient, under certain laws, to activate the bodily machine from birth to death.

To illustrate my meaning it is necessary to cite one or two examples. It is a well-known fact that when for reasons of safety, a diseased kidney is extirpated, the other kidney grows larger in size until it is able to perform the functions of both. The loss of eyesight is somehow compensated by increased sensitivity of the ears or skin, in some cases almost to an extent which appears incredible. Likewise it has been noticed that in some cases of damage to a certain part of the brain, say by a tumor or accident, its function is taken over by other parts.

We see the working of this mysterious force very plainly in the desperate situations caused by serious accidents. The fracture of the skull or damage to any other vital organ is immediately followed by certain reactions and readjustment of the bodily rhythms and functions, imperative for safety and survival. We never know what marvelous intelligence takes the decisions in such sudden contingencies with lightning speed to determine what course it should adopt to repair the damage caused. All the extremely complex reactions that follow a serious infection or a serious accident emanate from this mysterious intelligence present in every cell and fiber of the human frame. This is the marvel of *prana-shakti*, the divine instrument of life.

Strictly speaking, the awakening of kundalini signifies a sudden or gradual change in the whole function of the brain. This involves the activation of a normally dormant area to add another channel of perception to the already existing senses with which our brain maintains contact with the outer world. The opening of this new supersensory channel, in turn, involves a transformation in the activity of the whole cerebrospinal system, culminating in a change in the very pattern of consciousness. The existing evolutionary process working in the brain is aimed to arouse the dormant area to activity and to create conditions of the body and the vital organs conformable to it. In other words, the body and the organs performing the functions of digestion, blood circulation, oxidation, elimination, etc., have to be adjusted to maintain a tempo concordant with the demands of the new activity in the brain.

The sudden forced arousal to activity of this hitherto inactive center creates a condition analogous to that created by a serious accident. In fact, some of the practices of hatha yoga, as for instance *kechari mudra*, are virtually deliberate attempts to create a serious situation in the metabolic activity of the system. In this practice, the tongue is rolled back into the air passage to stop the flow of air into the lungs, creating a condition of diminished oxygen, threatening life.

The same condition supervenes when, with prolonged stoppage of breath in *pranayama*, the supply of oxygen to the blood is seriously impeded. This desperate situation forces the body to drastic responses in order to save one's life. The methods of hatha yoga are designed to force these extreme measures, one of which can be the arousal of the Serpent Power, to avert disaster to the brain. But such drastic responses can prove highly dangerous or abortive and instead of leading to beatitude and cosmic consciousness, bring calamities in their wake. This is the main reason why drastic forms of hatha yoga have never been viewed with favor by the illuminati of India.

It is a grave error to suppose that the arousal of kundalini can be achieved with impunity by anyone who applies himself to the discipline. The popular idea that the practices result simply in the activation of a new force in the body is fallacious. Those who believe that the arousal and mastery of the force can be achieved by one's willful effort alone live in a paradise of fools. Properly speaking, the position has to be viewed the other way round. It is actually the pressure exerted by the slowly opening supersensory channel in the brain on one's mind which acts as the root of the religious impulse, driving one to seek expedients to satisfy the longing.

All those who experience spiritual hunger in some form would be wiser if they ascribe it to this impulse coming from their subliminal depths, based on a certain transitional condition of the brain, rather than to their own wish or desire. Speaking more precisely, the impulse for God-realization or the urge to gain occult powers, in its psychosomatic origin, is parallel to the growing erotic impulse and its satisfaction in the mind of the adolescent. It is not a motivation subservient to our will, to be channeled as we choose, but a deep-rooted impulse coming up from the unfathomable depths of the psyche in which the brain, too, plays a vital part. The thrust of kundalini actually comes from the depths of consciousness and its instrument of expression, namely the brain.

There is nothing more important in our search for spiritual knowledge than the recognition of the fact that religious thirst is the outcome of a certain organic urge and that in order to relieve this thirst it is very necessary to know where this natural impulse is designed to lead. Without this knowledge we would be at a loss in assessing the correctness of our own desire and in determining the path we must follow to satisfy it.

It is evident that there is a close connection between the evolving center in the brain and the so-called abode of kundalini, meticulously described in the ancient texts. Analyzed in the context of present knowledge, the proximity of kundalini to the reproductive organs signifies its command over a source of surplus energy available to meet the demands of the system when the silent chamber in the brain begins to operate.

A settled way of life enabled human beings to obtain nourishment much more easily and in greater abundance than the nomadic forbears of the past. It provided them with a richer and more balanced diet in greater measure and with more regularity than they could procure before. Civilized individuals often eat much more than needed, causing obesity and other ill effects of surfeit. This full satisfaction of hunger leads to the storage of much more energy in the reproductive system than is needed for propagation alone.

It is this surplus store of sex energy which one often wantonly dissipates for pleasure under the mistaken belief that this waste does not recoil on the system in any adverse way. Since there is little awareness, even among the learned, of the evolutionary transformation of the brain and its demands on the body, this senseless expenditure of the precious energy causes ravages in the system of which the whole extent is impossible to gauge at the present level of our knowledge of the whole evolutionary mechanism involved in this sinful waste. Immoderation in erotic pleasure is a sin against Nature that can have far-reaching consequences. It is a colossal blunder to yield unrestrainedly to the demands of sexual desire. The cost paid for the momentary thrill of the erotic sensation, when it exceeds a healthy limit, is so high that generations can suffer for the unbridled lust of one libidinous ancestor.

A depleted store of reproductive energy in an individual can prove seriously detrimental when kundalini is suddenly aroused. In fact, one of the reasons why a spontaneous activation of the Serpent

Power often ends in mental disorder is the fact that, in addition to a faulty genetic heritage or unhealthy organic structure of the body, the excess expenditure of the reproductive essences can cause ravages in the system which make adaptation to the new activity of the brain impossible.

Among the millions of lunatics on the earth, whether in mental homes or at large, we see the unhappy result of our lack of knowledge of the evolutionary mechanism and lack of understanding about the twofold activity of the reproductive system. Much of our current knowledge of psychology is based on assumptions dangerous for the sanity and survival of the race. The main reason why mental and nervous disorders have shown an alarming increase in the industrial and advanced countries in the West rests on the fact that with all-round improvement in the standard of living, the tempo of evolution shows a corresponding increase, calling for appropriate changes in the environment and the way of life of the evolving multitudes.

TWO

Life in the Village of Gairoo

AFTER I HAD READ up to the third primary class in the village school we moved to Srinagar. I was just a village urchin, fond of outdoor play and sport in the company of other children. I went barefoot, walked and squatted on bare earth without any regard to my body or my clothes. I still bear the marks of injuries caused to my feet, one by a chilblain while walking barefoot in snow and frost and another by the abrasion caused by a pointed stone splinter on which I stepped while running on the road. My school life continued both in the village and the city. My mother always engaged a tutor for me during the early years. In the village her brother had performed this duty, but I was never steady or laborious in any studies and liked more to play than to read. It was only at examination time that I devoted some attention to my books to pass with credit and to keep my teachers pleased with me.

On return from Lahore, I joined the seventh class in a high school. I was never jealous of students who excelled in the examinations and almost always ascribed my own inability to achieve distinctions to my own neglect. I came poorly dressed to the school. There were well-dressed students from rich families in the class. But, as far as I remember, I never envied their rich clothes nor their wealth. Whenever we went to visit a rich relative, living in affluence in Srinagar or Lahore, I never made any effort to compare our condition with theirs or to sigh at our penury. In fact, from an early age I evinced a disregard for riches or position which helped me to maintain my self-respect and integrity in later years. My father's indifference towards wealth and status was somehow imprinted on my nature from the beginning. Had I been in the least covetous or even moderately ambitious, my life would have been very different and I might not have been able to write these pages. There are certain basic characteristics which should be either inborn or must be cultivated to meet the demands of inner transformation brought about by kundalini.

There are two incidents of those days which I still remember. One was an abortive attempt on my part at smoking a cigarette. One day, while walking with two of my class fellows in a narrow, lonely street, one of them offered me a cigarette he had lit for himself. I took a deep puff, filling my lungs with smoke as I saw him and others doing. Instantly I found myself reeling with giddiness and a sick condition of the stomach. I could stand only with difficulty and, what was worse, my head began to ache terribly. The pain lasted for several hours. From that day onward I never tried the experiment again.

I also recall that in the village my hobby was to climb trees, even huge walnut trees, with an agility that made the villagers wonder. There was a peach tree close to our building in Gairoo. The building was three stories high, covered by a thatched roof. The slant of the roof was fairly steep and it needed great care and skill to walk over it from one side to the other. A tall walnut tree flanked the other side of the building. In the walnut season it was my practice to climb the peach tree, which was comparatively easy to scale. From it I stepped onto the roof and, walking across, plucked walnuts from the branches of the tree hanging over the roof on that side. My sister, fond of green walnuts, waited below in the compound collecting the fruit that I threw down for the family. But all through the operation the onlookers displayed marked signs of agitation and fear at the risk that I was taking. It was comical for me to see them waiting keenly for the walnuts and at the same time wringing their hands while their eyes expressed signs of acute alarm and fear.

After the shock caused by the death of my elder brother, my father became more and more inaccessible and unresponsive. With this change in habits, his appetite became irregular and his tastes erratic.

Special vegetarian dishes had to be prepared to tempt him to eat. He became extremely austere in his dress and preferred to walk barefoot or, at times, when pressed to do so, with a pair of flimsy grass sandals on his feet. He took long walks every day and never hesitated to go out in even the coldest and most inclement weather. But, in spite of his irregular and scanty intake of food or unbalanced food combinations, he became wiry and vigorous, able to withstand hunger and fatigue or the rigor of climate to a remarkable degree. But his behavior became more and more eccentric and unpredictable. He became increasingly prone to visionary experiences and confined his study to a few ancient volumes, including *The Laws of Manu,** which he read over and over again.

The way in which my mother attended to his needs and served him during this phase of his life is beyond description. His premature self-enforced retirement from service brought only a meager pension of about fifty rupees on which the family had to live. Even this became possible after many months due to the hard efforts of his maternal uncle who lived in Lahore. The cost of commodities and the standard of living were lower in the days when my father bid adieu to his service, and the family could make ends meet within the amount of the pension.

But there were other heavy expenses to be met. How my mother managed to marry my two sisters, to help her needy brothers and to educate me with this meager income is a story of heroic battle against adversity.

My mother arranged the marriage of my two older sisters at the same time that I was made to wear the sacred thread. This function is attended by certain rituals lasting for two or three days. I was about seven years of age at the time, the younger of my two sisters was about eleven and the odler about fifteen years old. My mother had chosen the matches after a keen search and investigation. The would-be husbands belonged to respectable middle-class families with the promise of a bright future before them.

*Manava-Dharma-Shastra or *Manu Smrti,* an ancient code of life ascribed to a period circa fifth century B.C.E.

The husband of the younger sister was about twelve and that of the older twenty-five years old. The latter had lately entered service in the Forest Department of the state. The marriages and the sacred thread ceremony took place at Gairoo, where we dwelt in those days. The whole village was agog with excitement and every grown-up villager came to help at the function out of love and respect for my mother.

The marriage of a daughter amongst families in our society is a heavy responsibility. Not only the parents but all their kith and kin draw a deep sigh of relief when it is over and the bride leaves with the bridegroom for her new home. It is almost always a taxing and nerve-racking task. There are so many purchases to be made, so many arrangements to be completed and so many problems to be solved that for poor parents who lack resources or friends it becomes a nightmare for the entire time of the function.

Several months before the day of marriage, my mother went to Srinagar to arrange the preparation of gold ornaments and to make other purchases. It was a distance of about twenty miles from our village to the city. The journey was usually done on foot and sometimes on horseback. We stayed in the house of a relative and my mother worked hard every day to complete the purchases as speedily as possible. When the ornaments were ready, we had to return to the village with them. We left the city in the afternoon on horseback, accompanied by one of her cousins, a good-natured young man who followed us later to Lahore. I sat on the horse in front of my mother and her cousin walked along, matching his pace with that of the horse.

The sun began to set when we had traveled less than half the distance from the city. It was dusk when we came to a part of the highway notorious for the bands of thieves who made their haunts in the surrounding villages some distance from the road. The road at this place passed over a broad plateau about five miles long with a deep depression in the middle. There is no habitation close to the road in all this stretch. The soil of the plateau is rich for the cultivation of saffron and is used for this purpose even to this day. The small square saffron beds, with the tiny flowers peeping out, look very beautiful during the day and enchanting in the moonlit night. During the saffron season they fill the whole area with their fragrance.

We had just entered this lonely, low-lying lap of our journey when the thickening shadows of the evening made my mother pause for awhile to say to her cousin that it had been a mistake to leave the city so late and that the only alternatives now were either to turn back and pass the night in the small town of Pampur, about three miles away, or to proceed trusting in the mercy of heaven to keep us safe.

The way back was also not free of danger, so it was decided to move on to Latipura at the end of the plateau. Mother stopped the horse for a moment and, unwrapping the scarf from around her head, rewound it in the shape of a turban to present the semblance of a man in the dim light, when seen from a distance. All the gold ornaments, a fortune in those days, were tied round her waist, under the loose dress which she wore. Urging her cousin to quicken his pace, she spurred the horse to a faster speed. It was pitch dark when we reached Latipura on the descent from the plateau. The young cousin ran as fast as the horse the whole distance in order to cover the dangerous stretch in the shortest possible time.

At Latipura we sought the hospitality of a Moslem cowherd whose house stood on the road. They welcomed us with warmth and served us with fresh milk for our evening repast. We slept on a bed of dry grass in one of their rooms, covered with their homespun blankets. They all came to see us off in the early hours of the morning. I remember their warm hospitality and kindness to this day. The inner wealth of the spirit is not determined by affluence, climate, creed, or class. It is a gift from heaven and we have to know much more about the spirit before we can determine how the gift can be won.

The marriage ceremony was performed with becoming pomp and show. It was customary in those days for the bridegroom's party to arrive with a band playing at the head of the procession. Sometimes dancing girls attended the party and were munificently paid for the performance. In the evenings there was often a fireworks display to celebrate the occasion. Fireworks and the orchestra attend the function even today.

In our community, marriage is not a simple social or religious function but an occasion for merrymaking and festivity, often entirely beyond the means of the parties. The lavish displays and feasts in many cases leave the families impoverished and in debt for a long time to come. Most often, the victim of this outrageous thirst for false show of wealth and status is the family of the bride.

The marriage party of the elder bridegroom had brought with it a huge store of fireworks which they let off in the evening, entertaining the large crowd of villagers who came to witness the novel show. Among other things, there were a few hot air balloons that were sent up after kindling a flame in each of them. Carried by the wind, the lighted balloons traveled far, floating over distant villages that had never seen an object of this kind before. In a few days, the rumor went round that at least two of the villages had made religious offerings for having been preserved from this visitation from the other world. Nowadays, mammoth airplanes cause no surprise. The party of the other bridegroom had brought two dancing girls to entertain the guests. A large crowd gathered when, dressed in gaudy attire, they gave a performance in the morning in the large compound decorated for the purpose. I remember many details of the wedding and the ceremony, in which I had to participate, as vividly as if they had come to pass yesterday.

Between the younger of my two sisters and her husband there was a difference of about one year only. It was a child marriage of the sort current in those days. The bridegroom, only about twelve years of age, tried to look serious as the couple participated in the ceremony held to make them man and wife. They had to sit before a small ceremonial fire while the priests chanted mantras and poured clarified butter and other offerings into it.

The most beautiful part of this ceremony is witnessed when both the bride and the bridegroom are made to sit under an improvised canopy made of a large length of rich cloth which covers both of them. All the members of the family stand up to form a circle round the couple, still sitting in front of the sacred fire, and shower flowers on them to the chant of the priests until a heap forms on the small canopy covering their heads.

At that time they are no longer a man and a woman but incarnations of Divinity, uniting themselves into a solemn relationship to propagate the race. We often forget the fact that every conjugal union, leading to procreation, signifies a stage on the path of evolution that is slowly tending towards the superman and -woman. Modern knowledge, still largely unaware of this law, has no knowledge of the mighty god-like race to come.

There was a comic episode during the performance of the ceremony that drew peals of laughter from the guests assembled in the room. It is customary during the course of the ceremony for the bride and bridegroom, while they hold each other's hand, to try their skill at a hidden game aimed at taking off the ring from the other's finger without letting their hand out of one's grasp. It is held that the one who succeeds in snatching away the ring of the other becomes the real master in the life led by the two.

Both my brother-in-law and my sister prepared for this show of skill, no doubt instructed by their families about it. Unfortunately, my brother-in-law, to his dismay, found his ring slipping away from his finger, held by the more nimble fingers of my sister. Turning to his father, who was sitting close by for the ceremony, he cried, "Look father, she has taken away the ring from my finger. What am I to do now?" There was a loud outburst of laughter as his father turned to chide him for his weakness, bidding him to be silent and not make his incompetence known to the guests.

On our return to Kashmir after the first trip to Lahore, I joined the high school in Srinagar to continue my studies. Both my sisters were married and lived in their husbands' parental homes in different parts of Srinagar. They both loved me with all their heart, and this affection continued unaltered all my life. Their husbands, too, were extremely loving and kind to me.

It was my elder brother-in-law who unwittingly alerted me to the possibility that kundalini could arise through either *ida* (the left-hand channel) or *pingala* (the right-hand channel) instead of the central channel, known as *sushumna*. When kundalini is aroused through *pingala*, he said, it could burn the body with the heat generated, causing irreparable damage or death. This he had learned from his own guru, a poor Kashmiri Brahmin, whose appearance showed nothing of the study he had made or the knowledge he had gained about kundalini. But as my later experience proved, the information he had given to my brother-in-law was based on oral tradition seldom mentioned in books. Through all his life, my elder brother-in-law treated me as his son and in every difficult situation came to consult me as a friend most close to him.

He had a deep thirst for spiritual experience and, having learned that I was regularly meditating, often consulted me about his own methods and practices from time to time. His deep desire to assuage his spiritual thirst changed his whole life and mellowed his nature to such an extent that those who knew him for many years came to regard him as a saint. Though elder, he was very frank and outspoken with me and never hesitated to discuss even his most intimate problems. His utter faith and belief in the professions of the sadhus and holy men with whom he came in contact and his readiness to follow the methods prescribed by them sometimes cost him dearly.

One sadhu, as he told me later, instructed him to gaze intently at a circle drawn on a wall for as long a period as he could without blinking his eyes. This practice is known as *rikti* by the hatha yogis. The successful practice of this method, the sadhu had said, would win for him all the psychic powers or siddhis, as they are called.

The exercise was started, but, after only a few days, my brother-in-law found that his eyes were aching and tears began to flow if he kept them open any longer without blinking. He narrated his difficulty to the guru, seeking his advice on how to overcome it.

"You should wear a folded cloth below your eyes," the sadhu had said, "so that all the tears that flow are absorbed into it." My brother-in-law scrupulously followed the direction for some days, but his condition grew worse. His eyes became red and swollen and the lids began to pain, making it impossible for him to continue the practice any longer. Fortunately this compelled him to give it up and to sever his connections with the teacher.

On another occasion he was asked to make *japa* (recitation) of a mantra (sacred word) a hundred thousand times in forty days, sitting on the bank of a stream in a lonely spot where none could disturb him. Being a Forest Officer, it was not difficult for him to fulfill the conditions and to find a secluded place to practice the discipline. On the fortieth day, he was told, he would have the *darshan* (vision) of a supernatural being invoked by the mantra. When this happened, he could beg whatever boon he desired from the superearthly visitor. The only contingency against which he had to guard was not to show any sign of fear when the apparition appeared as that would be disastrous for the practice.

My brother-in-law faithfully carried out the injunctions, going to the chosen spot exactly at midnight to do the *japa*. Everything went well for over a month. In his thought and action and in his food and drink, sleep and behavior, my brother-in-law meticulously observed all the directions given to prepare himself for the great event.

After the thirty-fifth day, as he told me, signs of fear began to appear during the recitation, and he felt a pressure on his heart. This feeling grew in intensity and volume until, on the thirty-eighth day, he found himself shaking and trembling while beads of cold perspiration rolled down his body and face. In despair he gave up the discipline, preferring his sanity and peace of mind to the favors which a superearthly entity could bestow.

The incident revealed to me at once that loss of sleep caused by the nightly peregrinations and several hours solitary stay on the bank of the stream in expectation of the nocturnal visitor had caused an abnormal mental condition of anxiety and fear which, to preserve his sanity, obliged him to give up the exercise at last.

This story of my brother-in-law confirms what I came to know or hear of from my friends in the years following my awakening. Another devout seeker, also a resident of Srinagar, was advised by his teacher to make the *japa* of a similar mantra to invoke Bajranga-Bali, the monkey general of the God Rama, to obtain from him fulfillment of whatever wish he had in mind. The same admonition was repeated. He should show no symptom of fear when the apparition was seen across the mountain on which the window of his room opened. The practice was to be started after midnight and continued until the rise of the sun.

After a few weeks of the practice, the signs of fear began to appear, and the devotee felt his heart thumping under his ribs. He persisted in the practice to the fortieth day. Opening his eyes and looking at the mountain through the window in the light of the dawn, he saw an awful apparition spread across the whole area of the mountain visible to him. The shock was too much and with a cry of fear he fell down in a swoon. He never recovered the balance of his mind to the time of his death some years after.

There is no limit to the concept of the intellect. We know that the human mind has no hope of knowing even as much about the universe as a moth has to know about the earth. All our knowledge gained during the past thousands of years does not comprise even a drop in the ocean that still lies beyond the human ken. It is amazing that knowing full well the complexity of the brain and the inconceivably profound nature of consciousness, even sensible people should lend credence to the stories circulated by teachers of the occult about the efficacy of their methods and practices to gain psychic powers or transcendence.

The attainment of cosmic consciousness involves a total revolution in the microbiology of every cell, tissue and fiber of the organism. The arousal of kundalini, in its true sense, does not simply imply the activity of a hitherto sleeping force, but actually the start of a new activity in the whole system to adapt it to a new pattern of consciousness by changing the composition of the bioenergy or subtle life force permeating the whole body. Any human-made method to achieve concrete results must therefore cover the whole psychophysical frame of a human being. The position does not even end there. The discipline must be practiced generation after generation, or there must have occurred already a partial adjustment of the organs, the nervous system, and the brain to allow the practice undertaken to bear fruit.

This is the reason why genuine mystical experience has been so rare. The rough and ready methods of professionals who make tall claims not only reveal the poverty of knowledge of those who prescribe them but also lack of wisdom on the part of those who practice them without a thorough and penetrating study of the subject.

There are crowds of people, both in Eastern and Western countries who pay dearly for their ignorance and lack of foresight in various ways, especially in abnormal and difficult conditions of the mind.

My mother never complained at the willful behavior of my father in driving the family from abundance to penury by his own stubborn behavior. I do not remember a single occasion when even under the pressure of the most grueling circumstances she ever upbraided him or held him responsible for her difficulties. She was always resigned to Divine will and, while attending to every detail of the household, kept her mind calm and her behavior unruffled. Even in the most trying circumstances she did this as naturally as if she had practiced for years and read a hundred books on the art of self-mastery.

One single instance is enough to show with what fortitude, resignation and courage she faced the harsh exigencies of her life. We were still in Lahore in the old house in the area known as Ekki

Darwasa. It was midsummer and the temperature ranged from 108 to 114 degrees Fahrenheit. Suddenly my father expressed a wish to pay a visit to his native town of Amritsar at a distance of about 30 miles from Lahore. His intention seemed to be to return in two or three days. My mother tried to dissuade him from this resolve on the plea that the heat was intolerable and it would be difficult to find a cool place to stay in Amritsar. We had a family of rich relatives there, but she knew that he would never agree to stay there with them.

From her meager store of money, she gave my father enough to meet the railway fare and the cost of his meals for those few days. But my father prolonged his sojourn in Amritsar far beyond this period. Some days later, I received a hurriedly scrawled letter from him informing us that he was staying in a temple and had run completely short of money. The letter made my mother frantic with anxiety and, making her preparations in a few hours, she left for Amritsar on the same day.

She went directly to the house of our relatives, who warmly welcomed her and did all in their power to make her stay comfortable. They drove her in their carriage to the temple to meet my father and to settle the time of departure for Lahore with him. She later told me that she saw him reduced in weight, looking pale and weak as for several days he had subsisted only on a few handfuls of parched grain and water drawn from the well. The next day in the forenoon they drove in the same carriage to the station on the way to Lahore.

I did not attend the college that day and remained at home in expectation of their arrival. At about two o'clock in the afternoon I heard the front door open and soon the sound of steps mounting the staircase. I ran to the door and saw my father as he stepped into the open space in front of our kitchen. He was perspiring profusely and looked exhausted. Touching my shoulder with his hand, he went straight to his room without uttering a word. Soon after, I saw my mother stagger inside with the large bundle of clothes and bedding of my father on her head. She was reeling and her face was crimson.

I had never seen her in such a condition. Sweat poured like rain from every pore of her skin and she looked so exhausted, weak, and faint that I was shocked and could only gaze stunned and bewildered at her face. I could find no explanation for her condition. Taking the bundle from her head and putting my arm around her, I carried her gently to the inner room, where she collapsed on the floor gasping for breath and trembling in every limb. I fanned her gently for a while until the sweating ceased and then rushed into the kitchen to prepare a glass of sherbet for her, which I soon held to her lips. She took a few sips and then, burying her face in her hands, burst into tears. I continued to fan, stroking her arm gently with my hand without saying a word until the fits subsided and she was calm again.

Sensing my anxiety and perplexity about what had occurred, she said in a low tone that at the Amritsar railway station she had handed all the money she carried to my father to buy two tickets to Lahore and with the balance to pay the cab from the Lahore railway station to our house. He went to the booking office and returned soon after with two tickets in his hand. Without telling her anything he conducted her to a lady's compartment and seating her there, entered a male compartment nearby. The train moved and in due time arrived in Mian Mir, the station next to Lahore on the way to it from Amritsar.

As soon as the train stopped there my father, stepping out of his own compartment, came to my mother and asked her to come out, as he had bought tickets up to that station only, explaining that because of the rush at the sales window he had purchased inter-class tickets instead of third class and had to pay more for them. He asked for more money to purchase tickets from Mian Mir to Lahore on the next train, which would cost but a trifle. But she had not a single paisa in her pocket. Completely nonplused, she looked helplessly at the train as it moved out of the station, leaving the couple stranded there without the means to reach their destination.

It was an impossible situation. My mother would have died rather than beg for help, which might have been forthcoming if they had asked for it. Placing the bundle on her head and holding it with one of her hands, she motioned to my father to follow her. Inquiring their way from the passersby, they took the highway linking Lahore with Amritsar.

It was a wide asphalt road heated to an intolerable degree by the burning noonday sun, treeless and shadeless for long stretches, flanked by sand footpaths on either side in which the feet sank almost ankle deep. I had walked over this road for short distances more than once, but in winter when I was on a visit to my aunt who for some years dwelt in the area. At noon in midsummer, with a temperature well over 110 degrees Fahrenheit and a blistering sun overhead, it must have been hell to walk over this road for hours with sandals on their feet, sinking deep in the sand at every step. As usual during summer, men, women, and even children lay under the shade of trees or lazed in the shelter of their homes. They fanned themselves incessantly to keep cool. There were only a few other passersby who used the road only for short distances here and there.

It was a terrible ordeal for my mother with the load on her head, hungry and without even water, to drag herself over this road for a distance of over five miles to reach her home during the hottest hours of the day. I shuddered when my mother finished her story. Born and bred in the cool climate of Kashmir, the exposure could have easily led to a fatal sunstroke. In all probability, the bundle of clothes on her head, intercepting the rays of the blazing sun, saved her life. I looked fondly at her face and, embracing her, shed tears of joy at finding her safe and sound in the house after the risk she had undergone.

Even then she did not utter a single word of complaint against my father. As soon as she had recovered a little, she stood up at once, saying that she would not lie down like this any longer since my father had not tasted a cooked meal for several days and she must prepare one for him. She hurriedly went to the kitchen and within an hour my father had the simple meal he preferred, while she bustled around him to serve whatever he needed or wished for. I wonder to this day what had taught her this patience and this most angelic sense of duty.

The answer to this riddle, I believe, lies in the power of the spirit. We do not know whether it is the body which helps the spirit to express itself or if it is the spirit which fashions the mortal frame to play a part in the colossal drama of life. Or whether both are linked together in an inexplicable way under cosmic laws which lie beyond the reach of intellect and which we have to fathom during our sojourn on earth. Royal palaces of kings and the luxurious mansions of the rich quite frequently rear the poorest specimens of humanity—a disgrace to the blood to which they belong—but for some unknown reason thatched roofs, mud huts, and wooden shacks housing poverty and destitution give rise to some of the noblest characters in the history of mankind.

THREE
Memories of High School

MY SCHOOL AND COLLEGE LIFE was fairly uneventful. This was, in a sense, remarkable as for me it was a transition from the primitive atmosphere of a simple village and later, of a poor city to that of one of the richest capitals in India. But somehow I was preserved from company that could have proved disastrous for me in later years. The love of home and parents served as my strongest defense against vagrancy and association with truants. I had few friends, both in the school and the college. The one or two I had were sober and studious, whose company was of help and not of harm to me.

We lived poorly and in the later period I did not have the advantage of a private coach or guide. It was with great difficulty that my mother could find enough money to purchase even my essentially needed books and clothes. Denied the possibility of purchasing extra books, my study was confined to school classics, but when I was about twelve, at my aunt's house I accidentally came upon a slightly abridged translation into Urdu of *The Arabian Nights*.

This book for the first time created in me a burning thirst for fairy tales, stories of adventure and travel and other romantic literature which continued undiminished for several years. At the age of fourteen, starting with easy stories, I turned from Urdu to English, hungrily devouring every story book and romance that came into my hands.

From novels and other light material I gradually passed on to popular elementary books on science and philosophy available in our small school library. I read avidly, my developing mind eager for satisfactory replies to the questions which cropped up as the result of my own survey of the narrow world in which I lived and the stray glimpses of the broader one of which I came to know more and more from the graphic accounts contained in the books.

I was brought up in a strictly religious atmosphere by my mother, whose faith rested unshakably on each of the innumerable gods and goddesses in her crowded pantheon. She used to go to the temple long before the first faint glimmer of dawn streaked the horizon, returning at daybreak to attend to the needs of the household, in particular to keep our frugal morning meal ready for me. In early chidhood I followed implicitly the direction of her simple faith, sometimes to the extent of forgoing the sweet last hours of sleep towards dawn in order to go with her to the temple.

With rapt attention I listened to the superhuman exploits of Krishna, which my maternal uncle read aloud every evening until almost midnight from his favorite translation of the *Bhagavata Purana*, a famous book of Hindu mythology, containing the story of the incarnations of the god Vishnu in human form. According to popular belief, Krishna imparted the lofty teachings of the *Bhagavad Gita* to the warrior Arjuna on the battlefield before the commencement of action in a great war, as related in the *Mahabharata*. Wondering at the prodigious, supernatural feats of valor and strength recounted with a wealth of detail in the narrative, which carried my childish imagination into fantastic realms, I unquestioningly accepted as true every impossible and unbelievable incident with which the story abounds, filled with a desire to grow into a superman of identical powers myself.

About a year after our first visit to Lahore we returned to Kashmir and had our residence in a hired house in Srinagar where I passed my seventh class examination in the high school. On our second visit I joined the Dayal Singh High School, Lahore, in the eighth class and continued to study there until graduation, after which I was admitted to the college* of the same area.

On the first occasion, the family of my granduncle permitted us the use of a large room with a wide veranda in front which proved sufficient for our modest needs. On the second visit they again offered the use of the same place but now one of my sisters had

---

*Actually the equivalent of high school in the United States.

accompanied us and so we had to look around for a more roomy apartment for ourselves. It was then that we shifted to the place known as Ekki Darwasa near the outskirts of the city as mentioned in chapter 2. It was a three-storied building at the end of a narrow lane in which we occupied the uppermost floor under a flat roof. We had two medium-sized rooms, a kitchen open in front and an open space in front of the kitchen. This space I later transformed into a small flowerbed with dozens of flower pots which I watered and tended every day.

There was no water tap in our house nor, in fact, in any other house standing on this lane. There was a narrow well just a few houses away from which all of our neighbors drew their water. Accustomed to the spring water of Kashmir, the slightly salty taste of the well water was not easily palatable to me or my mother although father, accustomed to it from his childhood, felt no difficulty in drinking it. He always procured his drinking water from the well although our supply came from a water tap at a distance of about two hundred yards from our house. It was in a large bathroom constructed with public donations in the name of a saint who had lived and died in that house. The bathroom, with a number of taps, was open to all who cared to use it, fulfilling a very great need of the locality, especially in the scorching heat of summer.

My mother used to fetch one large pitcher of water in the early hours of the morning when the bathroom was almost empty. This sufficed for our drinking needs. Soon after, we engaged a man to supply us water for all purposes both from the well and the tap.

There was no electricity at that time in this part of the town. In the beginning I read and did my home tasks in the faint, mellow light of a small earthenware oil lamp. Later on I supplanted it with a kerosene table lamp which gave out a much better light and could be depended on for a steady flame. I never had a table or a chair for my studies, either in this house or another to which we shifted later before our return to Kashmir. I always did my reading or exercises seated on the floor with the lamp standing on a small wooden support. Most of our time in Lahore was spent in this house. My father occupied the larger of two rooms which had windows on two sides and two doors on the third, one opening on to the kitchen and the second on to the open space with the flower pots. The houses on two sides of our building were only one story high, which allowed us an open view of fields on one side and a part of the city with the railway station on the other.

A gentle breeze was always blowing through the two windows in summer which was a very welcome boon for me. It was hard to obtain the consent of my father to the use of a part of the room as my study. But on hot days I often sat close to one of the windows under an improvised tent made of fine cloth supported on a few sticks, to keep off the flies which swarmed all around. This device allowed me to read or to do my exercises in peace while the breeze blew through to keep me cool.

At other times of the year I used to study in the other room in which my books and belongings were kept in a small cupboard set into one of the walls. We all slept in the room occupied by my father.

The first and second floors of the house were also held by tenants. The occupants of the first floor kept a goat for milk. They used to bring it up to the roof where all the tenants slept in the summer.

The one constant object of fear in the house was a snake that had a hole somewhere in the passage leading from our entrance door to the staircase. It had been seen several times by the tenants on the ground floor but it never came up the stairs to the second or third floor. At least on two occasions the tenants alleged that they had to jump on their beds as they saw the snake slithering from the passage into one of the rooms.

Snakes in the hot plains of India can be very venomous. One of them in a house can be an endless source of terror for the inmates. But we carried on, trusting in the grace of God to keep us safe. Times without number I had to go down in the dark to open the door for a late caller or to cross the passage when coming late from my games in the college. On such occasions I was in a state of trepidation for the period I was in the passage but forgot it all afterwards, as soon as I had mounted the stairs.

What power preserved and protected me during the critical years of my adolescence in the vicious atmosphere of a modern town I cannot say. Except for my mother, I had no one to guide and instruct me at home. Born and bred in a village, she herself had no knowledge of the iniquities and vices common to a town. My father was not in favor of my study on the grounds that it tended to deflect from the traditional path of dharma (duty) prescribed by our faith. He was even more averse to the study of English and did not like to see me with such a book in my hands. I therefore had to depend on my own expedience to steer myself along the educational whirlpools and rapids that surrounded me in Lahore. My mother could not now afford a tutor to coach me at home. And I had to content myself with secondhand books and the cheapest exercise material in order not to strain the slender resources of the family too far. But somehow I was protected and guided in critical situations so that no harm befell me during this period.

My very path to the school led through a red-light district with gaudy disreputable houses on both sides of the road. But I passed them unconcerned, with the satchel of books in my hand, absorbed in my own thoughts, and I do not remember a single occasion when I looked keenly at the houses or at the brightly dressed pitiable creatures sitting in their windows looking for customers. I passed this area without the least interest or even curiosity twice a day, both on my way to and back from the school without ever allowing my thoughts to dwell on the people who resided there or in the social issues that arose from their existence.

Time after time I have asked myself how it was that, while living among the vices and temptations of a modern city at an impressionable age with no one to watch over my conduct or actions outside my house, I was able to preserve myself from evil and to wend my way unconcerned with all that happened round me.

The most powerful force that molded my life was the love of my mother, although even admitting the dominating influence of this attachment there must have been something in my own mental makeup also that threw, as it were, a protective wall around me and never allowed me to fall prey to those evil influences that end in the ruin of young lives. There must have been something discriminative and far-seeing in the subconscious depths of my mind that preserved me intact and whole during these critical years of my life.

Our mental bodies are swayed and influenced by a psychic environment in the same way as our gross bodies are affected by their physical surroundings. There are instinctive defenses in all human beings which come into play from early childhood. Parents in our time are now often more concerned with the intellectual progress of their children during their early years and seldom pay attention to the cultivation of those qualities that are much more important for them than the culture of the intellect. People cannot survive properly if their moral defenses are allowed to deteriorate for lack of parental or administrative attention, however tall they may grow in intellect.

At the high school which I joined on our first arrival from Kashmir, the teachers were pleased with me, and the boys were too young to intimidate a new arrival from a distant corner of the country who could not speak their language.

The position was different in the school which I joined on the second occasion. The boys there were older, ready to pick holes in a fresh addition to their class or to make him an object of fun for their own enjoyment. Unfortunately, I had enough material on me to provoke their humor.

In those days, a tuft of long hair on the crown of the head was the usual feature of a Hindu. But strangely enough I carried three more smaller tufts of long hair on either side of the crown tuft, in front and behind, which gave me a really bizarre appearance. Anyone who saw me with uncovered head was surprised at this singular display of these hairy tufts. My mother had added the other three at her own choice as an offering to three tutelary deities. I remonstrated on several occasions but she was adamant. I did not wish to cause her pain and so preferred to be the butt of ridicule to my fellow students rather than hurt her feelings by refusing to keep my hair tufts.

My classmates in the school began to make fun of me from the very first day I sat in the class. Their first target was the language. I had no knowledge of Punjabi and my pronunciation of Hindi was very defective. My inability to pronounce certain words correctly made the boys burst into roars of laughter in which even the teachers joined at times, in spite of their kindness towards me. Under the hail of sarcasm and ridicule I began to correct myself and to practice the correct pronunciation at home. This gave less occasion for laughter.

As ill luck would have it however, one day my classmates discovered the extra tufts of hair under my cap. Suddenly all eyes were focused on my head and they stared at me with wide-eyed astonishment, unable to find a reason for the strange spectacle. Then their loud roars of laughter began until the whole classroom shook with the concussion. I was speechless with discomfiture and dismay. Not to be daunted though, I put my cap on my head again and tried to look wholly unconcerned, while peals of laughter rang all around me.

From that day onward, the moment I entered the classroom in the morning I was greeted with giggles and laughter while fingers were pointed at my head. This was not all. Soon three or four of the students, emboldened by my silence, stepped close to me and made it a habit to take off my cap, holding the tufts of hair in one or both of their hands, and pulled them strongly from side to side, causing unbearable pain until tears came to my eyes.

This happened day after day for many weeks and I bore the torment silently without revealing my predicament to my mother. She was too shy and would not have had command of the language to come to the school to complain to the headmaster, nor did I wish to drag her into this affair. At the same time I wished to spare her pain which would be unavoidable as soon as she came to know of the torture I was suffering every day. It also seemed to me that it would have been a sign of unmanliness on my part to seek her help in a matter which I should have the courage to handle myself. It would be cowardice to involve my parents and ask them to extricate me from the difficulties I had to face in the school. Reasoning in this way, I never spoke of my humiliation and torment to my mother but continued to revolve the situation in my mind time and again to find a way of escape from my predicament.

I was fairly strong and robust for my age. Climbing trees, running, racing, and the game of *kabbadi*, which I loved, and played with the children of the village had made my body hardy and tough. I walked barefoot in the icy chill of the winter and leaped to long distances to outdo other children. I had almost unrestricted access to the store of buttermilk at home, which I drank avidly several times a day to replenish the energy I was spending in my daily bouts of strength. All this combined to give me a stamina and strength which helped greatly to meet the trials I had to face in later life.

The plan that came to my mind to save myself from this daily torment was to demonstrate my strength to the two or three mischievous students who usually came to pester me. I had already sized up their strength.

One day it happened. Catching around the neck the one on my right, who was holding a tuft of my hair in one of his hands, I put my right leg in front of both of his and with one strong pull threw him to the ground. He fell with a crash onto a bench and from there rolled to the floor, crying with pain and fright. Then, wrenching my hair free from the clutches of the other two boys with a surprise jerk of my head, I caught another on the left in the same grip, and in a moment threw him to the ground where he lay prostrate, too dazed to act for some time. The third, terror-stricken at the fate of the other two, took a sudden jump as I turned towards him and fled out of my reach.

There was a momentary hush in the class, but soon the discomfiture of my enemies was greeted with roars of laughter from the other students. They crowded round me and some of them patted me on the shoulders with words of encouragement and praise. I had won a victory. From that day onwards, the joking and the teasing ceased and I was treated as one of the elite of the class. The story went round the school in a few hours and the teachers and even the headmaster, a fine gentleman, came to know of it.

This change in position stood me in great stead later. Most of the students were now more kindly disposed towards me and took me into their confidence when there was some important boyish issue to decide.

One day, while returning from the school, I and some other students walking with me saw a crowd gathered on the road. In the midst was a poor Kashmiri laborer, almost in tears, disputing with a burly Punjabi about his wages. He had carried a heavy load of firewood for him from a distant store to his residence and the carriage charges had been stipulated between them. They amounted to a few annas only but it meant a great deal to the poor toiler who had come from a distant area, driven by hunger and cold, to try his luck in a warmer place. Many Kashmiri peasants and laborers even now migrate to the warmer towns in northern India to earn a livelihood with their labor in winter.

My young blood boiled at the cruel injustice and the outrageous conduct of the man who was trying to bully the laborer into accepting a lesser sum.

I knew that my classmates standing by me would stoutly back me if I took the side of the victim of this injustice. Turning to the laborer I asked him to relate his story, whch he did in a voice quivering with emotion. I then turned to the bully to enquire whether what the laborer had alleged was correct. He tried to browbeat me by saying that it was no affair of mine and I should mind my own business.

I made a rapid calculation in my mind and found that what he was paying for the carriage to the laborer was far less than the usual rate prevalent at the time. I knew this because I myself made all the purchases for the family, even at that young age, and knew the rates as well as anybody. Turning to the crowd I stated that the wage paid to the laborer was not at all fair or according to the current rates and that we should all see to it that he was paid what was in fairness due to him.

The crowd was impressed. My friends surged round me and with one voice demanded that full payment be made to the laborer at once. The Punjabi hesitated a moment but, seeing the determined look of the boys and the angry faces of the crowd, drew his purse and paid the balance to the laborer, grumbling the while that the wage demanded was too high.

I then continued on my way but the laborer followed me right up to my house. I talked to him in my own language and invited him to enter, which he did. My mother also was happy to talk to a fellow Kashmiri and offered refreshments to both of us. The laborer came several times to our house and finally made me the treasurer of the little sum he had been able to save, on the plea that it was unsafe in the room he was sharing with other fellow laborers in another part of the city. My mother accepted the responsibility and when he came to bid us adieu, she handed over his small savings to him to carry to his home and family.

I have not mentioned this episode to depict myself heroically. It was a trifling incident and I was only little more than a boy at the time. Many people stand up against injustices when they come across them in their life. But I have another purpose in relating this story. The trait in my character which made me stand up to secure fair treatment for the poor laborer became an integral part of my behavior in my official career also. I shall discuss this in more detail at another place in this work. At the time, this irrepressible impulse brought me into collision with official superiors who could make or break my career. On at least two occasions I ran the risk of losing my job. But I persisted in the belief that if one door was closed, another would be opened for me by fate.

The annals of the poor are thick with battles of this kind, but they are seldom made known to the world. The whole attention of chroniclers and historians is absorbed by the mighty, the strong and the rich. They lavish their talent to perpetuate the stories of those who are already widely known, without caring for the means by which notoriety or fame was gained. In the vast majority of cases, those famous figures of history extracted much more from the world than they gave to it. They occupied positions of power or distinction or honor not always by virtue of the merit they possessed but more often by tact, adroitness, strategy, intrigue, and even sometimes with murder, deceit, treachery, or betrayal.

History often makes no mention of the legions who, possessing the same or even greater merit, were put out of the way, suppressed, exploited, trodden down, deceived, betrayed, disabled, or killed to force the passage open for these so-called great ones to make their debut on the stage of fame.

For her supreme prize however, Nature has closed all the loopholes by which the ambitious, the adventurous, the power hungry, or the covetous could enter the arena. The laws of celestial justice circumvent all the machinations of men and women. And they live in ignorance of this fact. There is no distinction between mighty or weak, rich or poor, in the dispensation of heavenly grace. The intelligent forces of evolution take no account of position, power, wealth, or possessions. They may select a nonentity who conforms to the qualifications demanded in preference to the mightiest, the strongest, or the most informed, who more often than not attain to their height flouting the laws prescribed.

Values will change, new laws will come into force, new patterns of society will be devised, new criteria for merit and distinction will be framed, and the whole structure of history will be rebuilt when the implications of kundalini arousal become universally known.

At college there was no repetition of the bullying which I endured in the early school days when I joined the eighth class in Lahore. By that time I could speak Punjabi fluently and carried myself with assurance amongst the other students. I had a close friend in one of the boys from the school who joined the same college and was placed in the same section with me. He later entered the medical profession. I met him years later in Lahore where he had built a house for himself. On the partition of the Punjab he moved to Delhi and I never saw him again.

There was no other friend with whom I kept in contact after I had left the college. There was also no noteworthy event except the shock of failure in the house examination, which prevented me from going to university. It was this failure that became the turning point in my life and spurred me on to a more disciplined life than I had been leading before. But for the mastery gained during those years when the brain was more plastic and more amenable to control, I could have easily succumbed to the ordeals that I had to face on the arousal of the Serpent Power.

I remember one incident during my college period which is worth recording. I had so far stood the scorching heat of summer in Lahore very well. It was no trial for me to return at noon from my college to my home in the burning sun without an umbrella, covering a distance of more than a mile and a half from the college. On several days in the week I had to walk over again the same distance to the college and back to my home for games in the afternoon when the sun was still hot and bright. I never felt distressed, even when the heat was suffocating and walked unconcernedly in the hottest sun.

During my first summer in the college, for some inexplicable reason I lost my appetite. My food intake was so drastically reduced that, greatly alarmed, my mother sought the advice of physicians to cure the condition. There was no sign of any illness or fault in the system. But I lost all relish for food and would have liked to go without it altogether. For several years past my mother had been extremely careful with my diet. Some instinct told her that I should not be allowed to be with an empty stomach for a long time. She invariably thrust a small bottle of milk and a little round cake in my pocket before I left for school, both at Srinagar and at Lahore.

During the later years of the First World War, the prices of foodstuffs rose so high that the meager pension my father received was insufficient to cover the expenses. It became necessary to make drastic reductions in our daily diet. But my mother did not allow it to have the least affect on what I was accustomed to eating. When the price of rice became more than double, she purchased only half the quantity and contented herself and her cousin with the liquid drained off when the rice was cooking, reserving the solid portion for me and my father.

There was no diminution either in the daily cup of milk I was accustomed to drink or in the small measure of meat which she prepared for me almost every day. She cooked it without allowing my father to have the least awareness of it. He hated even the sight of flesh and would never allow it to be brought into the kitchen. In this way I continued to have the food which my mother believed was most healthy for my system, even during the days of high prices and scarcity which the family had to face.

During this summer, no amount of persuasion or coaxing on the part of my mother helped me to overcome the sudden distaste for food which I felt. We could not understand the reason for it nor could the kind physician who treated me explain it to us. He prescribed some medicines, but they did not help. My stomach revolted at the sight of food and I found it difficult to swallow even a few mouthfuls.

At last, my mother began to suspect that my long sojourn in the hot climate of Lahore had upset my system and that a trip to Kashmir might help to bring back my appetite for food. The doctor was consulted and after a brief examination he agreed at once, remarking that he was sure the change to a cool place would do me good.

The college summer vacation started soon and I left on the very first day at the insistence of my mother, who was in a state of great alarm about my condition. In order to travel to Kashmir in those days it was necessary to take the train to Rawalpindi and from there to hire a horse cart to Kashmir to cover the distance of about two hundred miles between Rawalpindi and Srinagar. But, only shortly before, motor lorries had started to ply between Rawalpindi and

Srinagar, reducing the time of travel to two days and even less. These lorries had solid rubber tires.

My aunt and her husband dwelt in Rawalpindi in those days. They had been transferred there from Lahore and Mian Mir. My uncle, who had been informed, came to meet me at the station and took me home. My aunt had prepared several delicious dishes for me to eat on my arrival. But I could eat only a few morsels and left almost all the delicacies untasted. On the next day in the morning I left for Srinagar in a lorry.

About seventeen miles from Rawalpindi the road to Srinagar starts the ascent of the Murree Hill. Because of its thick forests and low temperatures, the higher regions of the hill (over five thousand feet above sea level) provide an ideal resort for summer. We reached the Murree top at about noon and the lorry stopped for the passengers to have something to eat. I knew the state of my appetite but in order to have a few bites I asked the owner of a food shop to serve me a chapati (a small, thin piece of unleavened bread), with a little dhal (lentils) and vegetables.

But a change had already occurred in my system without my knowledge. I consumed chapati after chapati, eating with a hearty appetite for the first time in months. To my surprise and joy, even after eating more than my normal quantity and washing it down with cool fresh water from the spring, I still felt relish for more food. My appetite had returned, redoubled with the first caress of the cool mountain air on my body. I ate ravenously on the way and for some days after to make up for the deficiency suffered for months.

I passed all the months of that summer vacation in my native village, spending many hours in sports and games. I even extended my visit beyond the vacation with the consent of my mother, who wished me to be healthy and strong again. When the walnut season started, the temptation was too much for me. I was always fond of green walnuts from my childhood. On this occasion, I and three or four of my village friends, all of them almost of my own age, made a plan to climb the trees in a walnut grove close to our own house at midnight when no one was there to see us and to decamp with as many walnuts as we could gather. This was a risky undertaking as the trees were large in size and tall. To climb such huge trees in darkness was very dangerous as one could never be sure of his foothold in the tricky shadows of the night. But none of us was deterred by this consideration. In fact, we could not even realize the dimension of the risk in our youthful optimism. We went from branch to branch at great heights from the ground, trying to pluck as many walnuts as we could. The boy who gathered the largest number was acknowledged as the leader.

On one of these escapades I narrowly escaped serious injury. It was a moonless night and I had climbed a tall tree which bifurcated at some distance from the ground into two huge branches, each one a tree in itself. A certain nervousness was always present in us as the owners of these trees had come to know of our escapades at night and were acting to prevent it. Some of them actually tried to lay an ambush to catch us red-handed, but we always managed to outwit them and escape their clutches.

On this occasion we heard voices while we were up in the trees, indicating that some people were passing that way. Thinking that it might be an ambush to catch us, I and my friends flattened ourselves against the branches on which we were standing and stayed there without making the slightest movement till the voices grew faint and faded altogether. Fearing that the party might return, I hurriedly descended from the height to which I had climbed. But when I reached the trunk of the tree where it bifurcated into two I forgot in my haste that I was still on the tree a good distance above the ground.

Letting go of the branch that I was holding, I took a step in the air and fell on the hard gravel slope below, hurting my buttock, thigh, and knee by rubbing against the hard knotted trunk and impact with the small stones below. It took me quite some days to recover from the hurt, although after that we were soon at our nightly adventures again. The villagers whose walnuts we were stealing knew my mother very well and did not have the heart to be too harsh with me. Finally they gave up their attempts to catch us and even sent word that I need not risk my life at night and could have all the walnuts that I needed for the asking during the day. We now had all the walnuts we wanted but the excitement and adventure ceased.

On my return journey to Rawalpindi I had a rather unpleasant experience. We left Srinagar rather late and halted at Baramulla for the night. Among my fellow travelers there were two young students, older than me by a few years, who had come from some town in the Punjab. All the three of us hired a room for the night, and after that went to a nearby shop for our meals. When we returned to our room, the eldest of the two suggested that we make a round of the town before going to bed. As it was my habit to go early to bed after dinner I declined politely and went immediately to sleep. It was past midnight when they returned and knocked at the door. I awoke and opened the door to let them in. They walked heavily, with uncertain steps, towards their beds.

I saw their faces in the dim light of the lantern burning in the room and was shocked at their appearance. They had visited a house of ill repute and drunk heavily. I felt thankful that I had not agreed to their invitation and gone with them. They sank into their beds with all their clothes on and slept till morning. When we arose they tried to avoid my eyes, as if ashamed of their conduct. But later on that day with a guilty smile the eldest made the confession on the plea that sometimes it was good to have a little fun of this kind.

On my return to Lahore I felt even more healthy and strong than I was before. The few months of my stay in Kashmir in pastoral surroundings, indulging in vigorous physical activity for several hours every day, helped me greatly to regain my strength.

The next summer my brother-in-law invited me to pass the vacation with him. At that time he was serving as a Forest Ranger in Basant Garh, a hilly area in the Jammu province, two days' journey on foot from Udhampur. He sent his servant to fetch me. We went by rail from Lahore to Jammu and by bus from Jammu to Udhampur and thence on foot to Basant Garh.

It is a cool region, about five thousand feet above sea level, covered with tall pine and deodar (Himalayan cedar) trees interspersed with beautiful meadows that are a delight to the eye. I had already started the practice of meditation and applied myself to it regularly every day. The dense forest surrounding the large wooden shanty which served us as our residence provided me with beautiful secluded spots with charming natural settings for my daily practice. I took full advantage of the opportunity and exercised not only once but even twice or thrice every day. Fortunately a hint from within always came to caution me when I meditated too much. On such occasions I felt an instinctive reluctance to meditate for a day or several days at a stretch, which helped to restore me to my normal condition.

Excessive meditation, especially in the rush and hurry of modern urban life, can be very harmful instead of beneficial. A forced activity of the evolutionary mechanism can put a greater strain on the body than it can bear, leading to psychic imbalances of various kinds.

During the time of my stay in Basant Garh, my brother-in-law was much impressed by the change in my demeanor and my unbroken daily practice of meditation, to which I gave priority over everything else. Almost every day we sat talking for hours on this subject dear to both of us. He narrated to me his own experiences in the remote district in which he was serving at that time. One of the Forest guards, serving under him—a Rajput by birth—was a remarkable case of a double personality in one of which he displayed extraordinary psychic gifts.

Every Saturday, my brother-in-law told me, the guard invariably returned to his home from the place where he served. The spirit of a departed yoga adept manifested itself in him on the Sunday following. He rose early in the morning, completely altered from what he had been during the preceding week. A special room had been set apart for him to officiate as a yogi on that day. Besmeared with ash and wearing only a loincloth, he sat in asana in front of a small fire, which India's ascetics often keep burning before them. With a large pair of tongs on one side and a begging bowl on the other he looked every inch a sadhu seated in his ashram.

The rumors of the extraordinary miraculous feats he could perform in this condition had traveled far and wide. This led hundreds of visitors, some out of curiosity and some to seek a boon, to assemble in front of the door of his house each morning to seek answers to problems they had on their mind. They were not allowed to articulate their questions. He read their thoughts, one by one, as soon as they entered into his presence, and supplied answers suited to their questions. Singly, or in twos or threes the pilgrims to his shrine went in and came out, often astounded at his performance.

In his normal state, the conduct of the guard was unimpeachable. He was attentive to his duty, truthful and honest in his dealings. My brother-in-law never had a reason to find fault with him. One Sunday, drawn by curiosity, he went to the village of the guard. Without revealing his identity he mingled with the crowd standing in front of his house. No one knew him there and he did not talk or disclose the purpose of his visit to anyone. But he was visibly startled when, after a short time, the man standing at the door to control the entry of the crowd shouted his name at the top of his voice, saying that Shambu Nath, Forest Ranger, present in the gathering is ordered to the presence of the yogi. All eyes were turned towards my brother-in-law as he obeyed the summons without a word.

He had come with two questions prepared in his mind. One was "What is the nature of Divinity?" and the other related to his personal career. He had suffered a loss in his official position due to a false complaint made against him and wished to know what would be the decision of his superiors in the case. The guard, sitting cross-legged and erect in his posture as a yogi, did not show the least sign of recognition when he entered the room and instantly proceeded to answer his unspoken questions as he did with the others. "Your first question is unanswerable," he said. "What you wish to know has never been known and can never be comprehended in future as it is incomprehensible. About your second question, the matter will take a favorable turn soon and you will come to know of it." Shortly after, the complaint was proved false and the case was decided in his favor.

During my stay in Basant Garh, I too had an occasion to witness a psychic demonstration of another kind. The tutelary deity of the Hindu inhabitants of this hilly area is Goddess Chamunda. This is one of the names of Shakti (Kundalini). I had no knowledge then of the association of this name with a mighty force in the human body. There are small temples dedicated to the Goddess scattered over the whole region. The population is poor and, in those days was mostly illiterate, primitive, and superstitious, but good-hearted and friendly. There is a widespread belief among her worshipers that the Goddess can enter into chosen vessels among the dwellers in that region, who are known as chelas, or disciples. During the period of the possession, the disciples are transformed into clairvoyants, soothsayers, and healers. In that state they can provide evidence of extraordinary psychic or physical capacity not normally possible by other villagers. This puts the seal of confirmation on their claims that they are the chelas of the Goddess during the ceremonial performances.

In order to provide me with an opportunity to participate in one of these performances, my brother-in-law arranged our journey to Baskund, a mountain lake about 12,000 feet above sea level. To reach this lake we had just to climb to the top of the mountain known as Kaplas or Syoj to the local villagers, which rose to a height of about fourteen thousand feet above the sea. During the course of this journey, we had to pass through a village where a function of the Goddess was to be held on the day after our arrival.

On that day, from early morning onwards, the villagers began to assemble in a large square room with the effigy of the Goddess in a miniature temple built into one of the walls. There was a small square pit in the middle of the room to light the sacred fire. A small crowd of about thirty villagers had gathered in the room when we arrived there. Soon the fire was lit and preparations for the ceremony began. A group of five or six people, some with flutes to their lips and some with cymbals in their hands, began to play an eerie monotonous sort of music which swelled slowly until it filled the whole apartment. The worship of the Goddess had begun. A solemn hush fell upon the gathering and all eyes were turned towards the effigy in the temple.

In the dim light of the morning the whole ceremony wore a weird and uncanny aspect. There was an awed and fascinated look on the faces of the worshipers. I looked at my brother-in-law. His face looked pale and tense. The supernatural has a strange fascination for the human mind. It has always been in evidence since earliest times. After the ceremony was over, my brother-in-law said to me in confidence that the music and the atmosphere of the room had such a strange effect on him that his legs trembled and he felt urged to jump into the middle of the crowd. I felt no symptoms of the kind and stood unmoved to the end, watching the ceremony with a critical eye.

After the music had continued to play its plaintive strains for some time, an elderly short-statured man with a small gray beard on his round cherubic face suddenly jumped into the space left open round the sacrificial firepit for this very purpose. He was the headman of the village, and it was he who had arranged for our lodging and our other needs at the time of our arrival there. He seemed to be such a good-natured, artless human being that no one could easily associate trickery or deception with him.

With a sudden and unexpected jump into the open space in the middle of the crowd, he turned towards the temple in the wall and bowed low to the effigy of the Goddess with eyes closed and hands folded before him. While standing in this posture, he suddenly jerked himself erect and, as if galvanized to action by a powerful electric current passing through his body, at once began to shake from head to foot like a vibrating wire or a fast whirling machine. The movement from side to side was so rapid that his face appeared to be a blur, moving with a velocity that did not allow the features to be noticed. This vehement oscillation continued almost through the whole period of the performance, but slackened later to a degree where his face could be recognized and his voice heard. When the movement was still at its height, he took a small iron trident with a pointed handle from an assortment that rested on a projection of the wall, close to the image of the Goddess, and drove it into one of his cheeks, drawing it out from the other. The audience looked on in silence at the performance watching every movement of the man. The music had now ceased and all was still in the room.

There were other tridents also, with handles as long as three to four feet and thick as the middle finger of a man. After the ceremony was over, I was told that the longer tridents were used to pierce the stomach from one side to the other. They pointed to a younger disciple of the Goddess, stout and strong in build, standing there. "When possessed by the Goddess," they said, "he places the pronged end of the trident firmly on the ground and, bending over it, spits himself at the middle of the stomach until the other end projects out from the back. The wound heals immediately and there is no flow of blood."

The young man smiled when I looked at him, but I saw nothing in his appearance to conclude that what was reported about him could be a sleight of hand or trickery on his part, but I did not witness his performance. He had nothing to gain by it. In those poor, primitive surroundings the disciples had no chance of gain or lucre through their demonstrations. They performed their feats or acted as clairvoyants or healers merely as an offering to the Goddess. They did not use their gifts as a profession but only as a form of worship of the deity. I was mystified but not entirely convinced until I later came to read reports of the amazing feats of psychic healing and painless surgery claimed for the Brazilian José Arigo and for Philippine healers.

It seems to me now that there is a clear similarity between the disciples of Chamunda in the hilly districts of Dudoo and Kishtwar of Jammu in the north of India and the performances of the Philippine and other psychic healers. We can also trace a similarity to the well-known exhibitions of the American psychic Edgar Cayce.

The elderly chela soon also gave a demonstration of his clairvoyant and healing skill. There were several in the gathering who had come to seek his help. He prescribed herbal remedies and diet cures for their ailments, which they accepted on faith and heard with attention with the clear intention to follow. He also answered a few unspoken questions from others.

My brother-in-law had a question to ask which he did not actually articulate. This related to our contemplated pilgrimage to Baskund, the high mountain lake. It was the rainy season and the journey was at that time beset with difficulties and risks. The chela dispelled his fears with the assurance that, although the weather would be cloudy, we would reach our destination and return safely.

There are other shrines of the Goddess in that romantic, remote, far-flung, hilly region, in which the same kind of demonstrations are witnessed on certain festival days. One disciple, we were told, had the reputation of performing operations with a sword during the period of his possession without leaving any trace of blood or a wound after it was done. I refused to believe it then, but in the light of the stories now current about the surgical feats of psychic healers and my experience of kundalini, I am now of the view that an open-minded exhaustive study of such phenomena might reveal secrets and knowledge of forces still unknown to science. The fact that practices and phenomena of this cateogry have been current from earliest times is sufficient to expose the fallacy of the view which would summarily dismiss these exhibitions as superstition or faulty observation on the part of those witnessing them. There is such a close resemblance between these performances and those observed in some other parts of the world that the conclusion becomes irresistible that there is more behind these displays than we are able to explain at present.

Our trip to the sacred lake was uneventful and we returned

without encountering any obstacle on the way. This was the first time that I saw a mountain summit stretching for miles, forming a meadow of inexpressible charm and beauty, thickly strewn with small pretty flowers of different kinds and colors, all combining to present a glorious vista on which the eye never tired of feasting. Patches of melting snow, interspersed with the fresh green of the meadow, sent down tiny streamlets of water that sparkled and glistened as they meandered through the mosaic of flowers and the green turf. The scent coming from the flowers was overpowering. It was a wonderful sight and I stood lost in contemplation of the beauty which unadorned Nature can display, breathing the fragrant mountain air in large gulps to fill my whole being with its vitality and freshness. The scene is still vividly present in my memory. I can evoke the picture as fresh and clear as if I had seen it only yesterday.

This reminds me of a still inexplicable facet of my experience. I can recall the whole picture of the landscape on which my eyes lighted that day exactly as I saw it in my then-normal state of consciousness more than sixteen years before the kundalini awakening. But if I now imagine myself at the precise spot and try to visualize the panorama in the context of my present state of awareness, the picture is different. Magnified and bathed in silvery luster, the vision assumes a glorious and sublime proportion which was not there when I actually perceived it. In other words, I can recall the scene both in its original form as I saw it then, and also in the form as I would see it now. This exercise of my memory makes manifest, without the least shadow of doubt, the tremendous difference that had occurred in the pattern of my consciousness on account of the ministration of the Serpent Fire.

We were guided to the lake by a *gaddi*, a term applied to shepherds who dwell on these heights in summer to graze their flocks. They build small stone sheds with grass roofs for shelter and their ferocious dogs mount guard on the flocks day and night. Looking down from a rocky peak of the mountain we could see two lakes down below nestling in crater-like depressions, covered with ice. The slippery slope leading down to the edge of the lake was too steep for us to negotiate on foot. Both I and my brother-in-law, seated on folded blankets with an alpenstock in one hand, slid down the depression using the staffs to break the speed of the descent. The steep slope ended abruptly on the waters of the lake, making it necessary to slide down with caution. But two barefoot *gaddis*, one of them holding each of us by the arm, ran down on either side of us, supporting our weight when the speed exceeded a safe limit. They took a dip in the icy water at the same time as we did, and lit a fire for us to heat ourselves. On the way back, at places too steep for us to climb, they cut steps into the ice with the small axes they carried thrust into cloth girdles round their waists.

All this time they walked or ran barefoot with utter nonchalance, as if the icy wind that blew and the freezing cold of the snow under their feet had no existence for them. It is marvelous how Nature inures living creatures to the vigor of the climate in which they live. The strongest man alive not adapted to these conditions could never perform the feat which these unknown dwellers of a mountainous area did without even realizing the exceptional nature of the performance.

The whole prodigious load of the human race is held on shoulders which never come into the limelight, but which ache day and night with the heavy weight they bear. They never proclaim their greatness or are eager to be acclaimed great. They know their humble position and are content to pass their days in peace.

The sailor, the miner, the peasant, the laborer, the shepherd, the fisherman, the waiter, the scribe, the soldier or the domestic servant patiently toil on, relinquishing the place of honor to the ruler, the statesman, the general, the scholar, the rich trader, the intellectual, the teacher, and the priest. The latter do all the shouting and pushing, they cause all the ferment and fervor while the former provide them with all the necessities of life—shelter, food and clothes—and also the raw material for the work which they claim as their own. Where, then, is social justice when the clever brain takes all the credit and profit in everything while the others merely toil and sweat?

FOUR

Lessons Learned from My Father

I AM VERY HESITANT in discussing psychic powers. One reason for this is the fact that in a large percentage of cases those interested in the occult often show a greater predilection for psychic powers than for a divine state of consciousness. It is a tragedy that the real purpose of yoga or any other religious or occult discipline is not correctly understood. The aim is to attain a new dimension of consciousness and to build a new personality in rapport both with the visible and the occult worlds. If this objective is kept in mind there is absolutely no necessity for striving after psychic powers. They develop automatically when the objective is achieved.

Occult gifts without illumination are not a blessing. The studies of hundreds of mediums all over the world for the last century now make it clear beyond dispute that they have little or no control over the force which acts through them to cause the phenomena. In most cases they lie in a trance or semi-trance condition as if under the control of an external force entirely unknown to them. In others, they appear to be in a state of uncontrollable excitement and agitation as if forced to act in a manner in which they are normally incapable of acting. In either case the performances are neither elevating nor inspiring. They might be exciting and mystifying but this is only a transitory phase. A few months of constant attendance at the seance chambers is sufficient to cause satiation or attrition of the thirst for the phenomena.

The one advantage of mediumistic or psychic gifts is that they furnish evidence for the existence of other forces and planes than those which we perceive with our senses. They tend to revise or amend the picture of the universe presented by the intellect. The experiments conducted on psi phenomena during recent years have contributed not a little to diluting the entirely materialistic tendency of modern science. A large number of scientists now openly accept their validity, although their existence challenges some of the fundamental concepts of modern science.

Although I was slow to admit their existence, there is no doubt that my father was possessed of extraordinary psychic faculties. He never purposely demonstrated or exhibited them to cause curiosity or sensation. But sometimes they were evident spontaneously without any such intention on his part. No one who came in contact with my father could ever doubt that he lived and acted in another plane of consciousness. His whole behavior was a constant reminder of this fact.

It often happened that while talking with the family, which he did only rarely, he would suddenly pass off into another mood with a faraway look in his eyes, oblivious to those to whom he was speaking a moment before. The thread of the conversation was abruptly broken. When he came back to the present moment he was too overwhelmed by what he had witnessed during the interval to be able to continue the conversation.

According to Indian tradition, one of the signs of kundalini awakening is *vak-siddhi*. This means "prophetic utterance." What the tradition implies is that the words of an illuminated personality concern the future as easily as the present. This is the base from which the oracles and prophets drew their strength and their support from the masses. It was believed that the spirit or the power speaking through them had transcendental knowledge beyond the reach of the common folk.

The idea that human beings could officiate as the vehicle of expression for divine communications was more prevalent in the past than it is now. In this age too, there are many mediums and sensitives who evince faculties of this type to some extent. But in its real sense, *vak-siddhi* denotes a condition of transcendental knowledge in which the spoken word of an enlightened soul has the character of revelation and presage.

After his retirement, my father seldom evinced any desire for the company of his former friends and even relatives. He kept himself aloof from the activity and bustle of the world. The few friends who sometimes found a chance to talk to him often stayed in a state of awe in his presence. Even my mother and my elder sisters stood in awe of him. This was not because of his stern or severe attitude but because of an aura which he emanated and because the words he spoke at times, even in the course of ordinary conversation, proved so premonitory or prophetic that everyone who had this experience once was deeply impressed in their subsequent meetings with him.

At times it seemed as if he literallly read one's thoughts and answered them. But he never did this purposely. He was too much occupied in his own inner manifestations to be the least concerned with showing off his extraordinary gifts to make an impression. There was absolutely no desire either for fame or wealth. I can assert without hesitation that he was one to whom (according to the supreme test prescribed in the *Bhagavad Gita* [14:23–24] to distinguish the really enlightened) a lump of earth and a piece of gold were the same.

I am confident that my father had won to this state because once there occurred an event in the family which proved this beyond the least shadow of doubt. We were living in Srinagar in those days in a rented house close to the second bridge. This is the house where I was eventually married. There was a temple nearby on the bank of the river Jhelum, which I used to visit for my morning ablutions. The event occurred soon after my marriage.

A friendly neighbor who had lottery tickets to sell came one day to urge my mother to try the luck of the newly wedded bride and to purchase a ticket in her name. My mother immediately agreed and instead of one, purchased two tickets in her name. The result of the lottery was to be announced a couple of months later.

On the day of the announcement, the friend came running in great excitement to tell my mother that we had won the second prize, which amounted to fifty thousand rupees. My mother could not believe her ears and was profuse in her thanks to the friend for his advice to purchase the tickets. She could not contain herself for joy and at once sent word to my sisters to come and participate in her happiness.

My wife was in ecstasies. The lottery had proved that her entry into our family had the most auspicious augury for us. Since the retirement of my father, the family had been carrying on a hand-to-mouth existence. The mother, the daughters, and the daughter-in-law now sat together to discuss how this gift from Heaven should be utilized in the best possible way.

Not to leave my father out of this wonderful stroke of luck, my eldest sister went down to his room to convey the joyful tidings to him. He listened to her account in silence without making any comment. When I returned from the office in the afternoon I found the family almost dancing with joy and excitement. My mother and my sisters breathlessly told me the news of our great good fortune while my wife, filled with happiness, with bashful, downcast eyes, heard words most flattering to herself.

Suddenly I heard my father calling me down to his room. I hurried there at once and said, "They must have told you that we have won a lottery in the name of Bahurani [daughter-in-law]." He replied "I just heard of it from Janaki [my eldest sister]. I think it must be a mistake. But if it turns out true, do you know what we have to do with the money?" I replied respectfully that I did not know and would like to be enlightened. "Either spend the whole amount on charity," he answered, "or carry the sum with you to the bridge and drop it silently into the river at night when there is no one there to see you."

I looked at him in silence while he continued. "It is a gamble. Wealth not earned with hard effort can never be conducive to virtue or happiness. So you have to promise me that you will act on what I say."

I hesitated to give a direct answer. Fifty thousand rupees was a fortune for our poor family, and we had a hundred uses for it. We had no house of our own in the city. This was a pressing need for which, at least, a part of the sum could be utilized. My father clearly read my thoughts but said nothing. Finally I assured him that I would give full thought to what he had said and talk it over with him again before putting the money to use, when it was certain beyond doubt that our ticket had won the prize.

The next day the friend came again but crestfallen this time. He apologized for the false hopes he had raised. It was a terrible mistake. The number of one of our tickets was close to the one that had won the prize and that was the reason for his error. When I conveyed the news to my father I could see that he felt distinctly relieved of a load he had on his mind. The family was plunged into gloom at the news after having touched the height of jubilation for a short period.

A man of this caliber, risen so high above temptation, could not be expected to exhibit psychic gifts for petty human objectives. But they came to him as naturally as harmony flows from the fingers of a violinist. All the members of the family tried their utmost not to give the least cause for offense and implicitly obeyed his direction to carry out his wishes. It was not a difficult task as his wants were extremely few and he seldom interfered in our way of life.

I remember several incidents which clearly pointed to his extraordinary clairvoyant and prophetic gifts. I can recall every detail of these events since they made a powerful impression on my mind at that time. In spite of the fact that psychic faculties had become a normal part of my father's mental endowment, I was not at all happy either at the extreme degree of asceticism which he imposed upon himself or the utterly isolated life which he led. I never saw him bubbling with joy or beaming with happiness at the unbounded wonder and ecstasy of the inner world. He never experienced the beatitude of liberated consciousness. I feel this poignantly since he had done all that was humanly possible to conform to the disciplines which tradition prescribes for inner transformation. Perhaps he went too far in his efforts at self-denial and consequently was denied the prize which was otherwise due to him.

One incident occurred during the course of one of our journeys from Srinagar to Jammu. According to the practice still prevailing, the central offices of the government of Jammu and Kashmir have their headquarters in Srinagar during summer and in Jammu in winter. This is done for climatic and political reasons. The maharajas of the state shifted their residence from one to the other to keep themselves in touch with the people of each province and also to counter the inclemency of weather at either place.

We usually made the move to Jammu in the month of November and from Jammu to Srinagar in May. On this particular journey, we started rather late from Srinagar in a bus, which in those days used to take one and a half days for the distance of about two hundred miles which separates Jammu from Srinagar. We were on the other side of the upper Banihal tunnel when it began to grow dark. We were passing over a sharply winding road in the higher regions of the mountain. It is a barren slope traversed by furious winds at times and the path turned and twisted so abruptly that the driving had to be done with great caution.

Our destination that day was the village of Banihal, but it grew so dark before we could reach it that the driver thought it prudent to pass the night a few miles away rather than face the risk of night traveling with a furious wind beating in our faces. He halted at a place where no habitation was near and we had to pass the night in the bus the best way we could manage. There were no other passengers except ourselves since the bus was loaded with government records and had room for only a few passengers. We usually carried some cooked provisions with us on these trips. We dined in the interior of the vehicle. This done, each of us went to sleep with a blanket covering our bodies.

There were two other lorries traveling along with us, carrying only freight. They too decided to stop at the same place. Our driver and his assistant went to sleep with their comrades in the other lorries, leaving us all the room to accommodate ourselves. They came to wake us up while it was still dark next morning, saying that if we wished to reach our destination in good time we should start at once.

My father was still sleeping with the blanket covering his face. The rest of us awoke and were soon in our seats but my father did not stir and continued to sleep without paying any attention to the words of the driver. I hesitated to waken him but the driver, impatient at the delay, gently shook him awake. My father pulled the blanket from his face to know the reason for the disturbance. The driver repeated his words and motioned him to take his seat. My father looked in his face for a moment and then said: "Your haste will not help you to reach Jammu earlier, as there is a dead man across the road further on." The driver probably thought that he was still not fully awake and was repeating what he had seen in a dream. When my father was in his seat, he jumped into his own and the bus began to move.

When the sun began to rise about twenty miles further on, we were traversing a narrow stretch of the road with a gorge on one side and a steep, rocky slope of the mountain on the other. This narrow condition of the road continued for some distance at this place. After turning a corner, the driver saw a sprawling figure in the middle of the road and slowed down his speed. When we came nearer, great was our horror to see the body of a man lying at full length across the road with a load tied to his shoulders, his skull broken and brains scattered round. There were a huge boulder and a few smaller stones scattered close to the corpse obstructing the road on that side.

We could easily distinguish that the dead man was a Gujjor. He belonged to a community which subsists on herds of sheep and cattle, dwelling at high altitudes with their flocks in summer. They often migrate from pasture to pasture to feed their animals.

Looking towards the precipice on our left we could distinctly see the outline of a narrow footpath cut into solid rock about fifty feet above the road on which we were traveling. It could be that the man, while walking over this narrow track, had missed his foothold and fallen to his death on the road below, dislodging the boulder and the stones in the course of his descent. It could also be that the stones were dislodged by someone walking across the narrow path and that they descended with force, hitting the man on the head while he was walking on the lower road. The body and the stones lay across the highway in such a manner that there was no room to pass without running over some part of the corpse.

The drivers and their assistants conferred with each other. They were in a quandary. The position of the body left insufficient room on the river side of the road for the vehicles to pass. The boulder and the stones obstructed the other side. Removal of the corpse or the clearance of the stones would show clear signs of displacement and could involve them with the police as soon as an investigation was started. This they wished to avoid at any cost.

In the excitement of the moment the driver of our bus seemed to have forgotten all about the morning incident. He was a Sikh and, judging from his behavior, a good man. While conversing with the others, the whole memory of the morning suddenly came back to him in a flash. He changed color and, pointing to my father, whispered something to his comrades under his breath. They became fidgety and their eyes too turned to my father in wonder. Then, as if with one accord, all of them stood up and came close to us. Our driver, bowing to my father, touched his feet and asked for forgiveness for his behavior in the morning. My father, touching him on the shoulder, pointed to the other side of the road indicating that they could pass from that side. Encouraged by this gesture, the party pushed away the boulder and the stones to make room for their vehicles.

We never heard anything further about the incident. Obviously, the police did not care to investigate who had moved the stones to clear a passage for lorries to pass.

A second incident occurred in Srinagar. It was during the middle of summer. One day, after returning from his morning walk, father addressed my mother while we were all sitting together in a room and said: "Don't you hear the cries and lamentations? There is an epidemic in the city and scores are dying every day. But we are safe."

There was no epidemic and no outcry. Everything was functioning as usual. He repeated this warning several times, as if he actually witnessed the death and heard the cries. After about a month the first case of cholera was reported in the city. This was followed by a raging epidemic and hundreds died before the scourge could be controlled.

Another incident concerned my mother's cousin, who came to Lahore with us, found employment there and continued to stay when we returned to Kashmir. He was married and had a son. One summer he returned to his village home in Gairoo with his family, on leave from his office. We learnt this from a messenger who arrived with the news that he was ill and wanted to come to Srinagar for treatment.

I at once left for Gairoo to inquire after his health and to bring him with me to the city. He loved me dearly and had proven himself very affectionate and kind to all of us. He was a little hurt at my not coming up at once to meet him when he had arrived at the village, but we had not then known of his arrival. I explained the position to him and invited him to accompany me to Srinagar. We left for the city the next day.

At this time we occupied another house also close to the second bridge but on the opposite side. I put the cousin in our best room on the third floor. My father occupied a room on the fourth. He knew nothing about my cousin's illness or that I had brought him down from Gairoo. But he knew him very well as he had dwelt with us for years before we left for Kashmir.

My father was coming up the stairs when suddenly his eyes fell on our cousin sitting in the room assigned to him. He said nothing but on reaching the next floor called me by name and said, "Why have you put that corpse in the room below?" I was shocked and said that it was our kind relative, Baba Kak, naming him distinctly to bring him to the memory of my father. But he shook his head and said that it was a dead man whom I had placed in that room. There seemed nothing serious about the illness. It was an attack of chronic malaria and the condition of our cousin showed no symptoms of a grave nature. But during the next three days the illness took a sudden turn for the worse and he expired less than a week after the fatal prediction was made.

Clairvoyance and presage are common in the case of disoriented products of kundalini arousal. People in this category are known as *mastanas* or *avadhuts* in India. They are a class apart, and their disorientation is ascribed to miscarriage of spiritual practices or their failure to adjust themselves to the spiritual life on account of evil karma or some other cause. But they are venerated everywhere and crowds of people flock to them to have their *darshan* or to win their favor. They are often utterly indifferent to the world and its norms. But their remarkable psychic gifts are so amazing that they are regarded with awe and wonder by those who seek their company.

My father's predilection for this class of sadhus and saints had naturally a very unfavorable influence on his thinking and drove him to that extreme of asceticism which in all probability was the cause of hindrance to his harmonious transformation. Even before my own awakening, I was convinced by the example of my father that psychic gifts like telepathy, clairvoyance, premonition or presage were a reality, but there seemed to be no explanation for them. The clairvoyant observations and predictions made by my father could not be explained away.

Apart from this example, there is much evidence to show that prophecy, presages and premonitory dreams do sometimes come true. But to admit this involves a change in our whole concept of the universe and the laws of physics in particular. A single well-attested prophecy, coming true in every detail, is sufficient to question our assumptions about space, time and causality.

How can we know months or even years before that a certain

event will take place at a certain time without complete awareness of the whole causal chain leading up to it? But such absolutely certain calculation seems impossible since we can never have complete information of all the forces and all the circumstances, including the movement of atoms, that bring about the occurrence. This means that if such a precognition is possible there must be a higher Intelligence hidden within us that is latently aware of all that is happening or shall happen in the cosmos. In that case the explanation for these isolated precognitions could be that at times a hint from this Cosmic Intelligence penetrates into the mind of the psychic to convey the information given out as a premonition or a prophecy.

I was mystified by such clairvoyant and prophetic demonstrations by my father, but I never allowed myself to be carried away by them. What could it profit me, I reasoned with myself, if I could foretell what happened to a person or to myself at a certain period of time, when whatever I presaged was bound to happen even if I did not foretell it. It could have no effect on the fated event beyond a momentary sensation at my skill at prophecy.

On the other hand, a presage could have definite disadvantages. If the forecast pointed to a happy event, as for instance a sudden good fortune—addition to wealth, a high position, triumph over rivals, or recovery from an illness—its premature disclosure could tend to create a false sense of security and lead to the slackening of efforts to achieve what is foretold. On the other hand, if the forecast was of a misfortune or any evil threatening the individual, its premature intimation could prolong the agony that would otherwise be experienced only when the event actually occurred. Besides this, there is absolutely no guarantee that a prediction will really come true.

Out of hundreds of predictions made by clairvoyants and prophets, only a few turn out to be true. From an academic point of view, even a few predictions fulfilled in due course of time are of tremendous significance in enlarging our concept of the universe. But from an individual point of view, since the ratio of correct forecasts to those that turn out false is extremely small, those who depended on them to satisfy themselves about the future would always have to live in a state of uncertainty and suspense, in addition to their other worries. They could never be sure whether or not a particular prediction would turn out true. This uncertainty could seriously interfere with their peace of mind and even color their behavior.

I have never been able to understand why psychic phenomena should have such an exaggerated importance for so many people. In India I have seen crowds of people listening with rapt attention to the raving of hopeless lunatics, whom they sometimes confuse with disoriented *avadhuts*, in the hope of catching a word favorable to themselves or conveying an anwer to questions they have in mind.

It is a fact that some of the inmates of mental clinics evince paranormal faculties and show signs of behavior peculiar to those in whom kundalini, the Serpent Power, is aroused. This is not the place to enter into a detailed discussion of this matter. But there is no doubt that clairvoyance and telepathy are sometimes the possession of the insane who are not even aware of such faculties. In some cases such paranormal gifts are more pronounced than in others. In India, such individuals soon become the focus of public attention and crowds surround them when they walk through the streets.

I knew of one individual known as Lassa Mutoo in Srinagar. The name means "Lassa the mad." During the months of winter, he used to walk stark naked through the streets, with an earthenware pot on his shoulder filled with burning charcoal. The earthenware pot sometimes grew so hot that it literally burnt his flesh, causing streams of melted fat to pour down his body. He was totally immune to pain. His chest, abdomen, shoulders and the back of his neck were scarred with burns from the fire.

It was a horrible sight to see him, yet crowds followed him wherever he went. Whenever he stopped at a shop to ask for a loaf of bread or any other article of food he needed it was at once given to him. He spoke only rarely but his clairvoyant faculties, of which he occasionally gave sensational demonstrations, surrounded him with a halo of mystery and awe that caused people to stand and listen to him with reverent attention in spite of his loathsome appearance.

Anesthesia has often been a feature of mystical experience. The loss of sensation can occur not only in some forms of insanity but also in mystical ecstasy. Lassa Mutoo, it is very probable, was a case of a morbidly active kundalini which made him a clairvoyant on the one hand and an anesthetic maniac on the other. I have cited this example to show how the passion for psychic exhibitions can pervert taste to such an extent that even loathsome specimens of humanity can become objects of reverence and worship. People do not then stop to think that the individual whose feet they touch is a pitiable creature lost to his sanity and sense and that one who cannot cure himself of the terrible malady by which is gripped cannot help to tide them over their own difficulties.

This perverted taste is often the outcome of ignorance about the true aim of spiritual discipline and the nature of religious experience. It is for this reason that Indian masters have laid the greatest stress on *viveka*, or the power of discrimination between true and false or right and wrong. The mystical state, though extremely rare, has a peculiar character of its own. It has been confined to a class of men and women who found access to an inner world of beauty, grandeur and happiness, more captivating and satisfying than the physical world in which they lived. The connection with psychic phenomena should be studied.

Apart from the psychic faculties displayed by my father, there was another peculiar characteristic. Judging it on the basis of my later experience, I unhesitatingly assert that he had experienced the arousal of the Serpent Power. At times, he would burst into song in Punjabi, his native tongue, and continued singing for a spell in complete absorption. During these intervals his eyes turned upwards, revealing the whites through the half-closed lids, while his face assumed a sublime expression of intense happiness and peace. I was too young then to grasp the significance of this mood or to ask him any questions about it. I was surprised because on such occasions the expression on his face was so unlike its normal appearance.

The songs he usually sang were couplets from the verses of the well-known mystic of Punjab, Bulla Shah. They were touching pieces dwelling on the majesty and happiness of inner experience. After the last note of the song was over, a hushed silence used to follow for a few more minutes while the eyes still remained half open but completely withdrawn from the world. Then a torrent of tears rolled down his cheeks, enhancing the rare beauty of expression that his face wore at the time. After that, with a start, his eyes opened, looking vacantly at the objects around for a few moments before his face resumed its normal expression.

I was always struck by this sudden change in his moods which, though rare, presented his personality in an entirely different light. If he had been more communicative or if I had been a little more forward with him than I was, it is possible I might have picked up from him some hints about the condition he was in, which would have helped me in later life when I hovered between life and death on my own entry to the same state. But it was not destined to happen that way and I had to find my own path through trial and suffering to learn a few elementary facts about kundalini arousal.

It was only in after years that I could link these absorbed moods of my father with the ecstatic conditions normal to yogis and mystics. Sri Ramakrishna used to weep when his trance was over. Tears of gratitude and joy at the termination of the ecstasy are a common feature of the phenomenon. The mind is so overwhelmed by the wonder and the sublimity of the encounter that on return to normal experience, the gulf seems so great that the heart is melted and tears involuntarily flow down from the eyes at the sharp descent from the sublime majesty of the soul to the ego-bound awareness of individual mortal life.

FIVE
Mother Arranges My Marriage

IN MY YOUTHFUL STUDIES the information I accumulated from the high school texts and more extensively from the study of other literature had the effect of purging my mind gradually of irrational and fantastic notions I had gathered in childhood, replacing them with a rational and realistic picture of the world.

Occasionally, noticing an exact identity of thought between what I felt but could not articulate and the clearly expressed idea of a writer, I was so carried away by emotion that, dropping the book, I would stand up and pace the room for a while to compose myself before continuing to read. In this way my mind was molded by degrees as much by my own inborn ideas about the nature of things, developed by the exercise of reason in the healthy atmosphere of literature, as by the influence of the great thinkers whose ideas I imbibed from their works.

By the time I had completed my first year at college, the impact of the books, especially elementary treatises on astronomy and natural science, to which I had access in the college library, as well as my ideas, formed or confirmed by continued study, had become powerful enough to start me on a path contrary to the one I had followed in childhood, and it did not take me long to emerge a full-fledged agnostic, full of doubts and questions about the extravagant notions and irrational beliefs of my own religion, to which I had lent complete credence only a few years before.

Dislodged from the safe harbor which my mother's simple faith had provided for me, my still unanchored mind was tossed here and there, clinging to one idea for a time and then replacing it with another, found to be equally untenable after a period. I became restless and reckless too, unable to assuage the fire of uncertainty and doubt lit by my own desultory studies.

Without reading any standard book on religion or any spiritual literature to counterbalance the effect of the admittedly materialistic tendency of the scientific works I had gone through, I took up cudgels on behalf of the latter, wielding my weapons with such dexterity that in the college debates, as well as in private discussion, few adherents of the former could defend their points of view.

Although until that time I had not studied religion or tried any method of direct spiritual experience, nor acquired systematic knowledge of any science or philosophy beyond that provided by a few elementary volumes, the questions and problems which agitated my mind at that young age never found a satisfactory solution in any book on science, philosophy, or religion.

Study of the scriptures and also of the literature of the other religions did not suffice to quiet the restless element in my nature or to appease the hungry spirit of critical inquiry. Stray passages from the teachings of prophets and the expressions of sages found an echo in the depths of my being without carrying conviction to my uncompromising intellect. The very fact that the existing world religions, descended from prophets or inspired sages, while claiming to trace their origin to revelation from the Creator, differed radically in their cosmogony, mode of worship, observances, ritual, and even in some basic tenets, was enough to raise serious doubts in my mind about the authenticity of the claim that the revealed material was a direct communication from God, the infallible source of all wisdom, and not merely the creation of more advanced brains in occasional touch with a higher but sometimes still fallible plane of consciousness.

The total demolition by science, even in its very infancy, of some of the citadels of antiquated religions, especially on the cosmogonical side, was sufficient in my view to expose the vulnerability of their other fronts as well to the attacks of its now robust opponent at any time.

But science itself, though extremely useful in other ways and serviceable as a battering ram to smash religion, if not out of existence, at least out of shape, was not in my view fit to rule the domain where faith held sway. It had no satisfactory explanation to offer for my individual existence or for the infinitely complex creation around me. Confronted by a mystery, which grows deeper with the advance of knowledge, it was not yet in a position to be a source of illumination on issues admittedly beyond its present sphere of inquiry.

I thirsted for rationality in religion, for the worship of truth, whatever and wherever that might be. There was no spectacle more painful for me than the sight of a conscientious and intelligent man defending an absurdity which even a child could see through, simply because it formed an article of his faith to which he must hold at any cost, even if that cost included the sacrifice of reason and truth.

The conflicts and controversies going on between different faiths on the one side and between faith and philosophy on the other, made me wonder whether it would ever be possible to have a religion that possessed an appeal for all human beings, that would be as acceptable to the philosopher as to the peasant, and as welcome to the rationalist as to the priest.

Viewed in the context of a rigidly law-bound universe, as revealed by science, the miracles and supernatural manifestations associated with faiths appeared to me to be but isolated and as yet not correctly interpreted phenomena of a cosmic law, still shrouded in mystery, which had to be understood first to explain satisfactorily the apparent obscurities and anomalies of religion and religious experience.

More intent on demolition than construction, I read ravenously until in my second year I began to neglect my prescribed studies to the extent of giving preference to the library over the classroom. I was brought to an abrupt halt by my failure in the college examination towards the end of 1920. The shock demolished with one blow the seemingly invincible fortification of intellectual skepticism my immature judgment had created around myself.

I had grossly neglected my studies. The time I should have devoted to them had been recklessly spent in the reading of light literature, particularly novels and books, on subjects that had nothing to do with my college courses. Too late I realized that I knew next to nothing about some of the subject, and had no chance whatever of passing the test. I had no doubt gained a fund of information but it could not help me to pass the examination and bring joy to the heart of my mother, who centered all her hopes in me.

My guilty conscience reminded me that I had betrayed her trust in me and had taken advantage of her ignorance to read whatever books I liked while she was always under the impression that I was hard at work studying the college courses. It was impossible for me to make a clean breast of my dereliction and seek her forgiveness. It would have given her a great shock to know that I had been so neglectful of my duty and so callous of the expectations she had of me.

For days and nights I racked my brain for a plausible excuse to mitigate the effect of the painful news on her. She was so confident of my success that I simply had not the courage to disillusion her. I was a merit scholarship holder, occupying a distinguished position in the college, and was always highly spoken of by the teachers. I felt crestfallen, pierced to the quick by the thought that my mother, proud of my distinction and sure of my ability to get through the examination with merit, would be deeply hurt at this avowal of my negligence.

Instead of yielding or collapsing, I turned determinedly towards a path, actually aligned for me by nature, as it is at the moment for thousands of other men and women all over the world. I could not have visualized at that time what transpired afterwards, just as by no exercise of fancy can even an intelligent person form the least conception of what awaits on the superconscious plane.

Realizing that by my lack of self-control I had betrayed the trust reposed in me, I determined to make up for the lost opportunity in other ways. At no other time in my life should I be guilty of the same offense again. But in order to curb the vagrant element in my nature and to regulate my conduct it was necessary that I should make a conquest of my mind, which, by following unhindered its own inclinations to the neglect of duty, had brought me to such a sorry plight, a prey to poignant grief and remorse, fallen low in my own eyes.

Having made the resolve, I looked around for a means to carry it into effect. In order to succeed it was necessary to have at least some knowledge of the methods to bring one's rebellious self into subjugation. Accordingly, I read a few books of the usual kind on the development of personality and mind control.

Out of the huge mass of material contained in these writings, I devoted my attention to only two things: concentration of mind and cultivation of will. I took up the practice of both with youthful enthusiasm, directing all my energies and subordinating all my desires to the acquisition of this object within the shortest possible period of time. Sick with mortification at my lack of self-restraint, which made me yield passively to the dictates of desire to substitute absorbing story books and other light literature for the dry and difficult college texts, I made it a point to assert my will in all things, beginning with smaller ones and gradually extending its application to bigger and more difficult issues, forcing myself as a penance to do irksome and rigorous tasks, against which my ease-loving nature recoiled in dismay, until I began to feel a sense of mastery over myself, a growing conviction that I would not again fall an easy prey to ordinary temptations.

From mind control it was but a step to yoga and occultism. I passed almost imperceptibly from a study of books on the former to a scrutiny of spiritualistic literature, combined with a cursory reading of some of the scriptures. Smarting under the disgrace of my first failure in life, and stung by a guilty conscience, I felt a growing aversion to the world and its hopelessly tangled affairs that had exposed me to this humiliation; and gradually the fire of renunciation began to burn fiercely in me, seeking knowledge of an honorable way of escape from the tension and turmoil of life to the peace and quietude of a consecrated existence.

At this time of acute mental conflict, the sublime message of the *Bhagavad Gita* had a most profound and salutary effect on me, allaying the burning mental fever by holding before me the promise of a perennially peaceful life in tune with the Infinite Reality behind the phenomenal world of mingled joy and pain. In this way, from the original idea to achieve success in worldly enterprise by eliminating the possibility of failure owing to flaccid determination, I imperceptibly went to the other extreme. I was soon exercising my will and practicing meditation not for temporal ends, but with the sole object of gaining success in yoga, even if that necessitated the sacrifice of all my earthly prospects.

My worldly ambition died down. At that young age, when one is more influence by ideals and dreams than by practical considerations and is apt to look at the world through golden glasses, the sorrow and misery visible on every side by accentuating the contrast between what is and what ought to be tend to modify the direction of thought in particularly susceptible natures.

The effect on me was twofold: it made me more realistic, roughly shaking me out of unwarranted optimism based on the dream of a painless, easy existence, and at the same time it steeled my determination to find a happiness that would endure, and had not to be purchased at the cost of the happiness of others. Often in the solitude of a secluded place or alone in my room I debated within myself on the merits and demerits of the different courses open to me.

Only a few months before, my ambition had been to prepare myself for a successful career in order to enjoy a life of plenty and comfort, surrounded by all the luxuries available to the affluent class of our society. Now I wanted to lead a life of peace, immune from worldly fervor and free of contentious strife. Why set my heart on things, I told myself, which I must ultimately relinquish, often most reluctantly at the point of the sword wielded by death, with great pain and torture of the mind? Why should I not live in contentment with just enough to fulfill reasonably the few needs imposed by nature, devoting time I could save thereby to the acquisition of assets of a permanent nature, which would be mine forever, a lasting ornament to the unchanging eternal Self in me instead of serving merely to glorify the flesh?

The more I thought about the matter, the more strongly I was drawn towards a simple, unostentatious life, free from thirst for worldly greatness, which I had pictured for myself.

The only obstacle to the otherwise easy achievement of my purpose which I felt was rather hard to overcome lay in winning the consent of my mother, whose hopes, already blasted once by the sudden resolve of my father to relinquish the world, were now centered in me. She wished to see me a man of position and substance, risen high above want and able to lift her economically ruined family out of the poverty and drudgery into which it had fallen by the renunciation of my father, who had given away freely whatever my thrifty mother could save from their income, leaving no reserve to fall back upon in time of need.

I knew that the least knowledge of my plans would cause her pain, and this I wanted to avoid at any cost. At the same time the urge to devote myself to the search for reality was too strong to be suppressed. I was on the horns of a dilemma, torn between my filial duty and my own natural desire to retrieve the decayed fortune of the family on the one hand, and my distaste for the world on the other.

But the thought of giving up my home and family never occurred to me. I should have surrendered everything, not excepting even the path I had selected for myself, rather than be parted from my parents or deviate in any way from the duty I owed to them. Apart from this consideration, my whole being revolted at the idea of becoming a homeless ascetic, depending on the labor of others for my sustenance. If God is the embodiment of all that is good, noble, and pure, I argued with myself, how can He decree that those who have a burning desire to find Him, surrendering themselves to His will, should leave their families, to whom they owe various obligations by virtue of the ties He has Himself forged in the human heart, and should wander from place to place depending on the charity and beneficence of those who honor those ties?

The mere thought of such an existence was repugnant to me. I could never reconcile myself to a life which, in any way, directly or indirectly, cast a reflection on my manhood, on my ability to make use of my limbs and my talents to maintain myself and those dependent on me reducing me practically to the deplorable state of a paralytic, forced to make his basic needs the concern of other people.

I determined to live a family life, simple and clean, devoid of luxury, free from the fever of social rivalry and display, permitting me to fulfill my obligations and to live peacefully on the fruit of my labor, restraining my desires and reducing my needs, in order to have ample time and the essentially required serenity of mind to pursue calmly the path I had chosen for myself. At that young age it was not my intellect but something deeper and more far-seeing, which, building on the reverse suffered by me and triumphing at the end over the conflict raging in me, chalked out the course of life I was to follow ever after.

I was ignorant at the time of the awful maelstrom of superphysical forces into which I was to plunge blindly many years later to fish out from its fearsome depths an answer to the riddle which has confronted human beings for many thousands of years, perhaps waiting for an opportunity, dependent on a rare combination of circumstances to come in harmony with the modern scientific trend of human thought, in order to bridge the gulf existing between ingenuous faith on one side and critical reason on the other.

I can assign no other reason for the apparent anachronism I displayed at an unripe age, when I was not shrewd enough to weigh correctly all the implications of the step I proposed to take in adopting an abstemious mode of existence, to strive for self-realization while leading a family life, instead of tearing asunder the bonds of love, as is done by hundreds of frustrated youths in my country

every year in emulation of highly honored precedent and in consonance with scriptural and traditional authority.

As mentioned in an earlier chapter, we lived in Lahore in those
days, occupying the top part of a small three-storied house in a
narrow lane on the fringe of the city. The area was terribly congested,
but fortunately the surrounding buildings were lower than ours,
allowing us enough sun and air and a fine unobstructed view of the
distant fields. I selected a corner in one of the two small rooms at
our disposal for my practice and went to it every day with the first
glimmer of dawn, for meditation.

Beginning with a small duration, I extended the period gradually
until in the course of a few years I was able to sit in the same
posture, erect and steady, with my mind well under control and bent
firmly on the object contemplated for hours without any sign of
fatigue or restlessness. With hard determination I tried to follow all
the rules of conduct prescribed for the students of yoga.

It was not an easy task for a college youth of my age, without the
personal guidance of a revered teacher, to live up to the standard of
sobriety, rectitude, and self-restraint necessary for success in yoga,
amidst the gaiety and glamor of a modern city in the constant
company of happy-go-lucky, boisterous fellow students and friends.
But I persisted, adhering tenaciously to my decision, each failure
spurring me on to a more powerful effort, resolved to tame the
unruly mind instead of allowing it to dominate me. How far I
succeeded, considering my natural disposition and circumstances, I
cannot say, but save for the vigorous restraint I exercised upon
myself for many years, curbing the impetuosity and exuberance of
riotous youth with an iron hand, I think I should never have survived
the ordeal which awaited me in my thirty-fifth year.

My mother understood from my suddenly altered demeanor and
subdued manner that a far-reaching change had taken place in me. I
never felt the need of explaining my point of view to prepare her for
the resolution I had taken. Reluctant to cause her the least pain, I
kept my counsel to myself, avoiding any mention of my choice when

we discussed our future plans, considering it premature, when I had not even completed my college term, to anticipate a contingency due to arise only at the time of selection of a career. But circumstances so transpired that I was spared the unpleasant task of making my determination known to my mother.

After giving up my studies at the college, several courses were open to me. I could seek employment in one of the various departments of administration. In fact, my uncle once arranged a short-term assignment for me in a leave vacancy, and I did not have any difficulty in doing the work allotted to me. I was eager to supplement the slender income of the family with my efforts to help my mother to spend a little more freely on our needs. I had also the opportunity to apply for training to qualify myself for one of the professions. My eldest brother-in-law, always very kind and loving towards me, offered to help us financially during the period of my training. But he did not favor the medical profession for reasons of his own. He thought it was inhuman for a physician to demand fees in a case which he could not restore to health. I followed his advice and gave up any ideas of entering this profession. The outdoor life of a forest official had a greater appeal for me. I had had a taste of it on two occasions when I went to stay with my brother-in-law in his forest residences during summer vacations.

I applied for the training and was advised to appear in an interview and test to be held by the Conservator of Forests. He allotted me the second position among ten candidates selected for that session. His officer advised me to make preparations for my departure to Dehra Dun, as my nomination was certain. But that very year the Punjab government issued a directive that admissions to the training should be made on the basis of certain criteria laid down to provide due representation to the candidates of different communities. Contrary to expectations, my name was excluded from the list and a candidate from another community selected in my place. The Conservator of Forests, a short-statured stern man, as

I summed him up during my interview, lodged a strong protest at this overruling of the selection made by him, but to no avail.

It was a gloomy day for the family when I returned home and communicated the sad tidings to my mother. She wept bitterly, attributing my failure to the ill luck that had followed the footsteps of the family since the time of retirement of my father.

Looking back now at these happenings through the long vista of time, I cannot help thinking that everything that transpired during those days to push me into the events that followed later tended, in some way, to place me in circumstances favorable to me in the crisis I had to face later.

A strenuous course of training, followed by the demands of a profession in which I had to try my utmost to excel ahead of others, would have left me little time to attend to my regular practice of meditation, which was to become a part of my daily life. I had already started the practice when these events occurred. It was my attitude of detachment that I was steadily cultivating which helped me to keep unruffled and calm even in the face of the serious disappointments I had to face in those days. I never allowed ambition to have a place in my mind. Affluence also had no allurement for me. Our mind soon adapts itself to the luxuries provided by wealth and then starts to suffer from unsatisfied longings for more of the pleasures of earth, which can never be satisfied to the limit. From my point of view, destitution and overabundance were both detrimental to spiritual growth as both acted to disturb the even tenor of life. I was not therefore really grieved when my hopes for admission to the Forest College, after having been raised so high, were dashed to the ground. What really pained me was to see my mother's dreams of better days shattered, time after time, on account of my failures.

Meanwhile a sudden breakdown in my health due to heat created such anxiety for my mother that she insisted on my immediate departure to Kashmir, attaching no importance to my studies when a question of my health was involved.

She was happy when I finally succeeded in securing an appointment in Srinagar in the Public Works Department of the state. My health was more precious to her than my career. She drew a sigh of relief as she saw a modestly secure future for our small family. My earnings could now supplement our slender income and allow a better standard of life than we had been able to follow so far. A distant relative, holding a responsible post in the State government, helped me to secure this appointment. I went to Jammu from Lahore to seek help. The formalities were finalized in a few days when I returned to Lahore to convey the glad news to my mother. Preparations for my journey were soon made and I arrived in Srinagar to join the appointment well in time. I stayed with my eldest sister until my parents followed me after about a year. Soon after, my mother busied herself in finding a matrimonial alliance for me.

She did not have to search for long. Our relatives and a matchmaker whose services she engaged came with various proposals to her soon after she expressed her intention to them. In the settlement of marriage in our society the horoscope of the bridegroom and the bride are compared to see if the constellations tally to the benefit of each other. The other formalities are decided after this comparison is done. The responsibility for the reading of the horoscopes falls on the parents of the bride. It is they who have to signal their assent to the match after satisfying themselves about the astrological affinity of the couple.

There was a lot of excitement in our family at the time as our friends and relatives came with their offers to my mother. I left the whole issue in her hands, confident that whatever she decided would be best for me. The only wish I expressed was that the bride should be sound in health and pretty, of gentle blood and descent. Whenever she discussed an offer with me the only comment I made was that she should see the bride herself to make sure that we would be well matched.

In those days it was hard to obtain the consent of the parents to allow their daughter to be seen by anyone on the bridegroom's side. It was considered to be an affront to permit their daughter to be interviewed. The result was that the bride and the bridegroom did not usually see each other until the marriage day. In recent times conditions have now changed and the partners see each other and meet openly, often with the consent of their parents.

Finally, an offer made by a friend of the family appealed to my mother. It came from a gentleman who had served my father and knew our family very well. The Kashmiri Pandit family of the bride-to-be resided in Baramulla, a town more than thirty miles from Srinagar. The father of this girl was known to the gentleman as they both worked in the same department. He reassured my mother on every score and pledged his word that the marriage he was proposing satisfied her wishes in every way. My mother gave her consent, relying on his assurance that there was no need for her to see the bride, who was seven years my junior in age.

A date was fixed for the marriage and with her usual thoroughness my mother proceeded to make the preparations in which both my sisters participated. The responsibilities that devolved on me as the breadwinner of the family I shouldered myself to avoid putting too much strain on my mother. We had a little sum set aside for the function and a little more was willingly lent by my eldest brother-in-law and sister. It was a modest wedding in every way. We hired a bus to carry our relatives and friends to Baramulla, where a sumptuous feast had been prepared for us. My father-in-law was considered to be among the affluent residents of Baramulla and he had to live up to his reputation on this occasion.

Marriage functions in our society are considered to be the appropriate occasions for the display of one's wealth and position. This leads to a competition during the marriage sessions which must be seen to be believed. Families that can hardly live a hand-to-mouth existence sometimes become so lavish in their expenditure during the function that not infrequently the economic collapse suffered takes years to remedy.

During the ceremony, my wife tried to wrest the wedding ring from my finger but soon had to desist when I held her fingers between mine with a little force. The function came to an end as usual amidst the tears of the family at the time of the departure of the bride from her parental home to the home of her husband. This is always a pathetic scene.

Why it should be that it is the more delicately constituted and more sensitive woman who has to bid farewell to her ancestral home to join the bridegroom's family is rather hard to understand. Marriage institutions all over the earth need radical change and reforms to conform to the eugenic needs of the evolving race. This would be the first important issue that should come under scrutiny and investigation as soon as the evolutionary function of kundalini is empirically proven.

Meanwhile, our hosts lodged our party in one of the two buildings belonging to them. The bride was received by my mother in one of the rooms of this building while I, my father, and our guests sat and chatted in another part of the house.

A little while after the reception of the bride my eldest brother-in-law came to me in a state of perturbation which I could easily notice in his face. Putting his lips to my ear he said in a whisper that my mother, in a furious fit of anger, had lost all control over herself and was creating a terrible scene downstairs. I was dumbfounded. There was apparently no reason why she should behave in this outrageous way. She always kept herself well under control and her behavior, especially when in company, was perfect. I could not believe my ears. It was so unlike her to act in this manner that I thought at first that my brother-in-law had mistaken her for someone else. But soon another relative came up with the same story.

Leaving the place of honor reserved for the bridegroom during the function, I went hurriedly downstairs to learn the cause of the outburst. The room was full with men and women, some standing and some seated on the carpeted floor, many of them belonging to the bride's family. The outburst had occurred when my mother embraced the bride and lifted her veil to look at her face. I could never understand why she should have lost her temper so completely.

Probably the first look at my wife did not satisfy her about her comeliness. Perhaps, smitten with remorse that she had relied on the pledge of another and had not seen the bride herself as I had wished her to do, she felt angry with herself and gave expression to her feelings in a show of temper entirely out of keeping with her usual behavior.

The bride's people stood aghast, completely unnerved by this sudden explosion, unable to say a word, while my wife burst into a paroxysm of weeping. There was consternation in the bride's family as the outburst augured for them a bitter future for their daughter. But they dared not say a word. In those days the fate of the newlywed girls in our society depended so much on the mercy of their husband's family that their parents, sisters and brothers had to live always in submission to the other family. To some extent this is the position even now. But time, the great renovator, has brought a considerable change in the former position. My mother fell silent as soon as she saw me enter the room. The daily practice of meditation and my constant effort at self-discipline had built into me a sobriety uncommon at that age. My mother did not wish that my equanimity should be disturbed and so calmed herself with an effort. Walking straight to where she was sitting I put my arm around her neck and said in a whisper, without knowing the reason for her anger, that she need not disturb herself over trifles and should accept calmly what Heaven has ordained for us. That was sufficient to soothe her feelings. Within a few minutes calm was restored and my wife too ceased her sobbing. I returned to my place upstairs.

The next day our marriage party returned to Srinagar with the bride. At the time of our departure I asked my brother-in-law to convey word to my in-laws that they should not entertain the least disquiet in their minds about the incident and that their daughter would be treated in our house with the same love with which they had treated her to that day.

The bride's family never really came to understand the cause of my mother's sudden fit of anger. They probably attributed it to her disappointment with the dowry. But that was not the reason at all. The reason was that she thought I would be disappointed and unhappy at her choice and the thought was too much for her to bear with composure. Back at home she took me into her confidence and told me all about the cause of her displeasure. I made no protest and soothed her feelings. But in my heart of hearts I felt a keen disappointment, as I had all along counted on the fact that she would leave no stone unturned to see my wish fulfilled. She had promised to do so, but luck was against it.

At night my sisters conducted the bride to the nuptial chamber. It was a small room with a low ceiling and bare walls, a sorry place for a bride to sleep in on the first night of her marriage. But I never allowed my mind to dwell on our abject poverty. We had sufficient for our basic needs—shelter, food, and clothing—and that was enough for a happy inner life.

I entered the room after my sisters had left. My wife was sitting on the bed with her face buried in her arms. I sat by her side and gently lifting her face looked at her for the first time. She offered no resistance and looked at me bashfully under her half-closed eyelids. It was a homely face, but her eyes were beautiful and the whole atmosphere she breathed was of devotion and love.

What had upset my mother in the light of the room where she first saw my wife was the languor on her face. She looked weak and ill cared for. But the languor was mainly due to sleepless nights and nerve-racking strain and stress of the bridal days. She had a delicate constitution and the strain had been too much for her. She was very young, only fifteen years of age, ignorant of the world and its ways. She slightly trembled as I continued to look at her for a few moments with my hand on her arm.

Suddenly a sense of deep resignation swept over my mind and a feeling of assurance entered my heart. "She is the destined partner of my life," I said to myself. "I have pledged my trust to her and I must fulfill my duty towards her as best I can." Taking her gently into my arms, in a voice filled with emotion and love I calmed her fears and assured her of my love and care for all the time to come. In the early hours of the morning when I rose for my usual bath at the temple watertap followed by meditation, I repeated my assurance and left her with an embrace to follow my daily routine.

My mother was delighted when she saw that I made no complaint to her in the morning. We never discussed our brides before our elders in those days. I could not even talk to her in the presence of my mother, sisters, and other elders for many days to come. She had to sit with her face half covered with a veil or with one of the sleeves of her long dress.

The standard of decorum, decency and self-mastery of which our girls are expected to conform in the houses of their husbands is so exacting that, if applied to young men, they would rather forego their marriage than submit to it. The behavior of the bride must be perfect in every way when she sits from morning till evening surrounded by scores of women who come to see her in her new home at every hour of the day, without regard to her convenience. She must sit with her face half-covered without uttering a word except to answer questions with a sign from her head, exercising a measure of self-control which is hard to believe.

My mother was a strict disciplinarian, and her ambition was to see her daughter-in-law managing the household as well as she did. She found an earnest pupil in my wife, ready to learn, and this reassured her that the new member of the family was worthy of her trust and care. My wife never learned to read and write. She cannot even sign her name nor do addition or subtraction of even small figures. But for the last forty years now she has run the household in an admirable way, brought up her children, and cared for me in a manner beyond reproach.

My wife soon learned to awaken early and was up with me when I rose to leave for my bath. I startled her on our very first meeting by leaving the nuptial chamber at three o'clock in the morning for a bath under the copiously flowing water tap in the nearby riverside temple, returning after an hour to sit in meditation without a word until it was time to leave for work. She admirably adjusted herself to what must have seemed to her unsophisticated mind an eccentric streak in her husband. She was ready with a warm *kangri** when I returned from the temple, numb with winter cold. She had folded the bed, swept the room, and arranged my seat at the proper place for me to sit in meditation on my return. If it was too early she sat in the room awaiting my return and then left at once to work in the kitchen. She picked up her duties promptly without having to be reminded about the tasks she had to do and performed them to the satisfaction of my mother.

She admitted that she had seen me secretly from the window when I entered the compound of their house dressed in the finery of a bridegroom with a feathery crest on my head and loved me from that moment. The custom in those days was to dress the bridegroom in gorgeous clothes to make him appear like a prince. This manner of dressing is still prevalent, but the feathery crest on the turban is no longer used. In some parts of India the bridegrooms still come riding on a horse clothed in gorgeous attire, with a sword hanging on one side, and tresses of gold or silver tied to the headdress, hanging before their face.

I had a proof of my wife's deep attachment to me soon after our marriage. It was customary for our brides to be recalled to the houses of their parents and to stay there for varying periods, to allow a welcome break in the cloistered lives they have to lead at the husband's house. There is a formal procedure to regulate this movement of the bride between the two families. A word has to be sent through a messenger to seek the permimssion of the husband and his parents for the bride to return to her parental home. On her return to the husband's family, she must be accompanied with presents and a sum in cash according to the position of the family. On certain festive days or on the birthday of her husband or father-in-law or even a brother-in-law, costly presents in cash and kind

---

*A *kangri* is a small earthenware bowl encased in wicker in which burning charcoal is kept for heating the body. It is usually kept next to the skin under the long robe used by Kashmiris.

must arrive from her father or her guardian. This is a barbarous custom which causes unspeakable economic torture to parents who have several daughters to marry.

A word to my wife that she should not stay too long at Baramulla and comply with the wishes of my mother whenever she needed her presence back in our home was sufficient to elicit her compliance from the very beginning. She never tarried in her parental home a day longer than the period specified. A message or even a letter was enough to recall her at a moment's notice. She had a love for household work which was astonishing. From the very first day she realized that this was her home and she always tried her utmost to live up to the part which she thought was hers as the caretaker of the family. We rented the small house in which I was married and which we retained until I was transferred to Jammu a few years later to serve my term in that province. She followed me after a few months with my parents, to both of whom she endeared herself by her sense of duty and unremitting attention to their comfort.

Years passed, not without lapses on my part and interruptions due to circumstances beyond my control, but I never lost sight of the goal I had set before myself and never swerved from the path I had chosen, decreed in this manner to prepare myself to some extent, without having the least knowledge of the crisis I had to face in the great trial ahead.

SIX
Fighting Against Corruption

IN MY POST AT the Public Works Department in Srinagar I was new to the work assigned to me in the office but I picked it up quickly, assisted by the senior hands who were pleased with my behavior. After about a year I was transferred to Jammu in summer. As I did not wish to drag the family with me there in the unpleasant heat of summer I went alone on the understanding that they would follow me in autumn when the blistering heat was over. I and four of my office friends hired a commodious apartment and engaged a man to look after our needs. By the time my family arrived I had already rented another apartment sufficient for our needs in a different part of the city. We passed several summers in this house and became adapted to the simple surroundings, which I still remember with happiness. I usually had one or two of my nephews with us, to have lively youngsters to care for.

After a few years I was again transferred to a moving office which allowed us to shift to Kashmir in summer. In one of these trips my eldest child Ragina was born in Kashmir. That year the family stayed in Gairoo, our native village, while I resided with my sister in the city to be close to the office. Once or twice a week I passed the night at Gairoo, traveling the distance on my bicycle both ways. Once, before the birth of Ragina, my wife and I were invited to Baramulla, and her brother came to fetch us from Gairoo. We left the village rather late and had to wait at the roadside for another couple of hours before a bus picked us up and carried us to Srinagar. It was already evening when we arrived and so there was no chance of our traveling to Baramulla that same day. My wife and I passed the night at our sister's and her brother went to the house of a relative to pass the night.

There was a cholera epidemic in some parts of the valley and cases had occurred in villages close to Gairoo. There was no protected drinking water supply in the rural areas during those days and the streams were liable to contamination. I had told my mother to boil the drinking water but still the risk was not eliminated. Before we left for Baramulla my mother complained of pain in the bowels and decided to fast. When I was about to retire to rest in Srinagar that day the thought struck me with the force of a blow that I had been negligent and had not taken care to assure myself about my mother before I left with my brother-in-law. The prevalence of cholera in the nearby villages should have made me more cautious about the pain she had experienced. I was soon plunged into a frantic state of anxiety and remorse for my guilt. "How could I have acted so rashly and foolishly when maybe her life was at stake?" I said to myself over and over again.

It was nearly ten o'clock at night and the idea of returning to the village was impossible to put into practice. I did not say anything to my sister but went out into the street and thence to the market for medicine. Fortunately a chemist's shop was still open and I purchased a small phial of Amrit-Thara, which was then considered to be a specific for cholera. At three o'clock in the morning I quietly left the house carrying with me my brother-in-law's bicycle and in about two hours was at Gairoo again. It was still dark when I arrived there but soon saw my mother, who was an early riser, coming out of the house towards the stream for her morning ablutions. She was startled and surprised at seeing me but soon felt reassured when I disclosed the purpose of my early morning visit. She embraced me tenderly saying that she had now no pain whatsoever and that I had worried myself for nothing. In a few minutes she prepared a cup of hot milk for me. After a brief repast, I was soon on my way again and was back in the house before my sister had returned from her morning visit to the temple.

The birth of our first child was a happy event for my mother. She had been praying for it. My wife was husking rice for several hours

on the day prior to that on which Ragina was born. I came to
Gairoo that very day in the evening, after attending the office. The
husking is done by thrashing the grain placed in a large wooden or
stone mortar with a large heavy thrasher made of strong wood. It is
a fairly strenuous exercise when carried on for hours, but my wife,
like most other women in our society then, was accustomed to it.
The child was born easily the next day with only the help of the
village nurse. After a short period of rest my wife was up and active
again.

My official duties were now moved to the Bureau of the Divisional
Engineer in Charge of Irrigation Works, Kashmir. It was a new
office, as the appointment of a chief engineer for irrigation was
created for the first time. I was entirely unused to the work I now
had to do. Some of my colleagues had already served in other places
and had all the information they needed to make a selection of their
duties according to their choice. During those days, graft and corruption were widespread in the administrative offices, especially the
Public Works Department. My colleagues took care to install themselves in positions which provided better chances for illicit income. I
was at first ignorant of all these details and for a long time could
not even understand the artifices they adopted to gain opportunities
for graft.

I was assigned the duty of maintaining the records, of which I had
no experience at all. My ignorance allowed my colleagues to do as
they liked. Taking advantage of my newness, they had free access to
whatever files they liked to see. The Divisional Engineer himself,
unlike most of his colleagues, was an honest man. Slowly I became
familiar with the work and also began to gain more thorough insight
into the actions of my fellow clerks.

After only about a year, I was transferred to Jammu. Sometime
later the post of the Chief Engineer of Irrigation was abolished and
some of the clerks in that department, including myself, were transferred to the office of the Chief Engineer, who now controlled all the
Departments of Public Works, including Irrigation. Somehow my

work and behavior impressed the Superintendent of the office and he put me in charge of the administrative section to deal with the personal cases of the whole staff employed in the Department.

It was a responsible post with many avenues for illicit financial gain. What I came to learn afterwards showed me to what lengths greed for lucre can go to achieve its ends. The reason why it is so hard to eradicate corruption from government services rests on the fact that the position of power which even a petty official holds can provide a number of attractive channels for the practice which it is often not possible for even the most astute administrator to block. One single instance can serve to illustrate this.

The executive engineers of the Public Works Departments are placed in charge of sections, each of which is allotted a specified sum for the work it has to do in a year. With some honorable exceptions the executive officers in my time worked in collusion with the contractors to whom the works were assigned, to share in a part of the profits. This was possible by permitting inferior construction and inferior material, by overlooking faults, or by altering the specifications of the work done. The entire staff, from the lowest clerk to the executive officer, exerted their ingenuity more on finding ways to defraud the administration and the State than in the satisfactory discharge of their work. Secret meetings were held, code messages were sent and received, and many other devices were used to cut as large a slice for their own use as they could from the grants allotted to them.

The office of the Chief Engineer received its due share of the stolen gains, some of the officials more than the others. One of the methods to extort more than the due share was pure blackmail, though of an ingenious kind. When the budget figures became known, a mark was placed against the subordinate executive engineers who had the largest amounts to spend during the year. This naturally also assured for them a larger share of the budget. On an appointed day, rumors began to emanate from the office that large-scale transfers of executive officers were in the offing. This made the officers with larger budget grants more nervous than the rest. The rules of transfer were purposely kept loose and there was no prescribed limit before which a transfer could not be made in any case, except through complaint or inefficiency. Arbitrariness on the part of government services in the line of administration is the taproot of most evils that confront governments in the discharge of their responsibilities.

After some days a petty member of the office conveyed by some means a hint to one or two of the affected engineers that their transfer was almost certain and it was time that they did all in their power to avert it. This was a signal of despair for the latter. They knew what to do. Heavy sums of money secretly changed hands between them and the Superintendent or the Secretary of the office. The budget was shared by many, the superior officials retaining the largest share. This is but one out of a dozen disreputable methods that were used to keep the floodgates of illicit gain open in the Department.

It was in this maelstrom of corruption that I found myself when the charge of the Establishment section was entrusted to me. I had no prior knowledge of the dishonest practices that had been going on under my very nose during the period I had been in the office. It was only when I took over the section that both the victims and their extortioners began to come to my residence to unfold tales of villainy and trickery which it was hard for me to believe. Each affirmed his own innocence, putting the blame on the other to seek my help in some way. I listened to their stories in silence without committing myself in any way. Slowly I made up my mind about the course of action I had to follow to put an end to this abominable state of affairs as far as I could.

The Superintendent of the office and the Chief Engineer, an upright, pious man who gave up part of his own salary to charity, helped me to succeed in this endeavor. Every case that came for my opinion I studied thoroughly from every possible angle and then recorded my views without the least bias or prejudice. I picked out the resourceful intriguing officials, enjoying favors and concessions which were denied to others, and dislodged them from the positions where they had been entrenched for many years.

The very first few transfers of known favorites created a sensation in the Department. No one had dared to touch them before. No one had dared to bring in their place unsupported officials who had been stagnating on faraway, unimportant, and unrewarding posts on which no one else liked to work. Within a few months the situation was changed and a new atmosphere of fair play and strict regard to rules surrounded the Department. Every official knew when to expect his promotion or transfer and even the most influential started preparations for departure when their prescribed period of stay was over. I took the most humane view of every case consistent with rules as far as my limited judgment could allow.

Almost every day I was called upon to deal with a case to which justice had been denied for years. I never hesitated to take up cudgels on behalf of the unsupported and the weak. I pleaded for them with as much earnestness and force as if a heavy bribe had been paid to me to help them. It never entered my mind at that time that a strong advocacy of this kind might instill an entirely wrong idea into the mind of my superior that I too had been bribed. But my sincerity won. Every officer in the Public Works Department under whom I served reposed his trust in me and it was very seldom that a view expressed by me was not decided in my favor.

The system of blackmail current in the Department before the change allowed a certain proportion of the gain to filter to the Ministry as its share. The Superintendent in the office of the Public Works Minister was the largest beneficiary of this income.

An intrigue was soon hatched against our Superintendent—a relatively honest man—and he was retired. Later on, even the Chief Engineer fell victim to this conspiracy. It was reported that the Minister had declined to sign the order for his untimely retirement as his reputation for honesty and benevolence was very well known, but the paper was sent a second time by the Chief Minister and was then reluctantly signed. This is a painful story of plot and counterplot which is a common feature of administrative offices in India and abroad. The news of the premature retirement of the Chief Engineer was received with gasps of incredulity and astonishment by those who had known him but the conspiracy hatched to discredit him in the eyes of the Chief Minister was so consummately plotted and carried out that even his unblemished record and integrity of character could not save him from the blow.

With the transfer of the Chief Engineer and the Superintendent, who were my only bulwark against victimization, I was exposed defenseless to the attacks of my enemies. The Superintendent in the office of the Public Works Minister arranged the transfer of one his own brothers as the Superintendent in place of the one who was retired. A subordinate of the former Chief Engineer was now appointed as our chief. It appeared that at the time of his handing over the charge to his successor, our former Chief Engineer must have talked to him about me. They were friends and had worked for many years together in the State. This fact became apparent soon after taking charge, as the new Chief Engineer behaved like his predecessor and consulted me in every decision that he took with regard to the appointment of individuals.

It would make the story too long if I narrated all the ugly plots that were hatched to remove us from the office. One day, while taking an evening constitutional walk with his brother, the Superintendent in the Minister's office told him that he was surprised that it had not been possible for the latter to fabricate a complaint against me to encompass my dismissal. This was reported to me that very evening by a friend who had been one of the party that accompanied the Superintendent. But his brother had replied: "I cannot find it in my heart to fabricate charges against him when I see nothing that I could resent. Whatever he does, he convinces me about the properness of his actions." His brother gave an angry stare towards him and fell silent. But soon after, events occurred that at last gave him a pretext to contrive my transfer to another department.

Our storekeeper at Gilgit was due for transfer to a place near his home. He was to be replaced by another man who, according to the prescribed procedure, was due for transfer to the frontier. It took them two weeks to travel from Gilgit to Srinagar through a hazardous route on foot or horseback. Unfortunately the storekeeper eligible for transfer in this arrangement was the nephew of the Public Works Secretary. No one really believed that he would be shifted to such a far-off place against the wishes of the Secretary. But it was known that the decisions taken by our office were not easily influenced by such considerations. In fact, to make sure, word was sent to me by the Secretary to see him. He said it was a great honor for me to be taken into his confidence. He took it for granted that his wish would be obeyed without the least hesitation. High positions in administrative offices cause an inflammation of ego which often persists even after the high position is lost. The respect and obedience of the subordinates acts as an intoxicant to the mind. One who has once become tipsy with the effects of this wine never becomes normal again and can never reconcile himself to the fact that he is really an average man.

I listened to him in silence. He plainly said that his nephew was not in a position to shift to Gilgit at that time and that someone else should be sent in his place. I avoided a direct answer and said respectfully that I would convey his wishes to the Chief Engineer. But we had now gained a reputation for fair play, and I mentioned this to the Chief Engineer when I communicated the Secretary's wish to him. I could not commit an act of gross injustice and propose another storekeeper for transfer to keep the nephew at his place. The rules demanded that an employee transferred to Gilgit should in no case be made to stay there longer than three years, unless he voluntarily agreed to it.

The Secretary was furious when the news of the transfer was conveyed to him. Pressure was put on the Chief Engineer to rescind the order, but such a course would have put him into an embarrassing position in the Department. The order was executed and that was the end of the matter.

In addition to the Superintendent in the Minister's office who was ill-disposed towards me, I had now made an enemy of the Secretary too. But I continued to work with an unruffled mind and was not in the least disturbed by the thought that the hostility of these two influential officers could cost me my service. I continued to meditate in the morning and to attend to my official duties in the daytime as calmly as before. I did not even mention the risk I was running to my family or to any friend. In my heart of hearts I had made a plan that in case I was ousted from my post or forced to give it up, I would study and qualify myself as a physician in the Indian system of therapy.

An opportunity soon offered itself to both my opponents to put their designs into practice. Some posts of senior clerk fell vacant in the Department on which appointments were recommended by the Chief Engineer on the basis of seniority in accordance with the rules. The Minister in charge of Public Works, a stubborn man, had his own views on the score. He issued a directive for a revision of the proposal in accordance with his own ideas.

This was a flagrant act of injustice and I refused to be a party to it. I pointed this out to the Chief Engineer in a note and a strong, well-argued letter was sent to the Minister in reply to his directive. Angered at this flat disregard of his wishes, the Minister, rejecting the proposal of the Chief Engineer, issued the order of promotion in the way he desired. The Secretary and the Superintendent took this opportunity to poison his mind against me, putting the whole blame on me as being responsible for the violation of his directive. It is a common weakness in the management to lend an ear to what their subordinates, servants, or confidants whisper to them. This has been a tragedy throughout history. In this case, I was as powerless as a straw in the wind. Shortly afterwards an order was issued for my transfer to the Education Department without assigning any reason, and the Director of Education was asked to keep watch over me.

I actually welcomed the transfer since I was no longer happy in my existing appointment. The atmosphere there was too full of intrigues for my liking. My colleagues one and all deeply sympathized with me and helped to make the transfer of charge as easy for me as possible. Within a few days I gained the confidence of my new Superintendent and the Director, who was British. After only a couple of months he wrote a letter to the Minister, which was highly complimentary to my work, in reply to the latter's request that I should be watched closely.

The atmosphere in the Education Department was much more harmonious. There were no grants to be distributed and no bargains to be made with the contractors, although corruption on a minor scale was prevalent. Some time earlier, the Department had been a hotbed of intrigue due to rivalries and feuds among some officers. I was told that one of the inspectors had arranged to have a typewriter thrown into the river to escape being implicated in a case in which a false complaint was lodged against a rival. This complaint had been typed on this typewriter, and the government wanted to trace the complaint. But on the retirement of some of these intriguing officers the game of plot and counterplot had ceased to some extent.

Almost all the directors under whom I served were kind and considerate towards me. Although on several occasions I flatly refused to carry out their wishes, they were usually satisfied when I explained the merits and demerits of the case. I do not remember a single occasion in my whole service of more than twenty-six years when an officer under whom I served had to find fault with my work or suggest a course of action which was not according to the canons of justice and fair play or in conformity with the rules. But fair play and justice are not always palatable and can even create more foes than friends. It is a strange vagary of human character that when one is the victim of injustice, he promptly raises a hue and cry against the dispensers of law, but when he is the cause of injustice to another, he often exonerates himself and puts the blame on the victim.

I have had to face strange situations on account of this contradiction in the character of human beings. There were many whose rancor I evoked because they had to forego the favors and concessions they had enjoyed for years in usurping the rights of others without ever caring to acknowledge the fact. But they were in a minority and I paid no attention to their malice. The oppressed and the exploited won my sympathy with their cases as if they were my own, and I tried my utmost to see justice done for them.

On one occasion, the Headmistress of a high school for girls was suspended for unauthorized absence from the school. The complaint was lodged by the Second Mistress, who seemed to have a score to settle with the Headmistress. The complaint was that after remaining absent for a number of days the Headmistress had marked herself as present in the attendance register. The head of the girls' Education Department, an English lady, went to the school and confirmed the correctness of the complaint. She paid two visits for this purpose, and in addition, the personal assistant to the Director also visited the school and arrived at the same conclusion. At this stage the case was sent to me for presentation to the Director with my opinion for the issue of orders against the culprit.

I carefully studied the attendance register which accompanied the case. The period of absence extended to more than a week. The initials of the Headmistress appeared not to have been noticed or taken into consideration. They mainly relied on the allegation of the Second Mistress and their own impressions gained during the inquiry.

It was not easy to take a decision on the basis of the evidence provided by the witnesses who were examined by them. The Headmistress and the Second Mistress belonged to two different communities and the students and townspeople, belonging to either community, under the influence of religious bias, supported the teacher belonging to their own faith and put the blame on the other. This made an impartial assessment extremely hard, if not impossible, for the investigating officers.

But the telltale register related a different story. On all these eight or nine days a different shade of ink had been used on every day by all those who had marked their attendance in the register. The initials of the Headmistress appeared in exactly the same ink as had been used by the others. There was absolutely no variation. The reason for change in the shade of ink from day to day was due to the heat of the summer season when the event occurred. Every day the ink dropped into the ink pot dried up during the day and the next morning the ink pot had to be refilled or have water added to it to make fresh ink. Hence the exact shade of the color of the ink used was never the same on each following day.

To suppose that the Headmistress on returning from her absence changed the color of the ink to conform to the shade used each day for her initials was absurd. The shades were so peculiar and so different from each other that even the slightest variation in each one could be distinctly noticed. The inference was therefore clear that someone had initialed the attendance register each day on behalf of the absent Headmistress, naturally using the same ink as the others. This easily explained the mystery but who could this other person be who had signed the register in full sight of the others without implicating herself?

The circumstances of the case pointed to the complicity of the Second Mistress in the affair. Both she and the Headmistress had been in the habit of playing truant and initialing in place of each other during their absence. This fact did not come up in the inquiry because the class and the staff remained divided over the issue. Moreover, as the register went finally each day to the Headmistress and, in her absence, to the Second Mistress, the trickery might not even be noticed. The Director, a man of integrity, had formed a different opinion on the basis of the reports of the subordinate officers who had made the inquiry. But he soon changed his mind and passed a more equitable order on the case.

Almost once and sometimes even twice a week I had to deal with a petition or appeal from an aggrieved employee and to record my views on it. From the time I started to meditate, a conviction slowly grew in my mind that truth and the sense of identity with our fellow human beings are the two fundamental moral virtues on which a stable and equitable social order must be built. Concern for others is the basic factor for all charitable and benevolent acts. Placing oneself in the shoes of others to have a correct picture of their sorrows, suffering, or needs has been the basis of all the reform movements that took place in social, political, or religious fields. I believe that these two virtues are the first prerequisites in those who aspire to spiritual illumination. Compassion, commiseration, and pity have been the dominant virtues in all great mystics and saints. These are the driving forces which will ultimately triumph in building up a war-free, harmonious world.

A social order which makes material prosperity and a successful career the main objectives of life forms a barrier to evolution. The aim of the transformative processes in the human brain is to create a personality more in harmony with fellow human beings and more sensitive to their suffering and pain. Immoderate ambition or the desire to excel others blinds the mind to the fact that such a bent is unfair to others who have the same ambitions and desires. Fulfillment of ambition or the wish to excel over others entails a competition which can act as a poison to love and fellow feeling. This is the chief psychological malady from which the world is suffering today.

Before I started the practice of meditation, both in my childhood and teens, I was like the children and boys of my age, prone to mischief, untruth, and prevarication at times. My moral sense had not developed to an extent to inform me about the wrongful nature of my acts. But my untruth, fun, frolic, and mischief never exceeded a certain moderate limit. I instinctively avoided the company of known truants and mischief-makers. There was an inner urge to associate with those who were gentle and well behaved or distinguished for their study and intelligence. I wished to bring only happiness to my mother and sisters.

It was the shock of the failure in the examination that goaded me to take stock of myself, to know my faults and to correct them. It dawned on me for the first time that I had only a loose hold on myself and that it was highly necessary for me to tighten this hold and to remold myself to lead a perfect life.

Strangely enough, my resolve to improve myself did not center round my college career or a prosperous life after but found a different objective altogether. The ambition of a brilliant educational career followed by a high administrative appointment at which my mother aimed, and which too had been my earlier dream, also vanished completely. Contentment became the ruling note of my changed thinking about life. I had already gained the preliminary qualifications for a low-grade post in any government department or elsewhere and it was not necessary for me to pursue my studies further for the sake of securing a higher position. Even on a low order of service, I could honestly earn sufficient to make ends meet. I had passed my high school examinations with distinction and that was sufficient in those days to secure an ordinary appointment if I applied for it.

This shift from the idea of an ambitious career towards the more simple, though difficult, target of a homely perfect life to qualify myself for a spiritual career was not at all of my own making. Looking back at myself from this distance I can only say that this direction of my thoughts occurred spontaneously, as if welling up from within. The failure in the examination and the love of my mother merely acted as the stimulus to draw it out. I could just as easily have chosen any line of action, as for instance a more intensive course of study to prepare for academic distinction, or a professional career which, in all probability, I could have secured easily.

With the control over myself which I soon gained with the practice of self-discipline, I could have easily applied my once undisciplined mind to the hard study of any course I might have selected and probably completed it with distinction. I had the power of application and the intelligence to succeed. But somehow I lost the inclination to pursue such dreams further. My mind was now set not upon an ambitious wordly life but the knowledge of something more rewarding and lasting, something that could provide me with a clue to the Riddle of Existence.

The desire for self reform is the first sign of the activity of kundalini. The evolution of morals has not occurred either through the exercise of reasoning or through experience. The crude struggle for existence draws into play those resources of the body and properties of the mind which help one to overcome other competitors and rivals in the race for survival. The emphasis of this struggle would therefore seem to be on the strength of brain and muscle, on endurance and courage, cleverness and wit, strategy and cunning, deceit and trickery, planning and plotting, falsehood and sham or on violence and aggression, to achieve the dominating position in the battle. These are the traits that we see constantly at work in the animal kingdom everywhere—on land, in the ocean or the air. But the moral virtues that have been highly regarded since the dawn of civilization and are admired even today are the very opposite of these traits.

Innocence has a greater appeal to the heart than cleverness, frankness than duplicity, truth than falsehood, simplicity than sophistication, humility than pride, honesty than deception, self-denial than indulgence, pacifism than aggression, calmness than violence, artlessness than deceit and trickery, surrender than acquisitiveness, and so on. Some of these virtues are in direct opposition to the essential qualities needed in a ruthless battle for self-survival.

Yet an ordered life, free from immoderate ambition, desire, and lust, is a primary need of evolution. The transformative processes ceaselessly taking place in the brain of every normal human being become disorganized with uncontrollable outbursts of anger or passion, constant preoccupation with ambitious projects, greed, lust for power, and ignoble thoughts and actions. The basic teaching of all revealed scriptures aims to discourage human beings from yielding blindly to passion, desire, malice, envy, or other evil tendencies of the mind.

The purpose is always the same—the need for inner purification and discipline to allow the evolutionary processes to work unhampered by immoderate lusts or evil propensities of the individual. How could it be otherwise? If the aim of evolution is to bring into existence a loftier humanity, success can only be achieved if there is no daily friction between Nature's effort to elevate the brain and the individual's tendency to degrade it. The present-day disorientation of the intellect is the direct result of this conflict.

In my own case, the period of time intervening between my appointment in the service cadre of the State in 1923 to the day of the awakening in 1937 was an important period of preparation for me. Without the hard discipline that I imposed upon myself it might not have been possible for me to withstand the rigor of the years subsequent to 1937. My practice of meditation paved the way for the awakening, but it was the attempt I had made at self-mastery which enabled me to brave the hazard without even the guidance of a competent teacher.

As far as I can recall my mental state at the time, it was not a conscious effort but a sudden subconscious impulse that drove me to the practice of meditation and also to the exercises for the cultivation of my own will. I was not strongwilled by nature and had little control over my inclinations. I did not possess the gift of regular application with which some of my fellow students attended to their studies. They did their schoolwork regularly and reviewed their lessons at home. They were much better able to impress their teachers with their grasp of what they had learnt on the previous day. I tried to emulate them but could not. Constancy in the application of my mind was not possible for me. I did not read a lesson or touch a book for days and then, with a sudden spurt, tried to make up for the lost time. I could not completely overcome this habit, even in my later years. But there occurred a marked improvement with the exercises at self-mastery which I undertook.

I was not indolent, nor could I keep my mind idle doing nothing. Only I could not force it to a study that involved committing to memory the heavy material contained in the dry textbooks pre-

scribed by the college. A study of this kind somehow did not appeal
to me. I considered it to be drudgery.

But this dislike of textbooks did not extend to other reading
material. I was a voracious reader, and an interesting or an exciting
book held me spellbound until I finished it. I still remember vividly
almost whole nights spent with a book in my hand, poring over it
with tired, congested eyes in the dim, flickering light of a small
earthenware lamp with a flame so dim that I had to keep it so close
as to almost touch the book that I was reading. I used to place this
lamp on the parapet wall of the roof and would read lying down
close to it with the book held in both my hands. I could never read
so assiduously and with such concentration after the kundalini
awakening.

From this experience of my adolescent period, I am led to believe
that the distaste for daily exacting work, whether mental or physical,
the wanderlust, craving for drugs, and overmastering desire for
occult knowledge or spiritual experience which are an inexplicable
but marked symptom in a large proportion of modern youth denote
the strivings of an incipient inner transformation about which
science is still in the dark. The craze for meditation, the rush for
yoga, the keen search for gurus and masters, the widespread use of
drugs, and the hunt for occult powers which now capture the thought
and imagination of millions of young people in Europe and America
all point to such a departure from the thinking of the older generations in the first quarter of the present century. It would be negligent
to ignore the fact that a radical change has occurred in the psychological depths of the advanced nations of today.

With the practice of meditation and the control I started to
exercise over my thoughts and behavior, I felt a new vigor coming to
my mind. The languor and lassitude which I felt in applying myself
to the study of my texts began to disappear. A new self-confidence
was born in me. I became more sober in my conversation and
exchange of thoughts with others.

In the course of a few months, my personality underwent a change which did not fail to impress my people at home and my friends outside. At the same time, I became indifferent to dress and lost no time in trying to present a fine appearance. I preferred the simplest articles of attire and never allowed my self-respect to waver when, simply dressed, I found myself in rich company. In fact, it began to dawn on me that outer gloss and finery betrayed a lack of inner strength and a state of inward poverty which one tries to hide with outer display.

At this time, the boycott on foreign cloth and the preference for homespun, country-made articles of dress, advocated by Mahatma Gandhi, came as a sign from heaven for the confirmation of my own inborn trends, although I never used the prescribed homespun cotton dress and cap to conform to the changed atmosphere in the country as I was not in favor of regimentation. I wore homespun and other country-made cheap cloth for my costumes but not to fall from one kind of slavery to a prescribed fashion of dress into another from which I wished to keep myself free.

During this period, my granduncle celebrated the marriage of one of his sons in Lahore. The festivities started several days earlier. I was then wearing a coat made of homemade woolen cloth known in Kashmir as a *puttoo*. I had received this piece of cloth as a gift from my brother-in-law sometime earlier. It was a fine, durable piece of warm fabric, but with one defect: a part of it had a markedly different shade of natural brown color than the rest. The length of the piece was just sufficient for a coat and the tailor had made the mistake of using this differently colored piece to form part of the rear side of the coat. The result was that anyone looking at me from behind could not fail to notice the strange difference of shade in the two pieces of cloth, joined in the middle, which formed the back of my coat.

Two days before the day of the ceremony, my granduncle called me near to him and said, "This coat is not suitable for the marriage party. You know we have to take the bridegroom among strangers and all those who attend this party must be nicely dressed. Please change this coat for a better one." The first thought that came to me was to refuse compliance. But he was an old man, very affectionate and loving towards me. I went back to my home with a problem. To purchase a new coat was entirely beyond our means at the time. Luckily we had a still fresh, unused coat of my father. It was a bit too large for me but the tailor altered it to fit my size in a day, and I went to the marriage party wearing it.

After the marriage was over I continued to use the *puttoo* coat for a long time. I had very few clothes but with careful use I made them last for a long time. An overcoat which I had prepared for myself during the first year of my service in Kashmir I wore for nearly forty years. A bicycle purchased at the same time is still in good working order. A Gillette safety razor which I purchased in Lahore at the age of sixteen is still with me.

It was by devoting attention to minute details and by rounding the angularities in my life that I was able to harmonize my inner being. The transformation of consciousness does not take place through a miracle. It is a continuing process in which the conscious effort of an individual plays a decisive role. There must be a thirst to cultivate noble traits of character from the very start. The intellect must be able to discriminate between what is of lasting value and what is transitory in order to make life peaceful and happy. The choice of books, friends, food, behavior, and career must be subservient to the one supreme desire of self-knowledge.

A little reflection is sufficient to establish the need for attention to all these details in order to adjust one's mode of life to the transformtion sought. A glance at the lives of all great mystics of the past, both of the East and the West, is enough to convince us that all of them, without exception, can be included in one broad pattern of life, the main characteristics of which can be summed up thus: an insatiable thirst for knowledge of God, a constant preoccupation with the mystery of creation, absence of greed and ambition, detachment for the world, austerity, humility, truthfulness, simplicity, compassion, charity, and love of fellow beings. This is what the

Bhagavad Gita (16: 2–3) seeks to convey when it states, "Nonvio-
lence, truthfulness, absence of anger, renunciation of the idea of
doer in action, tranquillity, restraint from malicious gossip, kindness
to all creatures, detachment, mildness, sense of shame in doing
things not sanctioned by the scriptures, abstaining from idle pursuits, sublimity, forgiveness, fortitude, purity, absence of self-impor-
tance—these are the marks of one who is naturally endowed with
divine virtues, O descendant of Bharata."

The reason why there is repeated stress on the cultivation of these
virtues in the *Bhagavad Gita* and other religious scriptures lies in the
fact that they are an essential part of the path to higher consciousness. The inherent desire for self-mastery and cultivation of cardinal
virtues which is a regular feature of the hunger for self-knowledge
or longing for the vision of God can hence be considered to be the
corollary or the attendant symptom of a transformative process of
which a more harmonious, more exalted, and more perceptive
personality is the aim.

It was not, therefore, simply at my own will and choice that I
suddenly felt the desire to reform and master myself in the later
stages of my adolescence, but because some other psychic force had
begun to act in me, initiating a change in the direction of my thought.
This change in thinking has not been peculiar to me alone, and what
I have experienced is not an isolated case of this kind. It is fairly
common in young men and women to evince a thirst or urge of this
nature, provided they live in a healthy environment and there is a
hereditary element present in the system. This is an indication of the
fact that the transformative activity of kundalini starts at an early
age, probably close to adulthood, creating hidden urges and desires
for mental and behavioral changes conducive to its healthy manifestation at a more mature age.

The material supplied to meet the present demand of religious
experience or self-knowledge often do not take into account the
comprehensive nature of the change involved. Ascent to a transhuman state of consciousness implies a total transformation of the

whole personality, of all the mental and behavioral structure, so that a new human being emerges from the ashes of the old one.

It is not a little more calmness or relaxed condition of the mind nor a little more creative ability nor a feeling of euphoria nor visionary experiences nor a little more efficiency in work that determines whether or not a transformation in consciousness has occurred in an individual. Rather, it is a complete metamorphosis of the personality that points to it. Just as schizophrenia results in the formation of a distorted personality easily distinguishable from the average, so the alteration effected by kundalini results in mental and behavioral changes easily differentiated from the behavior of other human beings.

My exercises in self-mastery included scrupulous adherence to truth. At first sight this resolve appears to be easy to accomplish, but it is much more difficult than one can imagine before trying it in actual practice. In my official career, especially, it was a hard discipline to follow. When parties involved in a case came to seek my advice and help, it was extremely difficult to be open and frank with them.

It is a trait of human nature to justify one's actions. There were cases in which there was no justification for a complaint made or a claim put forward. Self-interest or a desire to make a nominated gain impelled many employees to make a regular round of the office with written petitions which they wished to be decided in their favor. Some of them even believed in the correctness of their own stand.

When I told them the plain truth that their case was hopeless and that, according to the rules, there was no chance for them to get what they had applied for, they felt aggrieved at me for throwing cold water over their hopes. Not infrequently I only succeeded in antagonizing them by my frankness. Not a few of them left my room as my enemies. There were some who sought undeserved favors to which I could never agree. My blunt refusal to help them frequently gave them the impression that I wanted to favor someone else. It took a long time before it became known in the Department that my real intention was to deal justice, as far as I could, and not to disappoint them because I wished to help someone else.

At first it was my habit when they came to seek my opinion to tell them frankly that they need not pursue their application any further as that would merely entail waste of time. This was the truth and it was frankly expressed in the hope that they would understand the position and be saved from the expense of time, energy, and even money lost in closely following the case from day to day. I was frank simply in their own interest, but often they misunderstood my well-meaning counsels and went away disgruntled, with bitterness against me in their hearts.

At last a friend advised me not to excite venom by my undiluted straightforwardness. "They would never believe that your advice to them not to follow their cases is motivated by honest intentions to save their time and labor. It is in the nature of human beings even to hope against hope that something would come out of their effort. Why do you nip their hope in the bud? Simply say that the application will be considered under the rules and every possible effort will be made to help if the rules permit it."

I saw the reasonableness of his advice and tried to act upon it. I no longer gave a blunt answer to the petitioners, but, at the same time, did not raise their hopes, as that too was sinful in my eyes. The result was that my visitors did not leave as dissatisfied as before. They made several visits to the office or to my home to inquire about the progress made and when I finally said that it had not been found possible to meet their request under the rules, and the application had been filed, they often accepted the verdict contentedly. They had, at least, the satisfaction that the application had been considered on its merits and they had the chance to follow it to the end. They were happy to waste their time in pursuing a lost cause which was hopeless from the very beginning.

SEVEN

Stumbling Blocks in the Path of Evolution

MY INTEREST IN THE STUDY and practice of yoga was not the outcome of any deep desire to possess psychic gifts. The tricks and deception sometimes practiced by men of this class, the exhortations against the exhibition and abuse of spiritual powers contained in the scriptures, and above all the utter futility of an effort useless as a means to secure lasting benefits either for one's own self or for others were all, to my mind, sufficient reasons to rise above the temptation to acquire the powers to flout the laws of matter without possessing at the same time the necessary strength of will to obey the laws of the spirit.

The emphasis laid in some of the books on yoga, both of the East and the West, on the development of psychic powers merely for the sake of gaining success in worldly enterprise invariably made me wonder at the incongruity in human nature, which, even in the case of a system designed to develop the spiritual side of man, focuses the attention more on the acquisition of visible, wonder-exciting properties of the body or mind than on the invisible but tranquil possessions of the soul. That some, at least, of the manifestations were genuine there could be little doubt. But how were they to be accounted for? It was only after many years that I was able to locate the source of the bewildering phenomena and trace it to a marvelous superintelligent power in man, which is both illuminating and mystifying—illuminating in the revealing flashes of genius and mystifying in the baffling masquerades of spirits and demons in mediums and the possessed; which is both blissful and awful—blissful in the enrapturing visions of ecstatics and awful in the appalling shadows of insanity.

The target I had in mind was far higher and nobler than what I could expect in the most attractive form of acquisition of the much coveted supernormal gifts. I longed to attain the condition of consciousness, said to be the ultimate goal of yoga, which carries the embodied spirit to regions of unspeakable glory and bliss, beyond the sphere of opposites, free from the desire for life and fear of death.

This extraordinary state of consciousness, internally aware of its own surpassing nature, was the supreme prize for which the true aspirants of Yoga had to strive. The possession of supernormal powers of the usual kind, whether of the body or mind, which kept an individual still floundering in the stormy sea of existence without carrying one any nearer to the solution of the great mystery, seemed to me to be of no greater consequence than the possession of other earthly treasures, all bound to vanish at the end of life.

When nothing tangible happened for nearly seventeen years, from the age of seventeen to thirty-four, I began to despair, at times led to doubt the method adopted and at others to suspect the whole science.

Spiritual illumination is not a marketable commodity easily available for a price. One reason why the founders of all great religions commanded such reverence for centuries is because illumination is so extremely rare. This was instinctively sensed all through the past until the intellect came to dominate the scene in our own time. Since then, there has been no agreement on a correct description of enlightenment. What happens to the individual during the course of transformation is now purely a matter of speculation. Before our time, illumination denoted an encounter with Divinity or an anthropomorphic God. Now, in the eyes of many scholars, it means a peculiar psychological condition, a trip to deeper regions of the mind or autointoxication brought about by altered chemistry of the body. This leads to the mistaken view that the drug experience has something in common with or is parallel to mystical ecstasy or enlightenment.

If we believe in the absolute wisdom, absolute knowledge, and absolute justice of the Godhead, can we heap a greater insult on Him than to suppose that He would demand of those who strive to reach Him an abnormal, unhealthy or eccentric way of life and behavior, irrationally different from other people?

Abnormality and mania have often been firmly linked to religion in the same way that eccentricity and madness have been associated with genius in other departments of knowledge or art. Of course, there have been many noble exceptions, as in the case of various secular geniuses. The founders of the leading world faiths also furnish examples of such immunity. In India the social environment and the code of discipline, particularly during the Upanishadic period (circa 800 C.E.), provided, to some extent, the conditions necessary for the healthy expression of a superior mind. Celibacy and monasticism were not a current feature of spiritual life in the Vedic age. Excesses and abnormalities entered later as the advance force of decadence.

The craziness of religious mania is similar to the eccentricity and madness of genius. Only the aberration takes a different form. It is only the highest luminaries, comparatively speaking, who have been free from it. Excessive penance, horrible self-mortification, utter seclusion, denial of love, renunciation of the world and family, abnormal ways of life and behavior, quaint appearance and dress are all part of this mania.

In their essentials, there is no difference between religious or secular genius. They are the twin fruits of the same tree. The tragedy is that while in the case of secular genius the eccentricity or madness was recognized as abnormal by the healthy common sense of the masses, the abnormalities of the religious genius were often accepted as a part of the divine way of life necessary in order to reach God.

It is not rational that the religious hierophants should behave differently from the elite in science or other branches of knowledge. Is it because they consider themselves, or are considered by others, to be superior to other human beings? Is it because they believe they are nearer to God than other human beings? In either case, spiritual exaltation should definitely tend to the deflation of the ego and dislike for earthly pomp and show. This is what is expressly stated in the religious scriptures of the world. Why then should they indulge in mannerisms or resort to actions which all point to a more inflated ego and a greater desire for name, fame, status, power, and even to wealth and possession than the ordinary ranks of the people whom they profess to teach?

The lives of all great spiritual geniuses of India, as for instance Sri Ramakrishna, have been models of humility, simplicity, unpretentiousness, brotherly feelings, and love. This has also been the case with Christian mystics and Sufis. The first change that should occur in the behavior of a mortal when his mind begins to mirror God is to perceive his *identity* with other human beings. The perception of this unity, in turn, should fill him with an ardent desire to make them sharers of his own sublime experience and overflowing happiness. How can he then consider himself superior to the crowds and see them groveling at his feet? How can he dress and adorn himself magnificently to look different on the outside if in his heart he is truly one with all others?

I have made this digression to emphasize the significance of inner transformation as distinct from outward show or behavior. The evolution of the brain towards a higher dimension of consciousness cannot proceed in total independence without the least deviation from the mode of life and behavior of enlightened individuals, but a distinction must be made between harmonious transformation and misleading appearances.

Environmental problems and hardships may also contribute to eccentricity in individuals in whom kundalini is active. In the case of my father, his three surviving issues were my two sisters, both elder to me, and myself. After my eldest sister, a pair of twins was born who died soon after. Then my second sister was born, and after her there was a male child who died while only a few years old, a victim to smallpox, a terrible scourge in those times. Indian tradition puts great store on a male issue. It is his offerings that propitiate the souls of the departed ancestors. In our community, as prescribed by tradition, a parent should expire with the head resting on the lap of a son. It is he who first pours the last few drops of the sacred Ganges water into the mouth of the dying parent before the jaw falls and the eyes close forever.

It is a terrible sight to see a beloved child dead of smallpox, his face and body ravaged by the dreadful disease. The death of his firstborn son caused such a shock in my father that he turned into a recluse, severing all his connections with the world. He refused to stir out of his room to mingle with the family, becoming irregular and capricious in his food and sleep. He applied for retirement and refused to attend his office anymore. The head of the department in which he was serving tried his utmost to change his mind and spared no effort to persuade him to resume his duties. But my father was adamant. All our relatives and friends sympathized with my mother from the core of their heart, smitten with pity at her young age and gentle behavior, but no one could revoke the decision taken by my father.

When I pieced together the stories that I heard later and weighed them in the light of my own experience, it became obvious that my father must have been passing through a critical state in his inner development as a result of a slow awakening of the Serpent Power. Evidently he had no inkling of the cause responsible for his altered mental state and behavior. It is frequent in such conditions to have visionary experiences, to nurture fantastic ideas and notions, to undergo constant change of mood for no apparent reason. Gnawing hunger for the ceaseless search often precedes the slow alteration.

It is not generally known that the unassuaged thirst for a master, adept, or guru springs from the activity of kundalini to draw attention to the mighty force waiting to leap to action if correctly understood and properly manipulated. But, alas, the general ignorance prevailing about the still unknown divine mechanism destroys the hopes of many men and women who, with proper guidance and efforts, could attain to the bloom of cosmic consciousness.

The real secrets of kundalini are not known even in India except, perhaps, to a few adepts who succeeded in awakening the power and leading it to the seventh center in the brain. Even well-known gurus and holy men, except for hints picked up here and there, are as barren of this arcane science as the average men and women who listen to their learned discourses. It is only prolonged research and the successful awakening of the Serpent Power in a few prodigies of the future that will add fresh, substantial material to that which is already contained in the ancient writings and the utterances of a few mystics of both East and West. It is therefore safe to presume that my father had no awareness whatsoever of the changes occurring within him or of the reasons for his radically altered behavior and mode of thought.

He was a hearty eater with no scruples against animal food, a confirmed smoker, and at times even sparingly partook of wine. In a sudden excess of asceticism, he stopped smoking and gave up eating meat, fish, and even eggs completely, renouncing also the occasional use of wine. He even refused to have anything to do with milk or its products anymore, on the ground that it was an outrage on the young calves to deprive them of their nourishment.

This extreme form of renunciation and austerity, at a time when a balanced diet was what he needed to calm the energy circulating within him, was the root cause for the secluded life and eccentric actions of his later days. Gradually his moods became more erratic and unpredictable, until aberrant behavior became a permanent feature of his personality, lasting to the end.

My mother related that she too had no knowledge of the factors responsible for this change and the behavior that followed. She ascribed it only to the tragic death of their son long before. After the tragedy, my father had sat at times gazing fixedly at the oil lamp at night without blinking. This practice must have been suggested to him by some holy man or he may have read of it in some book. Soon he began to show lack of interest in the affairs of the family and to frequent the haunts of ascetics, sadhus, and holy men of whose psychic exploits and penances he chanced to hear from his friends. He sought them out and sat in their company for hours at a time to satisfy his hunger for a master to guide him. But many of these sadhus and ascetics were strange and weird creatures, abnormal in their thinking and behavior, yet posing as enlightened knowers of the hidden secrets of existence.

One of them was given to occasional exhibitions of mind reading, always holding a small round piece of stone, known as *saligrama*, in his palm day and night, and never letting go of it, not using this hand for any other purpose whatsoever. This was a self-imposed penance to show his stubborn resolve to acquire occult knowledge. Smoking of hashish was a constant repellent feature of the haunts of these sadhus. Many of the daily visitors merely went to appease their craving for it. Even in modern times some of the ashrams of sadhus in India are undisguised dens for hashish or marijuana smoking. The habituated addicts to the drug can be recognized by the condition of their eyes and their jerky, irresponsible behavior. My father lavishly donated towards the expenses of these sadhus. In all probability most of this contribution went for the purchase of drugs and wine.

Unless the mind has been disciplined from an early age, a stimu-lated kundalini brings with it an irrepressible desire for the occult and the bizarre. It is incredible to what extent the victims of this desire can be duped by pseudo-Godmen, charlatans and imposters. It appears as if the mind has lost all its critical power of observing and judging the behavior of an individual whom people credit with psychic powers. They act in the most abnormal and revolting ways, which the duped audiences ascribe to mystical consciousness, tran-scending normal actions. In my own lifetime, one of these Godmen, residing in a village in Kashmir, used to urinate into a silver vessel in full view of the crowds that came to visit him and then sprinkled the liquid over the audience, both men and women. It is even said tht his admirers held up their faces and uncovered their bosoms to receive the sanctifying drops.

The thirst for bizarre stories is unassuagable. A whole library of books containing the most fantastic and bizarre stories, which no sane mind can believe, cannot extinguish or satisfy the widespread hunger for the irrational and fanciful.

This thirst, which appears inexplicable to a rational mind, is caused by the stimulation of kundalini in an undisciplined system as the first warning to show that the mind is in an unhealthy state. The desire for strange drug experiences, for erratic psychic phenomena, for fantastic messages received from mediums and sensitives, for the strange actions of gurus and occult teachers, springs from this unhealthy condition of the mind. Today, the Western world is in the grip of a mass hysteria which, if not remedied in time, will revive all those grotesque and orgiastic creeds and cults, including witchcraft, which have been a feature of all decadent cultures in the past.

One reason why I was reluctant to confide in and to consult sadhus and ascetics when face to face with the inscrutable mystery of kundalini arose from two experiences I had in Lahore. Once, while going to a well-known garden close to the zoo, I saw an ocher-robed sadhu sitting on the roadside. It was a solitary spot and there were few pedestrians on the road.

He had an impressive appearance and was sitting apparently in a state of absorption. While I was walking close by him he beckoned me nearer and said in a commanding voice: "Open your hand!" which I did. He then held his clenched hand above it and a stream of milk dropped from it on to my palm. I was startled. Before the sadhu clenched the hand I saw it was quite empty. Seeing my astonishment he said that this was a sign of extreme good luck for me and I should rest assured that an unexpected stroke of fortune was awaiting me in the next few days. He then demanded to have whatever I had in my pocket. I put my hand inside and found a four anna piece, which was all the wealth I carried with me at the time. I gave it to him and, making a salutation, went on my way. It was years after that I came to know that I had been the victim of a simple sleight of hand.

The second experience occurred in the narrow lane by our house and concerned our next-door neighbor, who was a moneylender. One day there suddenly issued a loud clamor from the house, which startled all the neighbors. Greatly puzzled and anxious, my mother went to inquire the cause. She returned after about an hour with a sorrowful face and related a doleful tale. A few days previously, a sadhu had entered the house to have a smoke and something to eat. The moneylender, impressed by his manner and appearance, seated him with honor, fed him and offered him a smoke from the hookah. After the ascetic had left, he rose to refill the small holder containing the burnt tobacco. Great was his surprise to find a heavy piece of yellow metal lying beneath the burnt residue in the holder. He cleaned and washed it. Being himself a dealer in precious metals, he saw at once that it was pure gold.

He ran out precipitately into the lane and then into the street, in the hope of finding the sadhu who, he had now ample reason to believe, had the fabulous supernatural power of transmuting base material into gold. But he was not to be found anywhere. The moneylender, whose name was Dina Nath, made a round daily through the neighborhood to find some trace of him. A few days later, he appeared unexpectedly again before their door and asked for a smoke. Unable to contain himself with joy, Dina Nath reverently fell at his feet and escorted him to his own cushioned seat, himself standing before him like a humble supplicant beseeching a favor. The sadhu bade him to be seated and after a few puffs from the hookah, remarked that he was highly pleased with his behavior and his service and would be glad to grant him any favor he would like to ask.

Dina Nath fell at his feet saying that he had two daughters to marry and that it would be most gracious of him if the sadhu were to help him to make their nuptials possible in an honorable way. "Bring a thousand currency notes of ten rupees each and I shall change all of them into genuine hundred rupee notes," said the sadhu. "You can then use them to meet the expenses on the marriage of your daughters. But you have to promise me that you will not breathe a word of it to anyone, including your family." The money-lender, overwhelmed with joy, clutched both the sadhu's feet and pressed his forehead on them. When the sadhu rose to depart he bade Dina Nath wait, soon after dusk, two days later, outside a temple close to the Lahore fort, then a desolate area where few people ventured at night.

The moneylender had to borrow from his friends to make up one thousand notes of ten rupees each and, forming them into a bundle, waited outside the temple at the appointed time. It grew darker and darker and soon it was too dark to discern anything. Dina Nath's heart began to beat wildly with fear caused by the darkness and the eerie stillness of the place. Soon he heard the sound of footsteps and in a few moments the sadhu stood before him. He could not see his face in the darkness but recognized his voice. After responding to his salutation, the sadhu asked if he had done what he had asked him to do. The moneylender replied in the affirmative and placed the bundle in his hands. Holding the bundle firmly, the sadhu began to chant a mantra when suddenly there was a noise of heavy footsteps close by and then a huge figure loomed in the darkness. It held a torch in its hand and flashed it full in the face of the moneylender. Dazzled for a moment, the moneylender could not see anything, but moving his eyes away from the light he was able to discern a tall, burly figure, naked save for a loincloth, with a heavy axe in one hand and then a voice thundered: "Run from this place at once and be thankful that I have spared your life. Do not speak a word to anyone of what you saw here tonight or I shall kill you, wherever you are!"

Almost swooning with fright, the moneylender took to his heels without casting a second look behind. Completely unnerved and out of breath, he reached his home and sobbed out the story to some of his neighbors drawn by his cries. Search was fruitless. The sadhu was never found again. Confidence tricks of this variety are still common in India. Out of a sense of shame at their own stupidity, the victims often refrain from reporting their loss to the police. But nevertheless, news of such occurrences still appears in newspapers every now and then.

There is a class of hatha yogis who resort to another type of deception to instill respect and awe among mostly rustic villagers in order to serve their own ends. *Vajroli mudra* is a hatha yoga practice which, it is alleged, confers on one the power to reabsorb seminal fluid after its emission and even to suck up the genital secretions of the female partner in the act of coition. In fact, there is a general impression prevailing both in India and the West that the exercises of hatha yoga contain methods for the prolongation of the pleasure experienced in the sexual act by retention of the seminal essence and its reabsorption into the system. Some modern books on hatha yoga profess to teach these methods. These books are avidly read by readers beguiled into the belief that such secret methods do exist.

How far this assumption is correct can be gauged from the demonstrations given by some unscrupulous yogis of this class. Their modus operandi is to sit at a conspicuous place in a village in a spectacular asana (physical posture) or to stand upside down with their head on the ground and legs towards the sky—a well-known asana of hatha yoga—and continue in this pose for a long time, sufficient to gather a curious crowd of spectators around them. When the gathering is large enough for them, they then assume a normal position and, taking out a vessel from the small bag they carry, they urinate in it in front of the audience. After this they pour the fluid into a small oil lamp with a wick in it. The wick catches fire at once and to the amazement of the spectators continues to burn. The feat is sufficient to establish the reputation of the yogi for supernatural powers, and crowds start to flock to him for spiritual instruction or some miraculous favor.

There are other methods by which they continue to retain the confidence and homage of the deceived folk for as long as they like.

In fact, there are regular professional secrets which allow pseudo-yogis of this class to impose upon the public in a way which is difficult to detect.

What the hatha yoga practice of *vajroli mudra* actually achieves is the ability to suck up fluids through the generative duct into the urethra. This does not at all imply the flow of the seminal fluid into the brain through the spinal duct. That is a natural process which can only occur on the arousal of kundalini and the opening of the supersensory center in the brain. This involves reversal of the action of the reproductive system so that seminal essence, instead of flowing downward and outward, is carried inward and upward by a new activity of the nervous system of which details can be ascertained only with scientific investigation of the phenomena.

This physiological process does not work at the will and choice of the individual in whom it starts to act. After a varied period it becomes a normal function of the autonomic nervous system, over which one has no control. In those cases where kundalini is perennially active in an organism, it is this state of upward flow of the seminal energy into the brain which is known as *urdhava-retas* in Sanskrit. This condition can occur in both the male and female. When the adjustment of the nervous system is complete this reverse action of the reproductive organs becomes a normal function of the body. But the initiate still retains the option of directing the energy at his will and choice downward and outward in coition.

Vajroli mudra is only an ill-conceived, crude, artificial method intended to duplicate this process. Attempts to imitate the behavioral and constitutional peculiarities of the illuminated have been current in India from very early times. In fact, the whole system of hatha yoga is designed to induce by artificial means the natural conditions displayed by an enlightened consciousness. Hatha yogis try to counterfeit the trance state with diminished breathing and heart action, which can be a striking and confirmative feature of the ecstatic state, by means of the arduous exercises of *pranayama* (yoga breathing techniques) resulting in perceptible slowing down of the metabolic processes for varying periods of time. This state of suspended animation can even extend to weeks and months, but it does not confer what is the priceless gift of yoga—namely, an illuminated consciousness.

In the same way, the capacity to suck up fluids through the penis or the vagina does not provide the possibility of transmitting the absorbed material to the brain. The very idea that this can happen is preposterous. The utmost that can be achieved when the suction is applied will be to draw up the fluid into the urethra in the case of males, or into the urethra and the fallopian tubes in the female. But from there, the gross secretions can find no passage to reach the brain. The utmost that can happen is that part of the material sucked up would be absorbed into the blood and part ejected out again at the time of micturation.

The futility of wasting precious years of life to gain this skill, highly extolled in some works on hatha yoga, is therefore obvious. This example is also sufficient to expose the fallacy of those writers who designate hatha yoga or tantric yoga as yoga of sex, pregnant with the promise of prolonged ecstasy or erotic pleasure, depending on the retention or the reabsorption of semen in the copulative act. The only harvest of such unnatural practices is to draw the individual further away from illumination by creating unhealthy habits with consequent morbid reactions in the system.

Any unnatural thirst or abnormal behavior can act as a stumbling block in the path of evolution. The existence of unhealthy appetites in a seeker after illumination can be disastrous. The least abnormality in thought or in the body is prone to become magnified when the new pranic energy begins to circulate in the system at the time of arousal of kundalini. The incessant and rapid natural suction of the reproductive secretions that occurs at this time is the only way open to Nature to save the brain from damage and to contrive the enhanced activity of the vital organs.

Energy is drawn from every part of the body through the nerves lining the genital organs to meet the highly increased demand without interruption. If interruption occurs, the consequences can be dangerous in the extreme. The newly activated chamber in the brain must be constantly fed by what is described by the ancient masters as a stream of ambrosia. But this vital stream itself must have a certain degree of purity. For this purpose a normal, healthy condition of the body and the blood stream is absolutely necessary. It is to maintain a healthy condition of the psychic system that the gross tonic material contained in the reproductive fluids is diverted to the vital organs—heart, liver, stomach, kidney, etc.—partly through the blood stream but mainly through the nerves or other ducts, to vitalize them.

The whole complex mechanism that comes into play on the awakening of kundalini can only be determined through sustained research on the phenomenon. Here it is sufficient to mention that any unhealthy or morbid tendency of the system can be fatal to the proper functioning of this extremely complex mechanism, with a devastating effect on the brain when the power is aroused. The primary aim of the elaborate system of physical yogic exercises, devised in ancient times, was to create a healthy condition of the body and the mind conducive to a safe arousal of the Serpent Power.

The need for a highly balanced and regulated life, as a prerequisite for cosmic consciousness, was recognized in India from very early days. The emphasis of all great religions on a chaste, consecrated life stems from the same necessity. Divested of the supernatural and the magical, the aim of all healthy religious disciplines is to create a highly supple and resilient psychophysiological state able to withstand the tremendous pressure and strains consequent on the arousal of the kundalini power in the initial stages until the nerves and the tissues become habituated to the new and more potent vital currents circulating in the system.

Every sensible aspirant to higher consciousness must, therefore, learn to make a clear distinction between the claims of the pseudo-yogis and the sensational results they promise and the true yogic disciplines, which demand a balanced life, regulated behavior and appetites, self-subdual, devout application, and a keen power of discrimination between right and wrong or good and bad. Side by side with the counterfeit, there are noble sadhus and ascetics in India whose lives are an example of purity, saintliness, and renunciation. But since they are unpretentious and humble, choosing solitude and simplicity to ostentation and display, they are seldom known or accessible to the seeking crowds. The rise from human to trans-human consciousness is an extremely arduous exploit and wil need all the resources of science for its achievement in the ages to come.

In the eyes of scholars the difficulties in acceptance of the views I am expressing about kundalini lie, firstly, in my assertion about the change in the pattern of the bioenergy and, secondly, about the reverse action of the reproductive system. Since this is the first time that these strictly physiological factors have been introduced into discussion of the phenomena of mystical ecstasy and genius, the skepticism and incredulity expressed are understandable.

But it is against the spirit of scientific enquiry to reject a hypothesis summarily without any effort at research. This attitude becomes all the more incomprehensible when it is recalled that what I assert is backed by the unimpeachable testimony of hundreds of veracious Indian savants who have themselves been firsthand witnesses to the phenomenon. The tragedy is that the same scholars and scientists are prepared to accept and investigate the counterfeit conditions, deliberately induced to create a sensation, but not the genuine states which are of paramount importance. For instance, they are ready to study a case of suspended animation brought about by *pranayama* or the control gained over the autonomic nervous system or physical feats like *vajroli mudra* but not the genuine transformation that results in the emergence of mystical consciousness or genius.

This paradoxical trend of the human mind can prove an endless source of wonder for those who detachedly view its behavior. The most striking example of this paradox is the radical difference in values during peace and war. What is a more heinous act in the former becomes a highly praised exploit in the latter. The instinctive love for children and respect for women and old age are transformed into virulent hate and the lust to kill. Beautiful landscapes and habitations which we love to see and admire in other lands during peacetime become targets for our vandalistic fury in war. It is not one man or a hundred men who are responsible for this shift from one state of mind to the other. But a sweeping wave of hate and malignancy overwhelms the minds of a whole mass or a whole nation. A hysterical condition settles on minds impervious both to reason and sanity. Confronted with the picture of atrocities committed during warfare, a dispassionate observer can only treat peace as a period of respite from a state of fury which is also as normal to the human mind as the former.

I had many occasions even during my early life to witness this contradictory tendency of the human mind. Once, during my stay at Gairoo in the summer vacation, strange rumors began to float in from the town. It was said that a mysterious supernatural creature was at large and had struck terror in every quarter of the city of Srinagar. Every day, it was alleged, disfigured and mutilated victims testified to its presence at one place or the other. All efforts made to capture the creature or even to identify it had failed. Only the wounded and dismembered victims were there, the rumors said, to tell about its ravages. Every day travelers between the city and the village brought bloodcurdling tales about the monster, but no one ventured any accurate description of its appearance.

Some said it was a gigantic bird with swordlike claws, others that it was a vampiric creature, half human and half beast, others that it was a prehistoric animal that could both fly and run, and so on. The villagers of Gairoo began to whisper to each other, and signs of fear were visible on many faces. It could well be, they said to one another, that the grisly monster might take it into its head to make a flying visit to their village.

At this very critical juncture a sudden call from my sister brought me posthaste to the city. She had heard that the creature had now started to cause devastation in the villages close to Gairoo. Sick with fright, she sent a messenger to fetch me to Srinagar. Soon after my arrival, I found the city almost in a state of siege. People hesitated to move out of their houses and the shopkeepers looked apprehensive about their safety. Rumors ran hot from one place to another. News about the depredations committed by the horror were rushed from one part of the city to the other.

My sister's house was three stories high, and there was a small wooden cabin on the roof from which one could have a view of the city. That cabin had formed my study room more than once. I knew the occupants of the surrounding buildings very well. But when I came up this time a strange sight met my eyes. It was nearing sunset and there was enough light to see clearly for a distance. On roofs here and there that could provide the facility, small groups of men and elders were seated scanning their surroundings with attention. They held strange objects—small drums, cymbals, gongs, large empty tins, wooden mallets and the like—in their hands and whistles close to their lips.

Suddenly a clamor rose from one side and at once all the groups on the roofs jumped to activity, beating the drums, clashing the cymbals, hammering the tins, and shouting at the top of their voices to drive away the monster. I had reasoned myself into the conviction that such a creature could not be possible and the whole uproar was the result of superstition and mass hysteria. But when I heard the pandemonium with my ears and saw hundreds of people gathered in groups at many vantage points shouting and gesticulating, I felt my confidence forsaking me. After all, I said to myself, it is not possible that so many people can take leave of their senses and raise such a hue and cry at the fear of a murderous creature that does not exist at all.

I descended from the roof revolving the whole affair in my mind. That very night a rather frightening incident, closely linked to the rumors, occurred in our own house. The father of my brother-in-law, an old man but courageous for his age, was also skeptical about the whole story. He denounced the episode as the creation of mischief-mongers who wished to plunge the town into a state of panic to amuse themselves. After the evening meal, when the family members were just retiring to their beds, a noise was suddenly heard from the opposite house less than twenty feet from their building. My sister cautiously opened the window and saw a large object flapping its wings on the opposite roof. She gave a cry of fear and at once shut the window and bolted it. Rushing to her father-in-law, she described to him what she had seen. The whole family, with fear on their faces, trooped into the room of the old gentleman for protection.

With undaunted courage he rose to investigate, chiding the others for their causeless fright. There was no electric light that evening. Taking a lantern in one hand and a heavy stick in the other, he opened the door slightly and looked out. In order to have better light to see, he thrust the hand holding the lantern through the opening in the door. Seeing the light the creature on the roof made a dive towards it, hitting the door with violence. Terrified at this unexpected attack, the old man reeled backwards and collapsed in the passage. One of the family who had followed after him when he went down the stairs rushed to the door and bolted it to keep the terror from entering into the house. Next morning they found that it was only a large kite (hawk) which had somehow lost its bearings in the darkness and taken shelter on the roof opposite to them.

The hue and cry slowly died down, and after some days normalcy and calm were restored in the city. The people began to realize that there had been nothing supernatural to cause the panic. It was only the circulating rumors of a nameless monster preying upon the unwary that had excited the imagination of the more receptive, while stories of horrible happenings traveled from one part of the city to the other. There had actually been no mutilations, no injuries, and no deaths. All the reported incidents were mere creations of fancy which were avidly seized upon by easily excitable minds, who in turn invented further tales of terror which others swallowed, only to fabricate even more dreadful episodes until the whole city was saturated with fear.

The factional fights going on at this moment in many parts of the world, resulting in damage, bloodshed and suffering, are the outcome of this very frailty of the human mind. When the passions are roused at some unsavory incident, the rival faction suddenly assumes the appearance of a monster and rumors run from house to house of the atrocities committed and the indignities heaped, until the whole atmosphere is saturated with hate and violence erupts between the antagonists. Once started, it becomes difficult to quell the disorder, as excited imaginations continue to invent tales and stories or to exaggerate minor occurrences into atrocious episodes, creating a vicious circle which becomes hard to end.

I had another experience of this type in a factional riot some years before the kundalini awakening. Within a few hours, neighbors who had been living close to each other for generations, sharing each other's joy and sorrow as deeply as the nearest kith and kin, always happy to sit, smoke, and chat together, were suddenly transformed into implacable foes, thirsty for the blood of others.

The disturbance had started in Srinagar. A number of deaths had occurred, some shops were plundered, and some households looted and ravaged. All shops were closed and the city presented a deserted appearance. My elder brother-in-law came to pay us a visit, mainly to assure himself about our welfare. The streets were empty, and no one had molested him. When he rose to depart I offered to accompany him, and we left the house together.

There were two routes open to us to reach his residence. One led through narrow streets and the other through a road, flanked with shops on either side. I suggested the narrow street, as a measure of safety, but he insisted on our taking the main road as he had just come that way without encountering any danger. I acquiesced and we took that road. He had come on a bicycle which he now pushed with his hand. We were close to a double bend in the road when the noise of an approaching angry crowd and stones hitting the houses close by suddenly smote our ears. At the other bend of the road, about one hundred feet away, a huge crowd burst into view hurling stones and bricks at everything that came in their way. A policeman standing about fifty feet in front of us in the middle of the road suddenly collapsed with blood pouring from his head. A stone had struck him in the middle of the forehead and another in the face.

My brother-in-law became so nervous that he found it hard to turn the bicycle round to enable us to flee. He hurled it to one side, but I picked it up and we made a dash in the direction from which we had come to escape the hail of stones and the fury of the crowd. Unfortunately, another group hearing the cries had, within minutes, gathered on that side too, to face the oncoming fury. We were literally caught between two fires and prepared for the worst. All at once I saw the entrance to a narrow lane on the right. We dashed into it, pushing the bicycle along, and after sprinting a short distance looked back. A portion of the crowd had stopped at the end of the lane and were debating among themselves whether they should pursue us further or continue on their way with the others. The doors leading to the houses on both sides of the lane were closed and they could have easily brought us down with the stones they were carrying. Thankfully, as luck would have it, they decided not to follow us in the lane and, turning round, disappeared from our sight.

The same inexplicable behavior of the mind which lets a trifling incident assume the catastrophic proportions of wholesale massacre, plunder and arson, with the inundation of pent-up feelings of fear, suspicion, and hatred, is also at the base of the tense situation of the world today. Partly on historical grounds and partly to preserve their identity, culture, and assets, many nations regard their neighbors or rivals with mistrust, fear, and suspicion. The excited imagination of the people then has ample opportunities to create bugbears which keep the entire population in a state of fright and panic.

Often we do not give sufficient thought to the colossal task which evolution has to accomplish. It represents a rise from the earth to the sky. A clod of earth has to gain the power of thinking, of awakening to the knowledge of itself and then of the universe round it. A handful of insensitive matter has to win a state of awareness where it can mingle with a consciousness which pervades the universe, from a handful of dust to be one with the All. It is a stupendous transformation, a mighty drama which only an absolute power could design, stage, and play. We tend to underestimate the inconceivably vast dimensions of creation and the stupendous proportions of the power of it because our mind and senses, like the brain and the eyes of an ant on a leaf floating upon the surface of an ocean are not able to register our own insignificant position compared to the titanic forces by which we are encompassed.

EIGHT

Living Through a Prolonged Nightmare

AT THE TIME OF my extraordinary kundalini awakening in 1937, I was serving as a clerk under the Director of Education in our state. Prior to that, as mentioned earlier in this narrative, I had been working in the same capacity in the office of the Chief Engineer, from which I had been transferred for having the temerity to question an unjust directive from the Minister-in-charge, who often took morbid pleasure in bullying subordinates. I had no liking for the work in either office, although from the point of view of my other colleagues I held enviable positions. I maintained the classified lists and service records of senior-grade employees, formulated proposals for their promotion and transfer, dealt with their petitions and appeals, and attended to their requests. In this way I had to deal with a large section of the personnel in both departments, many of whom, detecting chances of undeserved favors at the cost of unsuspecting fellow employees, frequented the offices regularly, hunting for easy gains, obliging colleagues to do likewise to save themselves from a possible loss.

By the very nature of my duties it was utterly impossible for me to escape comment and criticism of my acts, which influenced the life and career of someone or other. But some of these acts also had the reverse effect of confronting me with my own conscience on behalf of a poor and supportless but deserving candidate. Because of a desire to deal equal justice in all cases, I was frequently brought into conflict with hidden influences surreptitiously at work behind the apparently spotless facade of government offices, which every now and then created insoluble problems and odious situations for me. I had a strong partiality for the underdog, and this trait in my character worked equally against my own interests, and on at least two occasions impelled me to refuse chances of promotion, out of turn, in preference to senior colleagues.

Temperamentally I was not suited for a profession of this kind, but possessing neither the qualifications for another nor means nor inclination to equip myself for a better one, I continued to move in the rut in which I had placed myself on the first day. Although I worked hard and to the best of my ability, I was more interested in the study and practice of yoga than in my official career. The latter I treated merely as a means to earn a livelihood, just sufficient to meet our simplest needs. Beyond that it had no value or significance for me. I had a positive dislike of being drawn into controversies with crowds of disputing contestants on every side, as happened almost every day, creating at times disquieting ripples in my otherwise placid mental pool, which I strove to keep unruffled and calm, indispensable to my yoga practices.

In the Education Directorate the conditions were more reassuring for me. There were no chances of corruption on the scale that had existed in the Public Works Department. Consequently the distracting play of plot and counterplot, which had been a regular feature of the former office, was also absent. Here my path ran more or less smoothly until 1947. It was in no small measure due to the sense of security and the congenial atmosphere in the new office that I was able to retain my link with it in spite of the ordeals I had to face and the suspense I had to bear for a long period while attending to the day-to-day work at my table.

The sudden awakening of kundalini in one whose nervous system has reached the ripe stage of development as a result of favorable heredity, correct mode of living, and proper mental application is often liable to create a most bewildering effect on the mind. The reason for it, though extremely simple, may not be easily acceptable to the present-day intellect, which treats the human mind as a finally sealed product, dependent, according to some, exclusively on the activity of the brain cells, beginning and ending with the body; according to others, on the responsiveness of the bone-shielded gray and white matter to the extremely subtle all-pervading cosmic mind or Universal spirit; and according to still others, on the existence of an immortal individual soul in the body.

Without entering into a lengthy discussion of the correctness of these hypotheses advanced to account for the existence of mind, it is sufficient for our purpose to say that according to the authorities on yoga, the activity of the brain and the nervous system, irrespective of whether proceeding form an eternal self-existing spiritual source or from an embodied soul, depends on the existence in the body of a subtle life element known as prana, which pervades each cell of every tissue and fluid in the organism, much in the same way that electricity pervades each atom of a battery.

This vital element has a biological counterpart, as thought has a biological complement in the brain, in the shape of an extremely fine biochemical essence of a highly delicate and volatile nature, extracted by the nerves from the surrounding organic mass. After extraction, this vital essence resides in the brain and the nervous system, and is capable of generating a subtle radiation impossible to isolate by laboratory analysis. It circulates in the organism as motor impulse and sensation, conducting all the organic functions of the body, permeated and worked by the superintelligent cosmic life energy, or prana, by which it is continuously affected, just as the sensitive chemical layer on a photographic plate is affected by light.

The term *prana*, as used by authorities on yoga, signifies both the cosmic life energy and its subtle biological conductor in the body, the two being inseparable. At the very moment the body dies, the rare organic essence immediately undergoes chemical changes, ceasing to serve as a channel for the former in the previous capacity. Normally, the work of extraction of prana to feed the brain is done by a limited group of nerves, operating in a circumscribed area of the organism, with the result that the consciousness of an individual displays no variation in its nature or extent during the span of life, exhibiting a constancy which is in sharp contrast to the continuously changing appearance of the body.

With the awakening of kundalini, the arrangement suffers a radical alteration affecting the entire nervous system, as a result of which other and more extensive groups of nerves are stirred to activity, leading to the transmission of an enormously enhanced supply of a more concentrated form of pranic radiation into the brain drawn from a vastly increased area of the body. The far-reaching effects of this immensely augmented flow of an intense form of vital current into the cephalic cavity through the spinal cord before the system becomes fully accustomed to it may be visualized by considering the effects of a sudden increase in the flow of blood to the brain, such as faintness, complete insensibility, excitement, irritability, or in extreme cases, delirium, paralysis, or death.

The awakening may be gradual or sudden, varying in intensity and effect according to the development, constitution, and temperament of different individuals; but in most cases it results in a greater instability of the emotional nature and a greater liability to aberrant mental conditions in the subject, mainly resulting from tainted heredity, faulty modes of conduct, or immoderation in any shape or form.

Leaving out the extreme cases, which end in madness, this generalization applies to all the categories of those in whom kundalini is congenitally more or less active, comprising mystics, mediums, men and women of genius, and those of an exceptionally high intellectual or artistic development only a shade removed from genius. In the case of those in whom the awakening occurs all at once as the result of yoga or other spiritual practices, the sudden impact of powerful vital currents on the brain and other organs is often attended with grave risk and strange mental conditions, varying from moment to moment, exhibiting in the beginning the abnormal peculiarities of a medium, mystic, genius, and madman all rolled into one.

At the time, I had absolutely no knowledge of the technicalities of the science or the mode of operation of the great energy or of the spheres of its activity, as vast and as varied as humanity itself. I did not know that I had dug down to the very roots of my being and that my whole life was at stake. Like the vast majority of people interested in yoga, I had no idea that a system designed to develop the latent possibilities and nobler qualities in human beings could be fraught with such danger at times as to destroy the sanity or crush the life out of one by the sheer weight of entirely foreign and uncontrollable conditions of the mind.

On the third day of the awakening I did not feel myself in a mood for meditation and passed the time in bed, not a little uneasy about the abnormal state of my mind and the exhausted condition of my body. The next day when I sat for meditation, after a practically sleepless night, I found to my consternation that I completely lacked the power to concentrate my attention on any point for even a brief interval and that a thin stream of the radiant essence, which had impinged on my brain with such vivifying and elevating effect on the first two occasions, was now pouring into it automatically with a sinister light that, instead of uplifting, had a most depressing influence on me.

The days that followed had all the appearance of a prolonged nightmare. It seemed as if I had abruptly precipitated myself from the steady rock of normality into a madly racing whirlpool of abnormal existence. The keen desire to sit and meditate, which had always been present during the preceding days, disappeared suddenly and was replaced by a feeling of horror of the supernatural. I wanted to fly from even the thought of it. At the same time I felt a sudden distaste for work and conversation, with the inevitable result that being left with nothing to keep myself engaged, time hung heavily on me, adding to the already distraught condition of my mind.

The nights were even more terrible. I could not bear to have a light in my room after I had retired to bed. The moment my head touched the pillow a large tongue of flame sped across the spine into the interior of my head. It appeared as if the stream of living light continuously rushing through the spinal cord into the cranium gathered greater speed and volume during the hours of darkness. Whenever I closed my eyes I found myself looking into a weird circle of light, in which luminous currents swirled and eddied, moving rapidly from side to side. The spectacle was fascinating but awful, invested with a supernatural awe which sometimes chilled the vary marrow in my bones.

Only a few days before, it had been my habit, when in bed at night, to invite sleep by pursuing a pleasant chain of thoughts which often led me, without revealing the exact moment when it happened, from the waking state into the fantastic realm of dreams. Now everything was altered. I tossed restlessly from side to side for hours without being able to bring my agitated mind to the degree of composure needed to bring sleep. After extinguishing the lights, instead of seeing myself in darkness wafted gradually to a delicious state of rest preparatory to sleep, I found myself staring fearfully into a vast internal glow, disquieting and threatening at times, always in rapid motion, as if the particles of an ethereal luminous stuff crossed and recrossed each other, resembling the ceaseless movement of wildly leaping lustrous clouds of spray rising from a waterfall which, lighted by the sun, rushes down foaming into a seething pool.

Sometimes it seemed as if a jet of molten copper, mounting up through the spine, dashed against my crown and fell in a scintillating shower of vast dimensions all around me. I gazed at it fascinated, with fear gripping my heart. Occasionally it resembled a fireworks display of great magnitude. As far as I could look inwardly with my mental eye, I saw only a brilliant shower or a glowing pool of light. I seemed to shrink in size when compared to the gigantic halo that surrounded me, stretching out on every side in undulating waves of copper color distinctly perceptible in the surrounding darkness, as if the optic center in the brain was now in direct contact with an extremely subtle, luminous substance in perpetual motion, flooding the brain and nervous system, without the intervention of the intermediary channels of the retina and the optic nerve.

I seemed to have touched accidentally the lever of an unknown mechanism, hidden in the extremely intricate and yet unexplored nervous structure in the body, releasing a hitherto pent-up torrent which, impinging upon the auditory and optic regions, created the sensation of roaring sounds and weirdly moving lights, introducing an entirely new and unexpected feature into the normal working of the mind that gave to all my thoughts and actions the semblance of unreality and abnormality.

For a few days I thought I was suffering from hallucinations, hoping that my condition would become normal again after some time. But instead of disappearing or even diminishing as the days went by, the abnormality became more and more pronounced, assuming gradually the state of an obsession which grew in intensity as the luminous appearances became wilder and more fantastic and the noises louder and more uncanny. The dreadful thought began to take hold of my mind that I was irretrievably heading towards a disaster from which I was powerless to save myself.

To one uninitiated in the esoteric science of kundalini, as I was at that time, all that transpired afterwards presented such an abnormal and unnatural appearance that I became extremely nervous about the outcome. I passed every minute of the time in a state of acute anxiety and tension, at a loss to know what had happened to me and why my system was functioning in such an entirely abnormal manner.

I felt exhausted and spent. The day after the experience I suffered loss of appetite, and food tasted like ash in my mouth. My tongue was coated white, and there was a redness in my eyes never noticed before. My face wore a haggard and anxious expression, and there were acute disturbances in the digestive and excretory organs. I lost my regularity and found myself at the mercy of a newly released force about which I knew nothing, creating a tumultuous and agitated condition of the mind as the sweep of a tempest creates an agitation in the placid waters of a lake.

There was no remission in the current rising from the seat of kundalini. I could feel it leaping across the nerves in my back and even across those lining the front part of my body from the loins upward. But most alarming was the way in which my mind acted and behaved after the incident. I felt as if I were looking at the world from a higher elevation than that from which I saw it before.

It is very difficult to express my mental condition accurately. All I can say is that it seemed as if my cognitive faculty had undergone a transformation and that I had, as it were, mentally expanded. What was more startling and terrifying was the fact that the point of consciousness in me was not as invariable nor its condition as stable as it had been before. It expanded and contracted, regulated in a mysterious way by the radiant current that was flowing up from the lowest plexus. This widening and narrowing were accompanied by a host of terrors for me. At times I felt slightly elated with a transient morbid sense of well-being and achievement, forgetting for the time being the abnormal state I was in, but soon after was made acutely conscious of my critical condition and again oppressed by a tormenting cloud of fear.

The few brief intervals of mental elation were followed by fits of depression much more prolonged and so acute that I had to muster all my strength and willpower to keep myself from succumbing completely to their influence. I sometimes gagged my mouth to keep from crying and fled from the solitude of my room to the crowded street to prevent myself from doing some desperate act.

For weeks I had no respite. Each morning heralded for me a new kind of terror, a fresh complication in the already disordered system, a deeper fit of melancholy or more irritable condition of the mind which I had to restrain, to prevent it from completely overwhelming me, by keeping myself alert, usually after a completely sleepless night; and after withstanding patiently the tortures of the day, I had to prepare myself for the even worse torment of the night.

A man cheerfully overcomes insurmountable difficulties and bravely faces overwhelming odds when he is confident of his mental and physical condition. I completely lost confidence in my own mind and body and lived like a haunted, terror-stricken stranger in my own flesh, constantly reminded of my precarious state. My consciousness was in such a state of unceasing flux that I was never certain how it would behave within the next few minutes. It rose and fell like a wave, raising me one moment out of the clutches of fear to dash me again the next into the depths of despair.

It seemed as if the stream of vitality rising into my brain through the spinal cord, connected mysteriously with the region near the base of the spine, was playing strange tricks with my imagination. Also I was unable to stop it or to resist its effect on my thoughts. Was I losing my mind? Were these the first indications of mental disorder? This thought constantly drove me to desperation. It was not so much the extremely weird nature of my mental condition as the fear of incipient madness or some grave disorder of the nervous system which filled me with growing dismay.

I lost all feeling of love for my wife and children. I had loved them fondly from the depths of my being. The fountain of love in me seemed to have dried up completely. It appeared as if a scorching blast had raced through every pore in my body, wiping out every trace of affection. I looked at my children again and again, trying to evoke the deep feeling with which I had regarded them previously, but in vain. My love for them seemed to be dead beyond recall. They appeared to me not better than strangers.

To reawaken the emotion of love in my heart I held and caressed them, talked to them in endearing terms, but never succeeded in experiencing that spontaneity and warmth which are characteristic of true attachment. I knew they were my flesh and blood and was conscious of the duty I owed to them. My critical judgment was unimpaired, but love was dead. The recollection of my departed mother, whom I had always remembered with deep affection, brought with it no wave of the deep emotion which I had invariably felt at the thought of her. I viewed this unnatural disappearance of a deep-rooted feeling with despondency, finding myself robbed of that which gives life its greatest charm.

I studied my mental condition constantly with fear in my heart. When I compared my new conscious personality with what it had been before, I could definitely see a radical change. There had been an unmistakable extension. The vital energy which lighted the flame of being was pouring visibly inside my brain; this had not been the case before. The light, too, was impure and variable. The flame was not burning with a pure, imperceptible and steady luster as in normal consciousness. It grew brighter and fainter by turns. No doubt the illumination spread over a wider circle, but it was not as clear and transparent as before.

It seemed as if I were looking at the world through a haze. When I glanced at the sky I failed to notice the lovely azure I used to see before. My eyesight had always been good and even now there was nothing obviously wrong with it. I could easily read the smallest type and clearly distinguish objects at a distance. Obviously my vision was unimpaired, but there was something wrong with the cognitive faculty. The recording instrument was still in good order, but something was amiss with the observer.

In the normal man, the flow of the stream of consciousness is so nicely regulated that he can notice no variation in it from boyhood to death. He knows himself as a conscious entity, a nondimensional point of awareness located more particularly in the head with a faint extension covering the trunk and limbs. When he closes his eyes to study this entity attentively, he ends by observing a conscious presence, himself in fact, round the region of the head. As I could easily discern, even in that condition of mental disquietude, this field of consciousness in me had vastly increased. It was akin to that which I had experienced in the vision but divested of every trace of happiness which had characterized my first experience. On the contrary, it was gloomy and fear-ridden, depressed instead of cheerful, murky instead of clearly transparent. It seemed as if prolonged concentration had opened an only partially developed center in the brain which depended for its fuel on the stream of energy constantly rushing upward from the reproductive region. The enlarged consciousness field was the creation of this hitherto closed chamber, which was now functioning imperfectly, first because it had been forced open prematurely, and secondly because I was utterly ignorant of the way to adjust myself to the new development.

For weeks I wrestled with the mental gloom caused by my abnormal condition, growing more despondent each day. My face became extremely pale and my body thin and weak. I felt a distaste for food and found fear clutching my heart the moment I swallowed anything. Often I left the plate untouched. Very soon my whole intake of food amounted to a cup or two of milk and a few oranges. Beyond that I could eat nothing. I knew I could not survive for long on such an insufficient diet, but I could not help it. I was burning inside but had no means to assuage the fire. While my intake of food was drastically reduced, the daily expenditure of energy increased tremendously. My restlessness had assumed such a state that I could not sit quietly for even half an hour. When I did so, my attention was drawn irresistibly towards the strange behavior of my mind. Immediately the ever-present fear was intensified, and my heart thumped violently. I had to divert my attention somehow to free myself from the horror of my condition.

In order to prevent my mind from dwelling again and again on itself, I took recourse to walking. On rising in the morning, as long as I possessed the strength to do so, I left immediately for a slow walk to counteract the effect of an oppressive, sleepless night, when, forced to lie quiet in the darkness, I had no alternative but to be an awed spectator of the weird and fearsome display visible inside myself. On the way, I met scores of my acquaintances taking their morning constitutional, laughing and talking as they went. I could not share their enjoyment, and passed them in silence with merely a nod or gesture of salutation.

I had no interest in any other person or in any subject in the world. My own abnormality blotted out everything else from my mind. During the day I walked in my room or in the compound, diverting my attention from object to object without allowing it to rest on one particular thing for any length of time. I counted my steps or looked at the ceiling or at the wall, at the floor or at the surrounding objects one by one, at each for but a fleeting instant, thus with all the willpower at my command preventing my brain from attaining a state of fixity at any time. I was fighting desperately against my own unruly mind.

But how long could my resistance last? How long could I save myself from madness creeping upon me? My starving body was becoming weaker and weaker; my legs tottered under me while I walked, and yet walk I had to if I was to rid myself of the clutching terror which gripped my heart as soon as I allowed my mind to brood upon itself. My memory became weaker and I faltered in my talk, while the anxious expression on my face deepened. At the blackest moments, my eyebrows drew together into an anxious frown, the thickly wrinkled forehead and a wild look in my gleaming eyes giving my countenance a maniacal expression. Several times during the day I glanced at myself in the looking glass or felt my pulse, and to my horror found myself deteriorating more and more.

I do not know what sustained my will so that even in a state of extreme terror I could maintain control over my actions and gestures. No one could even suspect what was happening to me inside. I knew that but a thin line now separated me from lunacy, and yet I gave no indication of my condition to anyone. I suffered unbearable torture in silence, weeping internally at the sad turn of events, blaming myself bitterly again and again for having delved into the supernatural without first acquiring a fuller knowledge of the subject and providing against the dangers and risks of the path.

Even at the time of greatest dejection, and even when almost at the breaking point, something inside prevented me from consulting a physician. There was no psychiatrist at Jammu in those days, and even if there had been one, I am sure I would not have gone to see

him. It was well that I was not able to do so. The little knowledge of
diseases that I possessed was enough to tell me that my abnormality
was unique, that it was neither purely psychic nor purely physical,
but the outcome of an alteration in the nervous activity of my body
which no therapist on earth could correctly diagnose or cure. On
the other hand, a single mistake in treatment in that highly dangerous condition, when the whole system was in a state of complete
disorder and not amenable to control, might have proved fatal.
Mistakes were inevitable in view of the entirely obscure and uniden-
tifiable nature of the condition.

A skilled physician bases his observations on the symptoms present in an ailment, relying for the success of his treatment on the
uniformity of pathological conditions in the normal human body.
Physiological processes follow a certain specific rhythm which the
body tries to maintain under all ordinary circumstances. In my case,
since the basic element responsible for the rhythm and the uniformity
was at the moment itself in a state of turmoil, the anarchy prevailing
not only in the system but also in the sphere of thought, nay, in the
innermost recesses of my being, can be better imagined than described.

I did not know then what I came to grasp later on—that an
automatic mechanism, forced by the practice of meditation, had
suddenly started to function with the object of reshaping my mind
to make it fit for the expression of a more heightened and extended
consciousness by means of biological processes as natural and as
governed by inviolable laws as the evolution of species or the
development and birth of a child. But to my great misfortune I did
not know this at the time. To the best of my knowledge, this mighty
secret of nature is not known on earth today, although there is
ample evidence to show that certain methods to deal with the
condition, when brought about suddenly by the practice of hatha
yoga, were fully known to the ancient adepts.

I studied my condition thoroughly from day to day to assure
myself that what I experienced was real and not imaginary. Just as a

man finding himself in an unbelievable situation pinches himself to make certain that he is not dreaming but awake, I invariably studied my bodily symptoms to find corroboration for my mental condition. It would be a fallacy to assume that I was the victim of a hallucination. Subsequent events and my present condition absolutely rule out that possibility. No, the crisis I was passing through was not a creation of my own imagination. It had a real physiological basis and was interwoven with the whole organic structure of my body. The entire machinery from the brain to the smallest organ was deeply involved, and there was no escape for me from the storm of nervous forces which blew through my system day and night, released unexpectedly by my own effort.

NINE

An Unearthly Radiance Filled My Head

DURING RECENT TIMES there have hardly been any instances of individuals in whom the Serpent Fire burnt ceaselessly from the day of awakening of kundalini to the last, bringing about mental transformations known to and hinted at by the ancient sages of India. But that there have been many cases of a sporadic type in which the Shakti* was active intermittently admits of no doubt. The mystics and saints of all countries, who from an early age are prone to transcendental visions and pass occasionally into ecstatic trances, thereafter reverting to their normal consciousness, belong to the latter category. The psychics and mediums and all those possessing the power of clairvoyance, mind reading, prediction, and similar supernormal faculties owe their surprising gifts to the action of an awakened kundalini operating in a limited way in the head without reaching the highest center, where it overshadows the whole consciousness. The same is true of the men and women of genius in whom the energy feeds certain specific regions of the brain, stimulating them to extraordinary phases of intellectual, literary, or artistic activity.

In all cases mentioned above, either the flow of the more potent vital current is so regulated and circumscribed that it does not create any disturbance in the system or, as in the case of mystics in whom the impact of the current on the brain is very powerful at times, the condition begins at birth so that the nervous system usually becomes accustomed to it from infancy, when one is not aware of the variations in consciousness nor able to place a meaning on the abnormal happenings in the body and feel the sense of fear.

*See page 177.

But even so, the latter often have to face many a crisis and to endure unusual suffering and torment before they acquire a stable and peaceful condition of the mind and are in a position to study and express comprehensively the experience which marks them as a class apart from the normal run of mortals. The individuals belonging to these categories, excepting mystics, do not perceive the luminosity and the movement of nerve currents, except in exceptional cases, as the flow of the vital energy is too restricted to create weird effects. Moreover, having been an integral part of the organism from birth, it becomes an inherent trait of their personalities.

The popular books on yoga that I had read years before contained no hint of such an abnormal development and nerve-shattering experience. The learned authors confined themselves to the description of various postures and methods, all borrowed from the ancient writings on the subject. Few of them claimed to have had the experience but were eager to teach to others what they had never learned themselves.

In some of the books there was a passing reference to kundalini yoga. A couple of pages or a small chapter was all that the authors thought sufficient for describing this most difficult and least-known form of yoga. It was stated that kundalini represents the cosmic vital energy lying dormant in the human body which is coiled round the base of the spine, a little below the sexual organ, like a serpent fast asleep and closing with her mouth the aperture of the *sushumna*, the hairlike duct rising through the center of the spinal cord to the conscious center at the top of the head. When roused, kundalini, they said, rises through the *sushumna* like a streak of lightning, carrying with her the vital energy of the body, which for the time being becomes cold and lifeless, with complete or partial cessation of vital functions, to join her divine spouse Shiva in the last or seventh center in the brain. In the course of this process, the embodied self, freed from the bondage of flesh, passes into a condition of ecstasy known as samadhi, realizing itself as deathless, full of bliss, and one with the all-pervading Supreme Consciousness.

In only one or two writings were there vague hints of dangers to be met on the path. The nature of the danger and the methods to prevent or overcome it were not explained by the authors.

From the vague ideas I had gathered from these works or picked up in the course of discussions or talks about yoga, it was only natural for me to infer that the abnormal condition I had brought upon myself was the direct outcome of my meditation. My experience had corresponded in every respect with the descriptions given of the ecstatic state by those who had attained this condition themselves; there was therefore no reason for me to doubt the validity or the possibility of my vision. There could be no mistake about the sounds I had heard and the effulgence I had perceived.

Above all, there certainly could be no mistake about the transformation of my own consciousness, the nearest and the most intimate part of me, that I had experienced more than once, and the memory of which was so strong that it could never be effaced or mistaken for any other condition. It could not be a mere figment of my fancy because during the vision I still possessed the capacity to make a comparison between the extended state of consciousness and the normal one, and when it began to fade, I could perceive the contraction that was taking place. It was undoubtedly a real experience, and one that has been described with all the power of expression at their command by mystics and saints all over the world.

But in my case there was one particular and unmistakable deviation from the usual type of vision: the most extraordinary sensation at the base of the spine followed by the flow of a radiant current through the spinal column into the head. This part of the strange experience tallied with the phenomena associated with the awakening of kundalini, and hence I could not be mistaken in supposing that I had unknowingly aroused the coiled serpent and that the serious disturbance in my nervous system as well as the extraordinary but most awful state I was in, was in some way occasioned by it.

I made no mention of my condition to anyone save my brother-in-law, who came to Jammu during those days on a short business visit. He was many years older than I and loved me like a son. I talked to him unreservedly, aware of his deep affection for me. He had himself practiced meditation for many years under the guidance of a preceptor who claimed knowledge of kundalini yoga. Frank and noble by nature, he often narrated to me his own experiences in the simple manner of a child, seeking corroboration from me for the results he had achieved by his labors.

Without the least pretension to knowledge, he gave me every bit of information he possessed, and thus in a way was instrumental in saving my life. My wife knew nothing of the life-and-death struggle in which I was engaged, but alarmed by my strange behavior, lack of appetite, bodily disturbances, constant walks, and above all by the never-lifting cloud of anxiety and gloom on my face, she advised me again and again to consult a physician and constantly watched over me day and night, frantic with anxiety.

My brother-in-law could not fully grasp the significance of what I related to him but said that his guru had once remarked that if by mistake kundalini were aroused through any other *nadi* (nerve) except *sushumna*, there was every danger of serious psychic and physical disturbances, ending in permanent disability, insanity, or death. This was particularly the case, the teacher had said, if the awakening occurred through *pingala* on the right side of the spine when the unfortunate person is literally burned to death due to excessive internal heat, which cannot be controlled by any external means.

I was horrified by this statement and in desperation went to consult a learned ascetic from Kashmir who had come to spend the winter at Jammu. He heard me with patience and said that the experience I had undergone could not at all be due to the awakening of the Serpent Power, as that was always blissful and could not be associated with any agency liable to cause disease or disturbance. He made another gruesome suggestion, heard from his teacher or picked up from some ancient work, to the effect that my malady was probably due to the venom of malignant spirits that beset the path of yogis, and prescribed a decoction, which I never took.

On the suggestion of someone else, I glanced through a couple of books on kundalini yoga, translations in English of ancient Sanskrit texts. I could not read even a page attentively, the attempt involving fixity of attention which I was incapable of maintaining for any length of time. The least effort instantly aggravated my condition by increasing the flow of the newborn energy into the brain, which added to my terror and misery. I just glanced through the books, reading a line here and a paragraph there.

The description of the symptoms that followed the awakening corroborated my own experience and firmly strengthened my conviction that I had aroused the vital force dormant in me; but whether the agony of mind and body that I was passing through was an inevitable result of the awakening or whether I had drawn up the energy through a wrong nerve, I could not be sure.

There was, however, one very briefly stated injunction—call it accident or divine guidance—I picked up from the huge mass of material in that very cursory glance. It was to the effect that during the course of the practice the student is not permitted to keep his stomach empty but should take a light meal every three hours. This brief advice, flashing across my brain at a most critical moment when I hovered between life and death and had lost every hope of survival, later saved my life and sanity and continues to do so to this day.

At the time I paid no attention to this significant hint which, based on the experience of countless people, many of whom had probably lost their lives in the attempt to arouse the Serpent Power, had come down through the ages as guidance for the initiates. Even if I had tried my hardest to do so, I could not have acted upon the advice at that time, as food was so abhorrent to me that my stomach revolted at the mere thought of it. I was burning in every part of my body while my mind, like a floating balloon, bobbed up and down and swayed sideways erratically, unable to keep itself steady even for a moment.

Whenever my mind turned upon itself I always found myself staring with growing panic into the unearthly radiance that filled my head, swirling and eddying like a fearsome whirlpool; I even found its reflection in the pitch darkness of my room during the slowly dragging hours of the night. Not infrequently it assumed horrible shapes and postures, as if satanic faces were grinning and inhuman forms gesticulating at me in the blackness.

This happened night after night for months, weakening my will and sapping my resistance until I felt unable to endure the fearful ordeal any longer, certain that at any moment I might succumb to the relentlessly pursuing horror and, bidding farewell to my life and sanity, rush out of the room a raving maniac. But I persisted, determined to hold on as long as I had a vestige of willpower, resolved at the first sign of breaking to surrender my life rather than lose myself in the ghastly wilderness of insanity.

When it was day I longed for the night, and during the night I prayed fervently for the day. As time wore on, my hope dwindled and desperation seized me. There was no relaxation in the tension or any abatement in the ceaselessly haunting fear, or any relief from the fiery stream that darted through my nerves and poured into my agonized brain. On the other hand, as my vitality ebbed as a result of fasts, and my resistance weakened, the malady was aggravated to such a pitch that every moment I expected the end.

It was in such a frame of mind that the holy festival of Shivratri, or the night of Shiva, came to pass towards the end of February. As usual every year my wife had painstakingly prepared some dainty dishes on the day and gently insisted that I, too, should partake of the food. Not to disappoint her and cast a cloud of gloom on her already anxiety-filled mind, I acquiesced and forcibly swallowed a few morsels and then gave up and washed my hands. Immediately I felt a sinking sensation at the pit of my stomach, a fiery stream of energy shot into my head, and I felt myself lifted up and up, expanding awfully with unbearable terror clutching at me from every side. I felt a reeling sensation while my hands and feet grew cold as ice, as if all the heat had escaped from them to feed the fiery vapor in the head which had risen through the spinal cord like the ruddy blast from a furnace and now, acting like a poison on the brain, struck me numb. I was overpowered by faintness and giddiness.

I staggered to my feet and dragged myself heavily towards my bed in the adjacent room. With trembling hands I lifted up the cover and slipped in, trying to stretch myself into a position of ease. But I was in a terrible condition, burning internally from head to toe, outwardly cold as ice, and shivering as if stricken with ague. I felt my pulse; it was racing madly and my heart was thumping wildly below my ribs, its pounding distinctly audible to me. But what horrified me was the intensity of the fiery currents that now darted through my body, penetrating into every part and every organ.

My brain worked desperately, unable to give coherence to my frenzied thoughts. To call in a doctor for consultation in such an unheard-of condition would be a mere waste of effort. His first thought on hearing of my symptoms would turn to a lunatic asylum. It would be futile on my part to seek help from any other quarter for such an affliction. What could I do then to save myself from this torture? Could it be that in my previous semi-starved condition, subsisting only on a few oranges and a little milk, the fiery current could not attain such awful intensity as it had done now with the entry of solid food in my stomach? How could I save myself? Where could I go to escape from the furnace raging in my interior?

The heat grew every moment, causing such unbearable pain that I writhed and twisted from side to side while streams of cold perspiration poured down my face and limbs. But still the heat increased and soon it seemed as if innumerable red-hot pins were coursing through my body, scorching and blistering the organs and tissues like flying sparks. Suffering the most excruciating torture, I clenched my hands and bit my lips to stop myself from leaping out of bed and crying at the top of my voice. The throbbing of my heart grew more and more terrific, acquiring such a spasmodic violence that I thought it must either stop beating or burst. Flesh and blood could not stand such strain without giving way any moment.

It was easy to see that the body was valiantly trying to fight the virulent poison speeding across the nerves and pouring into the brain. But the fight was so unequal and the fury let loose in my system so lethal that it seemed there could be not the least doubt about the outcome. There were dreadful disturbances in all the organs, each so alarming and painful that I wonder how I managed to retain my self-possession under the onslaught. The whole delicate organism was burning, withering away completely under the fiery blast racing through its interior.

I knew I was dying and that my heart could not stand the tremendous strain for long. My throat was scorched and every part of my body flaming and burning, but I could do nothing to alleviate the dreadful suffering. If a well or river had been near I would have jumped into its cold depths, preferring death to what I was undergoing. But there was no well and the river was half a mile away.

With a great effort I got up, trembling, with the idea of pouring a few buckets of cold water over my head to abate the dreadful heat. But at that moment my eyes fell on my small daughter, Ragina, lying in the next bed awake, watching my feverish movements with wide-open, anxious eyes. With the remnant of sense still left in me I could understand that the least unusual movement on my part at that time would make her cry and that if I started to pour water over my body at such an unearthly hour, both she and her mother, who was busy in the kitchen, would almost die with fright. The thought restrained me and I decided to bear the internal agony until the end, which could not be far off.

What had happened to me all of a sudden? What devilish power of the underworld held me in its relentless grasp? Was I doomed to die in this dreadful way, leaving a corpse with blackened face and limbs to make people wonder what unheard-of horror had overtaken me as a punishment for crimes committed in a previous birth? I racked my distracted brain for a way of escape, only to meet blank despair on every side. The effort exhausted me and I felt myself sinking, dully conscious of the scalding sea of pain in which I was drowning. I tried desperately to rouse myself, only to sink back again, deadened by a torment beyond my power to endure. After a while, with a sudden, inexplicable revival of strength marking the onset of delirium, I came back to life with a shred of sanity left, Almighty alone knows how, just sufficient to prevent me from giving way completely to acts of madness and self-violence.

Pulling the cover over my face, I stretched myself to my full length on the bed, burning in every fiber, lashed as it were by a fiery rain of red-hot needles piercing my skin. At this moment a fearful idea struck me. Could it be that I had aroused kundalini through *pingala*, the solar nerve which regulates the flow of heat in the body and is located on the right side of *sushumna*? If so, I was doomed, I thought desperately, and as if by Divine dispensation the idea flashed across my brain to make a last-minute attempt to rouse *ida*, the lunar nerve on the left side, to activity, thus neutralizing the dreadful burning effect of the devouring fire within.

With my mind reeling and senses deadened with pain, but with all the willpower left at my command, I brought my attention to bear on the left side of the seat of kundalini and tried to force an imaginary cold current upward through the middle of the spinal cord. In that extraordinarily extended, agonized, and exhausted state of consciousness, I distinctly felt the location of the nerve and strained hard mentally to divert its flow into the central channel. Then, as if waiting for the destined moment, a miracle happened.

There was a sound like a nerve thread snapping and instantaneously a silvery streak passed zigzag through the spinal cord, exactly like the sinuous movement of a white serpent in rapid flight, pouring an effulgent, cascading shower of brilliant vital energy into my brain, filling my head with a blissful luster in place of the flame that had been tormenting me for the last three hours. Completely taken by surprise at this sudden transformation of the fiery current darting across the entire network of my nerves only a moment before, and overjoyed at the cessation of pain, I remained absolutely quiet and motionless for some time, tasting the bliss of relief with a mind flooded with emotion, unable to believe I was really free of the horror. Tortured and exhausted almost to the point of collapse by the agony I had suffered during the terrible interval, I immediately fell asleep, bathed in light, and for the first time after weeks of anguish felt the sweet embrace of restful sleep.

As if rudely shaken out of my slumber I awoke after about an hour. The stream of luster was still pouring in my head, my brain was clear, my heart and pulse had stopped racing, the burning sensations and the fear had almost vanished; but my throat was still dry, my mouth parched, and I found myself in a state of extreme exhaustion, as if every ounce of energy had been drained out of me. Exactly at that moment another idea occurred to me; as if suggested by an invisible intelligence and with irresistible power came the direction that I should eat something immediately. I motioned to my wife, who as usual was lying awake in her bed anxiously watching my every movement, to fetch me a cup of milk and a little bread. Taken aback by this unusual and untimely request, she hesitated a moment, and then complied without a word. I ate the bread, swallowing it with difficulty with the help of the milk and immediately fell asleep again.

I woke up again after about two hours, considerably refreshed by the sleep. My head was still filled with the glowing radiance and, to my surprise, in this heightened and lustrous state of consciousness I could distinctly perceive a tongue of the golden flame searching my stomach for food and moving round along the nerves lining it.

I took a few bites of bread and another cup of milk, and as soon as I had done so I found the halo in the head contracting and a larger tongue of flame licking my stomach, as if a part of the streaming energy pouring into my brain was being diverted to the gastric region to expedite the process of digestion.

I lay awake, dumb with wonder, watching this living radiance moving from place to place through the whole digestive tract, caressing the intestines and the liver, while another stream poured into the kidneys and the heart. I pinched myself to make sure whether I was dreaming or asleep, absolutely dumbfounded by what I was witnessing in my own body, entirely powerless to regulate or to guide the current.

Unlike the horror I had experienced before, I felt no discomfort now; all that I could feel was a gentle and soothing warmth moving through my body as the current traveled from point to point. I watched this wonderful play silently, my whole being filled with boundless gratitude to the Unseen for this timely deliverance from a dreadful fate; and a new assurance began to shape itself in my mind that the Serpent Fire was in reality now at work in my exhausted and agonized body and that I was safe.

Here, while begging to be excused for digression from the main thread of my narrative, I wish to emphasize that I believe that the story of my life and family background has significant relevance to the extraordinary development that occurred in me twelve years later, when I was forty-six. Placing this kundalini awakening in its proper personal and cultural perspective should aid scientific inquiry in the much-disputed realm of the supernormal.

I hesitated for nearly twenty years in making the experience public because in the first place, I wanted to make myself completely sure about my own condition, and secondly, I was entirely averse to exposing myself to the criticism of well-meaning friends and the ridicule of opponents. The story I had to relate was so out of the ordinary and so full of strange episodes that I was very doubtful about its being accepted as a truthful account of an experience which, extremely rare, has always remained wrapped in mystery from times immemorial.

I thought there might be but few who would straight away believe what I had to narrate about the bizarre phenomenon, but the urge to make the hidden truth known prevailed at last. I knew that with the publication of this work I was exposing myself to criticism from various quarters, especially from those who should be more interested in the subject. Men of science on the one hand and those of faith on the other, some of whom instead of snatching at the chance of reconciliation now offered were likely to treat it as an encroachment upon the preserves of their idolized opinions and views, forgetting for the moment the fact that truth is an entity that grows richer in adversity and stronger in opposition.

I knew all this, but yielding to an irrepressible urge, which took shape in my mind soon after the appearance of the abnormal condition and which since then has never been wholly absent, demanding wide publicity for the experience as the first step towards organized research in all manifestations of the superconscious for which the time is now opportune, I have applied myself to the task of recapitulating the story of my life relevant to the subject, with a view to giving background and coherence to the subsequent surprising development, which, though existing in a certain class of people as a natural endowment, has so far eluded every effort directed to its investigation.

I have, at the same time, tried to draw attention to the mental and physiological conditions that precede the manifestation of such abnormal developments in human beings, bearing a resemblance in essentials, though differing in detail, to other phenomena of the kind in the past. But for the fact that the manifestations attending the awakening of kundalini are at present a sealed book to the world, barring perhaps a few exceptions, there is in actual fact nothing unique in my experience, as may be established by other similar occurrences in the future for which this work may create the necessary conditions.

The connection between food and kundalini is an important one, and ancient yoga treatises have stressed that the subtle prana that feeds kundalini is obtained from both food and air.

The sensitivity of my digestive system has been a marked feature of my life. It persists even today. During the first three or four years of my childhood, as my mother used to tell me, it was difficult for her to make me eat any solid food as the other children did. She had to coax me into eating. Sometimes she sought the help of neighbors to persuade me to eat. They carried me in their arms for some distance to put me into a good humor and then fed me from a small bowl containing cooked rice and other things which my mother wished me to eat. Even now, I have a faint recollection of being carried in the arms of one of our young neighbors, holding me with one arm and the bowl of rice in the other hand. I have also recalled the vagaries of my appetite, in chapter 3.

Until the day of the awakening, my average intake of food was rather less than normal. I usually combined my breakfast and lunch together in the morning repast, which I usually took a little after nine o'clock. We had to be in the office by ten o'clock, but I was often late because after this modest meal I used to take a few minutes rest before starting for the office. On returning from there, between four and five in the afternoon, I could never accustom myself to the regular habit of eating something or drinking a cup of milk or tea before my dinner. The latter I usually avoided unless pressed to take it at the house of a friend or relative. It was immaterial whether I did so or not. My mother always tried to instill in me the habit of a morning snack and an afternoon cup of milk, but I was never serious about it. This indifference towards a vital need of my body could be one of the reasons why, after the awakening, I had to be so meticulously careful in my diet. I have to be extremely attentive to it even now.

In spite of my faulty food habits I never suffered from lack of energy. I could stand the extremes of climate with impunity, as if I had a reserve of energy in me that came into play in exigencies. Only a few years before the awakening, an incident occurred to me in Jammu which showed how well my system was adapted not only to withstand the rigor of heat and cold, but also the deprivation caused by lack of food for several days.

It was summer and I was alone in Jammu, living all by myself in an apartment close to the office. I had sent my family earlier to Kashmir to save my wife and children from the inclemency of the heat of Jammu. The Superintendent of our office was on leave and I was asked to officiate in his place. He was expected to resume his duties in a couple of months, when I could have the opportunity to join my family in Srinagar.

During this period a case of cow slaughter caused an uproar in the town which, for lack of proper handling, assumed a serious proportion. There was a general strike in the whole city. The tradesmen refused to open their shops. Soon this resulted in a complete closure of business which lasted for several days. The hotels, restaurants, even tea shops, were closed and not a morsel of food could be obtained anywhere.

Since the departure of my family I was having my meals in the house of a friend who lived close by. Only a day before the strike he was obliged to leave for Kashmir with his family on account of ill health due to the heat, which he could not stand very well. His departure should not have created any problem for me as I was accustomed to cooking for myself when alone. But I had no provisions in the house as I had not been dining at my place. The closure of the shops, all of a sudden, before I could store the provisions, placed me in a predicament which I could not overcome.

Actually it was not such a difficult problem at all. Any one of my friends or colleagues in the office would have been happy to make me his guest. In fact, some of them who knew that my family was away in Kashmir did inquire what arrangements I had for food and readily offered their hospitality. But, reluctant to make my dilemma known to them, I returned evasive answers and did not allow them to have any insight into my difficulty. I supposed that the strike would not last for long. The usual period for closure of business, even in more explosive situations, was two or three days at the most. I thought that it would not be difficult for me to manage without food for this period. But the strike became prolonged and the shops remained closed day after day for a period of a week.

After the first three days, I felt hunger gnawing in my interior. Even then, I could have easily dined at the house of any one of my friends, and I had only to open my lips to apprise them of my position after my first refusal. But, as I had once declined their offer, it went against my grain to make my weakness known to them now. It was surely a fault in my thinking since I was exposing myself to a risk in the hot season.

I knew that my system could not stand fasting with impunity, but my false sense of self-respect in such a matter made me overlook even this consideration. Had lack of food at that time actually led to an attack of illness, it would have become necessary for me to seek the help of my friends. I could very well have sought it earlier to save myself from starvation and its consequences, but I persisted and continued to go without food for all the period of the strike.

During those days, I attended the office and did all my share of the work as usual. Until I revealed it to them months later, not one of my office colleagues had even a suspicion that every day during this interval I was coming to the office and working hard without a morsel of food in my body. But there were no ill effects, either during or after the fast. My health and sleep remained undisturbed.

From the knowledge that I gained later in life, I became convinced that kundalini was already slightly active from my birth but through the solar nerve *pingala* and not through the middle path, *sushumna*. I am led to this conclusion when I recall my habits, particularly in regard to the antipathy I had towards food from my childhood. There were other symptoms too that are mentioned elsewhere in this autobiography.

There are millions of people in whom the evolutionary organ is already slightly active. It is the men and women of this class who comprise the more dynamic and more intelligent section of the human race. But their temperaments are different.

The allopathic system of therapy in the West takes no account of the variations in temperament in different individuals. But it might have to revise its attitude in the course of time. Just as there are different types of blood, so there are also different constitutional peculiarities in human beings. These peculiarities spring from the activity of the particular channel—*ida*, *pingala*, or *sushumna*— through which the kundalini force is predominantly active.

The bioplasma which energizes all organic systems has a slightly different spectrum for every human being. The variations in the constitution of the kundalini force are also reflected in this spectrum. This is the reason why, on the awakening of the force, radical changes occur in the working of all the organs in the body, as there is now a change in the pattern of the force which energizes them.

In the case of a sudden, powerful arousal of the Serpent Power, the utmost care has to be taken of the following: (1) the state of mind, (2) the intake of food, and (3) erotic behavior. The will must have been already cultivated to exercise control over the now chaotic state of the mind. Like the pendulum of a clock, it oscillates between hope and fear, anxiety and assurance, joy and sorrow, for no apparent reason, as if pushed from this side to that and back again by an invisible force from within in a manner entirely unpredictable to the subject of the experience. If the will is not firm and lacks the strength to hold itself in check, the oscillations can lead to those irresponsible acts which are a characteristic of mental disorder.

Attention to diet is as necessary as attention to breath. The energy expended by the highly increased metabolism in the body must be replenished time after time to allow the brain to function in its altered condition. The awakening causes an upheaval in the whole system, throwing the normal rhythm of the body into utter disorder. It takes months and even years to bring order into this chaos so that the organs and the tissues get accustomed to the flow of the altered bioplasmic currents. Until then, the body acts in the same way that it does to counteract the effect of a sudden serious infection which threatens life.

The reason why the guidance of a competent guru has been

considered necessary at this time is because the exigency created needs careful handling, time after time, to avert disaster. The only way to allow the body to cope with the serious situation is to keep its store of energy from depletion. This can only be done through the intake of food at regular intervals in moderate quantities. But the combination of the various articles of diet is also of utmost importance. As in the case of infants, milk is the most appropriate body and brain building food for this transformation and, when combined with other articles of diet in proper proportion, provides the ideal nourishment for cases of this kind.

The veneration for the cow in India has a deeper significance behind it than is generally supposed. It could have sprung from cases of kundalini arousal in which milk literally acted as the savior of life. This property of milk does not depend merely on its chemical composition but also the quality of prana contained in it. Less than a century ago even expert physicians had no knowledge of vitamins and hormones. They are wiser now. They will be wiser still when they are able to detect prana and study it.

Classification of temperaments into four broad categories, namely the bilious, the phlegmatic, the sanguine and the melancholic* according to the ancient Greeks, and into three according to the Indian treatises, has a sound physiological reason behind it. More or less activation of kundalini through the three channels can be the cause of these different types of temperament in the individuals in whom the power is working. Preponderance through *pingala* can lead to the bilious, through *ida* to phlegmatic and through *sushumna* to sanguine temperaments. The permutations and combinations of these broad categories can lead to other areas of difference in the constitutions and temperaments of human beings. It is these hidden springs of human life and behavior which further research on kundalini is sure to bring to light.

─────────────

* The natures of the four temperaments, according to the Greeks, are (1) bilious— bad-tempered or cross; (2) phlegmatic—calm, cool, sluggish or dull; (3) sanguine— warm, cheerful, optimistic or passionate; and (4) melancholic—sad, sober, gloomy or depressed.

There is no doubt that a moderate amount of meditation in a balanced individual who avoids overstrain and is free from worry can prove of great help in inner unfoldment and the building of a harmonious personality. But excessive meditation in a system with a leaning either towards *pingala* or *ida* or under constant mental stress and strain can be harmful instead of beneficial. I am constantly reminded of this fact by other cases of those who have suffered harm with these practices.

Inert and passive types of meditation that induce a relaxed, daydream-like state are helpful in soothing tense or strained conditions of the mind. But they can also be a great disadvantage. Constant practice of this type of meditation (which is really reverie rather than meditation proper) can become a habit. It can then intervene even at times when alertness is needed and make concentration and one-pointed application of the mind very difficult. In certain cases even the power to apply the mind to the everyday problems of life can be lost, and unhealthy tendencies of withdrawal from the world become manifest.

Active meditation, moderately done without overstraining the brain, strengthens the will and adds to one's power to keep a grip on the mind when it is applied to a task. With regular practice the grip on the mind can become firmer until a stage is reached when it can be kept steadily occupied with a problem and absorbed in meditation without conscious effort of the will. This is the crucial point beyond which, with properly directed endeavor, samadhi, or mystical trance, can be achieved. Proficiency in meditation can allow the meditator to concentrate the mind easily without constant effort of the will in the same way that constant practice enables the nimble fingers of an expert typist to manipulate the typewriter while the mind is engaged in reading what is to be typed.

The aim of meditation is to increase the power of attention to a point where the conscious center in the brain is pressed to a greater and more sustained activity under the direction of the will. The ultimate effort of the constant exercise of the conscious center is the activation of the silent paranormal chamber and the arousal of kundalini. With the start of this new activity the normal strength and pattern of bioenergy becomes insufficient to feed the brain. Supply from a new source becomes imperative to preserve sanity and life. This new and most potent source of psychic energy is provided by the reproductive system. How the reversal of the action of the generative organs and the activity of the paranormal chamber comes into effect, only sustained research on kundalini will disclose.

TEN

Still No Sign of Miraculous Psychic Powers

BEFORE THAT FATEFUL MORNING in December when I had my first glimpse into the superconscious state and saw fabulous kundalini in action, if even the most truthful man on earth had narrated to me a similar episode, I should have unhesitatingly placed him in that class of intelligent but credulous individuals who, while most accurate and conscientious in all other matters, exhibit a streak of puerility in respect of the supernatural. As this sequel will show, I remained in uncertainty about my strange condition for a long time, utterly at a loss to put a meaning on the occurrence. It was only when, after years of suspense, the adventure culminated in the development of clearly marked psychic attributes not in evidence before that I decided to put the extraordinary episode on paper.

This resolve was further fortified by the realization that kundalini must be active in millions of intelligent men and women of all civilized nations, though in a lesser degree and imperceptibly, creating in the majority psychic and physical disturbances which modern therapy is incapable of preventing or curing because of absolute ignorance about the cause.

Considering the colossal nature of the physical and mental metamorphosis that has to be effected as a prelude to spiritual unfoldment, I do not wonder at the accompanying trials and tribulations, since the mystic state represents the last and most arduous lap of the journey which began with the human ascent from dust and terminates with tasting, after suffering and travail, the incomparable bliss of unembodied existence, not after death, but within the human span of life on earth. The path in front of us now is so difficult and of such bewildering alignment that it will need all our willpower and all the resources of our intellect to negotiate it safely step by step until the goal comes clearly in sight.

When I awoke the following morning, I found myself too weak to rise from bed without assistance, and I remained lying down, revolving in my mind the fearful incidents of the night, while profuse tears of thankfulness streamed down my face at what I thought was divine intervention at a most critical time to save me from a dreadful fate. The more I thought about it, the more convinced I became that a superhuman agency acting through my mind had conveyed the hint, which in that terribly agitated state I could never have thought of myself, by which I was able to extricate myself from an entirely hopeless situation absolutely beyond the reach of mortal aid. No power on earth could have saved me from death or insanity, nor could any medicine have alleviated my suffering.

As if planted in my mind from the very start to save me from submitting my body to experimentation by healers not competent to deal with my condition and to protect me from the deleterious effects of common drugs that would have acted as veritable poisons in that extremely sensitive and delicate state of my nerves, I felt from the first day of my affliction a deeply rooted aversion to taking medical men into my confidence about this extraordinary ailment, not that I had no respect for the profession, but because I had a feeling that my malady was beyond the grasp and power of the highest medical authority.

With a feeling of relief I at last rose weakly from bed like a man in whom an invisible but intense internal fire has burnt for hours and who finds that not only has the fire been extinguished but even the excruciating pain of the burns has disappeared miraculously overnight.

I looked at myself in a mirror and found my face pale and haggard, but the maniacal expression had nearly vanished and the gleam of madness was almost gone from my eyes. I was looking at a sane but terribly weak and anguished countenance that had borne, as it were, the torture of hell for days and days. My tongue was still coated and my pulse weak and irregular, but all other signs and symptoms regarding the condition of my organs were so reassuring that my heart leapt with joy and hope.

There was no diminution in the vital radiation which, emanating from the seat of kundalini, sped across my nerves to every part of the body, filling my ears with strange sounds and my head with strange lights, but the current was now warm and pleasing instead of hot and burning, and it soothed and refreshed the tortured cells and tissues in a truly miraculous manner.

For the proper understanding of my condition after the memorable night of my release, it is necessary to say a few words about my mental state as well as about the radiating vital current darting up and down my spine which was now a part of my being.

My mind did not function as before. There had occurred a definite and unmistakable change. At that time my thought images came and went against a somber background possessing vaguely the same combination of light, shade, and color as characterized the original objects which they represented; but now the images were vivid and bright, as if carved out of living flame, and they floated against a luminous background as if the process of thought was now done with another kind of lustrous mental stuff, not only bright itself, but also capable of perceiving its own brilliance.

Whenever I turned my mental eye upon myself I invariably perceived a luminous glow, both within and outside my head, in a state of constant vibration, as if a jet of an extremely subtle and brilliant substance rising through the spine spread itself out in the cranium, filling and surrounding it with an indescribable radiance.

This shining halo never remained constant in dimension or in the intensity of its brightness. It waxed and waned, brightened and grew dim, or changed its color from silver to gold and vice versa. When it increased in size or brilliance, the strange noise in my ears, now never absent, grew louder and more insistent, as if drawing my attention to something I could not understand. The halo was never stationary but in a state of perpetual motion, dancing and leaping, eddying and swirling, as if composed of innumerable, extremely subtle, brilliant particles of some immaterial substance, shooting up and down, this way and that, combining to present an appearance of a circling, shimmering pool of light.

The constant presence of the luminous glow in my head and its close association with my thought processes was not a matter for such bewilderment as its ceaseless interference with the normal working of my vital organs. I could distinctly feel and perceive its passage across the spine and nerves into the heart or liver or stomach or other organs in the body, whose activity it seemed to regulate in a mysterious manner.

When it penetrated the heart, my pulse became fuller and stronger, showing unmistakably that some kind of tonic radiation was being poured into it through the connecting nerves. From this I concluded that its penetration into the other organs had the same vivifying and invigorating effect, and that its purpose in darting through the nerves to reach them was to pour its tonic substance into their tissues and cells through the slender nerve filaments, stimulating or modifying their action.

The penetration was occasionally followed by pain, either in the organ itself or at the point where the linking nerve entered it, or at the point of contact with the spinal cord, or both, and was often accompanied by feelings of fear. It appeared on such occasions that the stream of radiant energy rising into the brain was sending offshoots into the other vital organs to regulate and improve their functions in harmony with the new development in my head.

I searched my brain for an explanation and revolved every possibility in my mind to account for the surprising development as I watched attentively the incredible movement of this intelligent radiation from hour to hour and day to day.

At times I was amazed at the uncanny knowledge it displayed of the complicated nervous mechanism and the masterly way in which it darted here and there as if aware of every twist and turn in the

body. Most probably it was because of its almost unlimited dominance over the whole vital mechanism that the ancient writers named
kundalini as the queen of the nervous system, controlling all the
thousands of *nadis*, or nerves, in the body and for the same reason
designated her as Adhi Shakti ("basic Shakti"), on which depends
the existence of the body and the universe, the microcosm and the
macrocosm.

During the next day and the days following, I paid scrupulous
attention to my diet, taking only a few slices of bread or a little
boiled rice with a cup of milk every three hours from morning until
about ten o'clock at night. The amount of food taken each time was
extremely small, a few morsels and no more. After the last meal,
when I laid myself down to sleep, I found to my great joy a gentle
drowsiness stealing upon me in spite of the shining halo surrounding
my head, and I fell asleep enveloped in a radiating and soothing
mantle of light.

I awoke next morning greatly refreshed in mind but still extremely
weak in body. I had no strength to walk and reeled when I stood up.
But my head was clear and the fear that had pursued me had
decreased considerably. I was able, for the first time after weeks of
anguish, to collect my thoughts and to think clearly.

It took me about a week to gain sufficient strength to walk from
one room to another and to remain standing for any length of time.
I do not know what reserve store of energy sustained me during the
terrible ordeal before the last miraculous episode, as I had taken
little food for more than two months. I did not feel as weak then as
I now felt, probably because in the poisoned state of my nerves I
was wholly incapable of assessing correctly the condition of my
body.

Days and weeks passed, adding to my strength and to the assurance that I was in no imminent mental or physical danger. But my
condition was abnormal, and the more I studied it with growing
clarity of mind, the more I wondered and the more uncertain I
became about the outcome.

I was in an extraordinary state: a lustrous medium, intensely alive and acutely sentient, shining day and night, permeated my whole system, racing through every part of my body, perfectly at home and absolutely sure of its path. I often watched the marvelous play of this radiant force in utter bewilderment.

I had no doubt that kundalini was now fully awake in me, but there was absolutely no sign of the miraculous psychic and mental powers associated with it by ancient tradition. I could not detect any change for the better in myself; on the contrary, my physical condition had considerably deteriorated and my head was yet far from steady. I could not read attentively or devote myself with undivided mind to any task. Any sustained effort at concentration invariably resulted in an intensification of the abnormal condition. The halo in my head increased enormously in size after every spell of prolonged attention, creating a further heightening of my consciousness, with a corresponding increase in the sense of fear now present only occasionally, and that, too, in a very mild form.

Perceiving no sign of spiritual inspiration and always confronted by the erratic behavior of an altered mind, I could not but be assailed by grave misgivings about myself after watching my condition for a few weeks.

Was this all that one could achieve after arousing the Serpent Fire? I asked myself this question over and over again. Was this all, for which countless individuals had risked their lives, discarded their homes and families, braved the terrors of trackless forests, suffered hunger and privations, and sat at the feet of teachers for years to know? Was this all that yogis, saints, and mystics experienced in ecstatic trances, this extension of consciousness accompanied by unearthly lights and sounds, carrying a man momentarily into an abnormal mental state and then dashing him again to earth, without creating any extraordinary talent or quality to distinguish him from the average run of mortals? Was this ebb and flow of a subtle radiant essence and the resultant widening and narrowing of consciousness which I witnessed day and night the ultimate goal to which the occult doctrines of the world pointed with confidence?

If this were all one could achieve, then surely it was far better not to delve into the supernatural but to devote oneself with undivided attention to worldly pursuits and to follow the common path, to pass an undisturbed, happy existence free from the uncertainty and fear which had now become an inseparable part of my life!

I continued to pay careful attention to my diet, as experience had now made me fully alive to the fact that my life and sanity depended on it. I did not eat in excess of the quantity I deemed proper for myself, fixing the amount according to the reaction of my digestive system, nor did I allow any delicacy to tempt me to depart from my self-imposed regimen. There was reason enough to make me extremely cautious on this score, as the slightest indiscretion in respect to the quantity or quality of the food consumed and any disregard of time created results and reactions so disagreeable and distressing as to make me upbraid myself severely for having committed the mistake.

This happened time after time, as if to impress indelibly upon my mind the fact that from now onwards I must not eat for pleasure or the mechanical satisfaction of hunger, but to regulate the intake of food with such precision as not to cause the least strain on my oversensitive and overstimulated nervous system. There was no escape from this forced regimentation, and during the first few weeks, even the slightest error was instantaneously punished with an intensification of fear and a warning disturbance at the heart and digestive centers. Usually on such occasions my mind lost its flexibility and I felt powerless to shake myself free of the gloom that unaccountably settled upon me all of a sudden after eating the offending morsel. In my anxiety to avoid those unpleasant visitations, I was meticulous not to commit the least error; but try as I might, mistakes did occur now and then, almost always followed by suffering and penitence on my part.

Excepting the abnormal physiological reactions and the existence and extraordinary behavior of the luminous vital currents in the body, which to uninitiated and unprepared subjects like me are sure to bring a host of terrors in their wake, there was nothing in my initial experience which approaches the uncanny and entirely abnormal phenomena witnessed in professional mediums and other psychic subjects.

What made me hesitate in according publicity to it is the unique nature of the phenomenon; it neither falls in line with the known manifestations observed in mediums, nor does it seem similar in kind to the recorded experience of any known mystic or saint, Eastern or Western. Its peculiarity lies in the fact that, in its entire character, the phenomenon represents the attempt of a hitherto unrecognized vital force in the human body, releasable by voluntary efforts, to mold the available psychophysiological apparatus of an individual to such a condition as to make it responsive to states of consciousness not normally perceptible before.

It is this particular aspect of my extraordinary experience which makes it remarkable and demands attention from quarters interested in the supernormal or in ascertaining the physiological basis of superorganic psychic phenomena.

It is an undeniable fact that the quest for the unknown was as unmistakable a feature of ancient civilizations as it is now. There was as persistent a search for the spiritual and the supernatural, and as strong a thirst in countless people for the acquirement of supernormal powers and for tearing aside the veil that hides the beyond. But either because of the fact that time was not ripe for complete unraveling of the mystery or because the human mind revels in keeping the subject dealing exclusively with its own nature enshrouded in uncertainty, fear, and superstition, the discoveries made in this domain were kept the closely guarded secret of a select few.

There is not a shadow of doubt that to the ancient adepts of India, China, or Egypt, the cult of kundalini was better known than it is to the foremost thinkers of today. On the basis of my own experience I can assert unhesitatingly that the phenomenon of the effulgent current, its circulation through the nerves, the methods of awakening the Power, the regimen to be followed, precautions to be taken, and the part played by the reproductive organs were, as is apparent from the ancient writings or from the nature of the ceremonial followed by the initiated, to some extent known to the experts, who, because of the risky nature of the experiment, the hereditary factors involved, and the required mental and physical qualifications, could be but few.

It must be said at once, to avoid misunderstanding, that the cult of kundalini was not the only path by which the ancients approached the difficult-to-reach domain of the supernatural; there existed contemporaneously other creeds, schools, and systems dealing with the mysterious and the supernatural. As happens even during these days, the followers of the various sects must have tried to tear each other down, belittling the methods of their rivals and extolling their own. The existence of this unceasing warfare, as is obvious, could not but be detrimental to the general acceptance of the kundalini phenomena, which in consequence was relegated to the background, especially because of the rigid physical regimen, the magnitude of the risk, and last but not the least, the rarity of a successful consummation, and in the course of time was consigned to the lumber room of obsolete creeds.

It can also be said without any fear of contradiction that the rise of all great religions of the world, in spite of the fact that each is rooted inextricably in the soil prepared and watered by this prehistoric cult, contributed not a little to eclipse the creed of kundalini as an honored and established system of mental and physical discipline for gaining approach to the transcendental. It does, however, continue to exist in India, although in form only, divested of its former importance and influence, though still retaining much of the fascination that it once exerted on seekers trying to reach the Unseen.

It is obvious that all religions, all creeds, and all sects, including even the bloody cults of savages and the self-torturing or self-mutilating creeds found up to recent times, owe their origin to the existence of an urge, rooted deep in human nature, which finds expression in countless ways, healthy and unhealthy, and has been the constant companion of the human race all through its ascent from the most primitive condition to the present state. The desire for resolving the riddle of existence, for supersensory experience, for establishing contact with the hidden forces of nature, or for gaining supernormal powers, present in many minds with overpowering and compelling effect, is but a mode of expression of this yet incompletely understood but potent impulse, which, rising from the depths of being, emerges as part and parcel of one's personality, often discernible in thought and action from an early age.

All religious observances, all acts of worship, all methods of spiritual development, and all esoteric systems which in one way or another aim to provide a channel of communication with the supersensible, the divine, or the occult, or offer an avenue for exploring the mystery of being, are all means, both effective and defective, to procure satisfaction for the deeply seated and universally present urge. The form taken may be of a heinous bloody sacrifice, self-inflicted wounds, the self-caused blindness of the sun-gazer, constant torture to the body on a bed of nails, melodious chanting of hymns, recitation of prayers, prostration in devout worship, the discipline of yoga, or any other spiritual exercise. The objective invariably is the occult, the mysterious, or the supersensible in divine, demonic, spiritual, or any other form.

From the very beginning, the urge has expressed itself in an infinite variety of religious beliefs and creeds, superstitions and taboos traceable to the remotest epochs of man's existence. The impulse to invest the inanimate forces of nature with intelligence, and to credit the spirits of the dead with continued existence beyond the grave, characteristic of the primitive mind and civilized man's attempts to postulate an Almighty Creator to worship, arose from the same source, and owe their existence to the presence in the human organism of an extremely complicated and difficult-to-locate mechanism, which the ancient Indian savants called kundalini.

Whether the aim be religious experience, communication with
discarnate spirits, the vision of reality, liberation of the soul, or the
gift of clairvoyance and prediction, the power to influence people or
achieve success in worldly undertakings by supernatural means or
any other mundane or supermundane objective connected with the
occult or divine, the desire springs from the same psychosomatic
source, and is a twig or branch of the same deeply rooted tree.
Kundalini is as natural and effective a device for the attainment of a
higher state of consciousness and for transcendental experience as
the reproductive system is an effective natural contrivance for the
perpetuation of the race. The contiguity of the two is a purposely
designed arrangement, as the evolutionary tendency and the stage of
progress reached by the parent organism can only be transmitted
and perpetuated through the seed.

Most people have never been able to understand the surpassing
efficiency which men and women of genius bring to bear on their
intellectual or manual creations, and still less are able to compre-
hend the mental condition of an ecstatic. The former are completely
engrossed in their problem or handiwork, and the latter are lost in
the rapt contemplation of a beatific internal display or an external
object of adoration. They are both carried for the time being away
from the world to a more alluring state of existence and present an
enigma for the solution of which it is necessary to look again
carefully inside the human frame in order to locate the hidden source
from which the brain in these conditions of extreme absorption
draws the nourishment required to maintain the highly developed
activity for long periods. The completely isolated nature of individual consciousness, caused by the segregating effect of the ego, makes
it difficult for anyone to look into the locked compartment of
another mind, even of one nearest and dearest to them. This lack of
access of one mind to another has given rise to certain common
misconceptions which it will take a long time to remove from human
thought.

The average person, when studying a genius, a mystic, or a

medium, is apt to presume, because of this inability to look into their minds as one does into one's own, that they are conscious entities like oneself, but with the difference that one has more intelligence and more skill in wielding the pen or brush or chisel with a greater power of sustained attention and application and a more observing eye. The other, one supposes, has more love and devotion for the deity, with a stronger control over passions and appetites and a greater power of sacrifice or an incomprehensible link with other minds or hidden forces of nature, with the power to create a condition of the brain that allows disembodied intelligences to act through it at times.

Without entering into a detailed discussion of the various hypotheses put forward to account for the existence of genius or of supernormal faculties in sensitives and psychics, it is sufficient for our purpose to say that whatever explanation is offered, it is invariably based on the supposition, tacit or expressed, that the individuals possessing these extraordinary gifts, in spite of surprising intellect or uncanny powers and the immense distance between them and the normal mind, have the same nature of consciousness as the average man and woman. This is a most erroneous conception which has always stood in the way of a proper understanding and investigation of the phenomenon.

On their side, the gifted, endowed by nature from birth, unable to peep into the minds of others, and often entirely in the dark about the real source of the remarkable variation in themselves, reciprocate the feelings of the common man about them, often attributing their own exceptional talents to the same causes to which they are traced by the latter, ignorant of the always overlooked fact that there exists a basic and fundamental difference in the nature of consciousness, in the very depths of the conscious personality tenanting their bodies, and in the very nature of the vital essence which animates them.

There exists at present a general ignorance about the demonstrable fact that the evolving human frame is tending to develop a higher personality endowed with the attributes which characterize seers and men and women of genius by the refining and development of the vital principle, with corresponding adjustments in the brain and the nervous system, somewhat in the same manner as a more powerful electric current passing through a more properly adjusted filament in a bulb leads invariably to brighter illumination.

The point has been merely touched here in passing in order to lend clarity to what is to follow in the succeeding chapters. The urge for knowing the unknown, for supersensory knowledge and religious experience, existing deep in the human mind, is the expression of the embodied and incarcerated human consciousness to win nearer to its innate majestic form, overcoming in this process the disabilities imposed on it by the carnal frame.

The evolution of human beings in actual fact signifies the evolution of their consciousness, of the vital principle inhabiting the body, by which alone the embodied self can become cognizant of its true immortal state. It does not signify merely the development of the intellect or reason, which are but instruments of the indwelling spirit, but of the whole personality, of both its conscious and subconscious parts, which involves an overhauling and reshaping of the organic machine to make it a fit abode for a higher intelligence, essentially superior in nature to that which resides in the normal human body.

It is for this reason that the mode of conduct or intellectual activity normal to a prophet appears entirely beyond the capacity of the average person, whose mind, flooded with passion at the touch of the beloved or assailed by desire at the sight of a coveted object, has seldom been able to live up to the standard of morality prescribed by the former, whose brain, fed by a higher form of vital energy permeating the whole personality, belongs more to heaven than to earth.

But I could detect no change in my mental capacity; I thought the same thoughts and both inside and out was the same mediocre type of man like millions of others who are born or die every year without creating the least stir on the surface of the ever-flowing stream of humanity. There was no doubt an extraordinary change in my nervous equipment and a new type of force was now racing through my system, connected unmistakably with the sexual parts, which also seemed to have developed a new kind of activity not perceptible before. The nerves lining the parts and the surrounding region were all in a state of intense ferment, as if forced by an invisible mechanism to produce the vital seed in abnormal abundance, to be sucked up by the network of nerves at the base of the spine for transmission into the brain through the spinal cord. The sublimated seed formed an integral part of the radiant energy which was causing me such bewilderment and about which I was as yet unable to speculate with any degree of assurance.

I could readily perceive the transmutation of the vital seed into radiation and the unusual activity of the reproductive organs for supplying the raw material for transformation in the mysterious laboratory at the lowest plexus, or *muladhara chakra*, as the yogis name it, into that extremely subtle and ordinarily imperceptible stuff we call nervous energy on which the entire mechanism of the body depends, with the difference that the energy now generated possessed luminosity and was of a quality allowing detection of its rapid passage through the nerves and tissues, not only by its radiance but also by the sensations it caused with its movement.

For a long time I could not understand what hidden purpose was being served by the unremitting flow of the newborn nervous radiation and what changes were being wrought in the organs and nerves and in the structure of the brain by this unceasing shower of the powerful vital essence drawn from the most precious and most potent secretion in the body. Immediately after the crisis, however, I noticed a marked change in my digestive and eliminatory functions, a change so remarkable that it could not be assigned to accident or to any other factor save the Serpent Fire and its effect on the organism.

It appeared as if I were undergoing a process of purgation, of internal purification of the organs and nerves, and that my digestive apparatus was being toned to a higher pitch of efficiency to ensure a cleaner and healthier state of the nerves and other tissues. I encountered no constipation or indigestion provided I refrained from overloading the stomach and followed strictly the regimen of eating which experience was forcing on me. My most important and essential duty now was to feed the sacred flame with healthy food, at proper intervals, with due regard to the fact that the diet was nourishing, containing all the ingredients and vitamins needed for the maintenance of a robust and healthy body.

I was now a spectator of a weird drama enacted in my own body in which an immensely active and powerful vital force, released all of a sudden by the power of meditation, was incessantly at work and, after having taken control of all the organs and the brain, was hammering and pounding them into a certain shape. I merely observed the weird performance, the lightning-like movements of the lustrous intelligent power commanding absolute knowledge of and dominance over the body.

I did not know at the time that I was witnessing in my own body the immensely accelerated activity of an energy not yet known to science, which is carrying the human race itself towards the heights of superconsciousness, provided that by its thought and deed it allows this evolutionary force full opportunity to perform unhindered the work of transformation.

I little knew that the chaste sacrificial fire, to which so much sanctity and importance has been attached by all the ancient scriptures of India, fed after being lighted with the oblation of clarified butter, dry fruits of the choicest kind, sugary substances, and cereals, all nourishing and purifying articles of food, is but a symbolic representation of the transforming fire lit in the body by kundalini, requiring when lighted the offering of easily digestible and nutritive food and complete chastity of thought and deed to enable it to perform its godly task, which normally takes epochs, within the span of a single life.

After only a few days I found that the luminous current was acting with full knowledge of the task it had to perform, and functioned in complete harmony with the bodily organs, knowing their strengths and weaknesses, obeying its own laws and acting with a superior intelligence beyond my comprehension. The living fire, invisible to everyone else, darted here and there as if guided unerringly by a mastermind which knew the position of each vein and artery and each nerve fiber and decided instantaneously what it had to do at the least sign of a hitch or disturbance in any organ.

With marvelous agility it raced from one spot to another, exciting this organ to greater activity, slowing down another, causing a greater or lesser flow of this secretion or that, stimulating the heart and liver, bringing about countless functional and organic changes in the innumerable cells, blood vessels, nerve fibers, and other tissues. I watched the phenomenon in amazement. With the aid of the luminous stuff now filling my nerves, I could, by diverting my attention towards my interior, discern clearly the outlines of the vital organs and the network of nerves spread all over my body, as if the center of consciousness in the brain, now always ablaze with light, had acquired a more penetrating inner sight by which it could look inside and perceive dimly the interior of the body as it could see its exterior in a hazy, uncertain light.

At times, turning my attention upon myself, I distinctly saw my body as a column of living fire, from the tips of my toes to the head, in which innumerable currents circled and eddied, causing at places whirlpools and vortices, all forming part of a vast heaving sea of light, perpetually in motion. It was not an hallucination, as the experience was repeated innumerable times. The only explanation to account for it that occurred to me was that on such occasions my undeniably extended consciousness was in contact with the world of prana, or cosmic vital energy, which is not normally perceptible to the ordinary individual, but is the first subtle immaterial substance to come within the range of superconscious vision.

Like a man suddenly transported to a distant planet, where he finds himself utterly confused by the weird and fantastic nature of the surroundings which he could not even conceive of on earth, filling him with awe and amazement, I was completely bewildered and unnerved by this sudden plunge into the occult. From the very first day I felt myself walking on a ground that was not only unfamiliar but presented such queer formations that, losing my bearings and self-confidence, I trod hesitatingly with utmost caution, fearing a pitfall at every step. I looked around desperately for guidance, only to face disappointment on all sides.

Without mentioning my condition, I talked to several scholars and sadhus well versed in Tantric lore, with the object of gleaning some useful hints for myself, but found to my sorrow that beyond a parrot-like repetition of information gathered from books, they could not give me any advice or authoritative guidance based on experience. On the other hand, not infrequently they admitted frankly that it was not easy to grasp the meaning of the texts dealing with kundalini yoga, and that they themselves had encountered difficulties at many a place. What was I to do then to set my doubts at rest and to find some sort of an explanation for and, if possible, some effective method to deal with my abnormal condition?

I made a mental survey of all possible sources in India of which I had any knowledge to decide which of them I could approach. There were the dignified heads of various orders with hundreds of devoted followers. There were the princely divines residing in cities, counting titled aristocrats, rajahs, and magnates among their disciples, and there were the silent ascetics living by themselves in out-of-the-way spots, whose fame brought large crowds from distant corners to pay homage to them.

Then there were the ordinary sadhus gathered in colonies or living alone or roaming about from place to place, diversely garbed or almost unclad, belonging to various sects, with striking peculiarities and quaint accoutrements and carrying with them an atmosphere of weirdness and mystery wherever they went. I had seen and talked to many of them from my boyhood, the most accomplished as well as the least sophisticated, and the impressions I had gathered provided no room for hope that there would be even one among them capable of advising me correctly about my condition. At least I did not know of any, and therefore the only alternative open to me was to make a widespread search for one.

But I had neither the means nor the physical capacity to travel from place to place looking for a yogi in the whole of the vast subcontinent of India, with all its endless variety of monastic orders and spiritual cults, its religious mendicants, sadhus, and saints, who might correctly diagnose my trouble and heal it with his own spiritual powers.

At last, mustering my courage, I wrote to one of the best-known modern saints of India, the author of many widely read books in English on yoga, giving him full details of my extraordinary state, and sought his guidance. I waited for his reply in trepidation, and when it failed to come for some days, I sent a telegram also. I was passing a very anxious time when the answer came. It said that there was no doubt that I had aroused kundalini in the Tantric manner and that the only way for me to seek guidance was to find a yogi who had himself conducted the Shakti successfully to the Seventh Center in the head.

I was thankful for the reply, which fully confirmed my own opinion, thereby raising my hopes and self-confidence. It was obvious that the symptoms mentioned by me had been recognized as those characterizing kundalini awakening, thereby giving to my weird experience a certain appearance of normality. If I were passing through an abnormal condition, it was not an isolated instance nor was the abnormality peculiar to me alone, but must be a necessary corollary to the awakening of kundalini, and with modifications suited to different temperaments must have occurred in almost all those in whom awakening had taken place. But where was I to find a yogi who had raised the Shakti to the Seventh Center?

After some time I met another sadhu, a native of Bengal, at Jammu and described my condition to him. He studied my symptoms for a while and then gave me the address of an ashram in East Bengal, the head of which was supposed to be a yogi of the highest order who had himself practiced kundalini yoga. I wrote to the address given, receiving a reply that I had undoubtedly aroused the Shakti but the man who could guide me had left on a pilgrimage.

I consulted other holy men and sought for guidance from many reputed quarters without coming across a single individual who could boldly assert that he actually possessed intimate personal knowledge of the condition and could confidently answer my questions.

Those who talked with dignified reserve, looking very wise and deep, ultimately turned out to be as wanting in accurate information about the mysterious power rampant in me as those of a more unassuming nature who unbosomed themselves completely on the very first occasion without in the least pretending to know any more than they really did. And thus, in the great country which had given birth to the lofty science of kundalini thousands of years ago and whose very soil is permeated with its fragrance and whose rich religious lore is full of references to it from cover to cover, I found no one able to help me.

The only thing I was sure of was that a new kind of activity had developed in my nervous system, but I could not determine which particular nerve or nerves were involved, though I could clearly mark the location at the extremity of the spinal cord and round the lower orifice. There undeniably was the abode of Kundalini, as described by yogis, the place where She lies asleep in the normal person, coiled three and a half times round the lowest triangular end of the spine, awakened to activity with proper exercises of which concentration is the main adjunct.

Had I been under the guidance of a qualified master my doubts might have been resolved on the very first day or at least on the day when I passed the crisis, but having neither the practical experience of a teacher to draw upon nor enough theoretical knowledge of the subject to enable me to form a conclusive opinion independently, I remained vacillating in my ideas about the condition. This wavering state of mind was further enhanced by the variations in and the waxing and waning of my consciousness.

Perhaps it was destined that it should be so and that I should be guideless and without adequate knowledge in order to allow me to form an independent judgment about the phenomenon without prejudice or prepossession. Perhaps it was destined also that I should suffer acutely for years because of my ignorance and lack of guidance, to enable me by suffering to make smooth the path of those in whom the Sacred Fire will burn in the days to come.

Before proceeding to narrate the incidents that followed, it is necessary to say a few words about this long-known but rarely found reservoir of life energy in man known as kundalini. Many informed students of yoga hear or read about it one time or another, but the accounts given in modern writings are too meager and vague to serve as helpful sources of authentic information. The ancient treatises exclusively dealing with the subject of kundalini yoga abound in cryptic passages and contain details of fantastic, sometimes even obscene ritual allusions to innumerable deities, extremely difficult and often dangerous mental and physical exercises, incantations and formulas technically known as mantras; bodily postures called asanas; and detailed instructions for the control and regulation of breath, all couched in a language difficult to understand, with a mass of mystical verbiage which, instead of attracting, is likely to repel the modern student. Truly speaking, no illustrative material is available either in the modern or ancient expositions to convey lucidly what the objective reality of the methods advocated is and what mental and organic changes one may expect at the end.

The result is that instead of becoming illuminative and pragmatic, this strictly empirical science has fallen into abuse and disrepute. Some of its practices, forming integral parts of a combined whole and serving as a means to a definite end, such as the asanas and *pranayama* (breathing exercises), are now being regarded as laudable ulterior ends in themselves to the neglect of the ultimate object for which the exercises were devised.

The real object of this system of yoga is to develop a type of consciousness which crosses over the boundaries confining the sense-bound mind, carrying the embodied consciousness to supersensory regions. Distracted by the tyrannical demands of modern civilization and discouraged by the generally incredulous attitude towards the possibility of such a development in oneself, the present-day aspirants often content themselves with a few postures and breathing exercises in the fond belief that they are practicing yoga for spiritual uplift.

The descriptions of chakras and lotuses, of supernatural signs and omens accompanying success in the practice, of the miraculous powers attainable, the genesis of the system, and the origin of the various methods, are so overdone and full of exaggeration that to the uninitiated the whole conception embodied in the ancient literature on the subject appears incredible if not preposterous. From such material it is extremely difficult for the modern seeker to gain plain knowledge of the subject divested of supernatural and mythological lore or to find clarification for his doubts and difficulties. Judging from the fantastic accounts contained in the writings, not only in the original ancient treatises but also in some of the modern books, kundalini for an intelligent, matter-of-fact individual can be no more than a myth, a chimera born of the innate desire in people to find an easy way of escape from the rigors imposed by a rigidly governed world of cause and effect, a kind of Philosopher's Stone, invented to satisfy the same desire in a different form by providing a shortcut for the acquisition of wealth. In India no other topic has such a mass of literature woven around it as yoga and the supernatural, and yet in no book on the subject is a penetrating light thrown on kundalini, nor has any expert provided more information than is furnished in the ancient works. The result is that except for perhaps a few almost inaccessible masters, as scarce now as the alchemists of yore, there is no one in the whole of India, the home of the science, to whom one can look for authoritative knowledge of the subject.

The system of complicated mental and physical exercises relating particularly to kundalini is technically known as hatha yoga, in contradistinction to other forms of yoga in vogue in India from very ancient times. Hatha in Sanskrit is a compound of two words, *ha* and *tha*, meaning the sun and moon, and consequently the name hatha yoga is intended to indicate that form of yoga which results from the confluence of these two orbs.

Briefly stated, the moon and the sun as used here are meant to designate the two nerve currents flowing on the left and right sides of the spinal cord through the two *nadis*, or nerves, named *ida* and *pingala*. The former, being cool, is said to resemble the pale luster of the moon; the latter, being hot, is likened to the radiance of the sun.

All systems of yoga are based on the supposition that living bodies owe their existence to the agency of an extremely subtle immaterial substance, pervading the universe and designated as prana, which is the cause of all organic phenomena, controlling the organisms by means of the nervous system and the brain, manifesting itself as the vital energy. The prana, in modern terminology "vital energy," assumes different aspects to discharge different functions in the body and circulates in the system in two separate streams, one with fervid and the other with frigid effect, clearly perceptible to yogis in the awakened condition.

From my own experience I can also unhesitatingly affirm that there are certainly two main types of vital currents in the body, which have a cooling or heating effect on the system. Prana and *apana* exist side by side in the system in every tissue and every cell, the two flowing through the higher nerves and their tiny ramifications as two distinct currents, though their passage is never felt in the normal state of consciousness, the nerves being accustomed to the flow from the very commencement of life.

Because of its extremely subtle nature, vital energy has been likened to breath by the ancient authorities on yoga, and it is maintained that the air we breathe is permeated with both prana and *apana* and that the vital currents flow alternately through the two nostrils along with the air at the time of inhalation and exhalation. As is well known, the air we breathe is composed mainly of two gases, oxygen and nitrogen. Oxygen is the chief agent in combustion, burning up the impurities in the blood by its action through the lungs, while nitrogen exerts a moderating effect on its fervor. In view of the fact that the old writers on kundalini yoga sometimes use the same term for prana or *apana*, namely, *vayu*, which is used for the air we breathe, there is a possibility of confusion being caused that breath and prana are identical.

This is absolutely not the case. Life as we know it on earth is not possible without oxygen, and it is noteworthy that this element is an ingredient of both air and water, the two essential requirements of earthly life. This is a clear indication of the fact that on the terrestrial globe the cosmic vital energy, or *prana-shakti*, utilizes oxygen as the main vehicle for its activity. It is possible that biochemistry, in the course of its investigations, may have to accept at some future date the instrumentality of oxygen in all organic phenomena as the main channel for the play of the intelligent vital force prana.

The earth has its own supply of prana, pervading every atom and every molecule of all the elements and compounds constituting its flaming core, the fiery molten regions below the crust, the hard surface layer with its mountains and seas, and the atmosphere to its outermost fringe. The sun, a vast reservoir of vital energy, is constantly pouring an enormous supply of pranic radiation on the earth as a part of its effulgence. The superstitions connected with eclipses may thus have an element of truth, as on all such occasions the pranic emanations from the sun or moon are partially or totally cut off for a time.

The changes in the weather and the vapor and dust content of the atmosphere, which have a marked effect on certain sensitive temperaments, might also be found to cause alterations in the flow of pranic currents. The moon is another big supply center of prana for earth. The planets and stars, both near and far, are all inexhaustible stores of prana, vitalizing the earth with streams of energy conveyed by their luster. The pranic emanations from the sun and moon, planets and stars, are not all alike, but each has a peculiar characteristic of its own in the same way that the light of heavenly bodies, when analyzed on earth after traveling through enormous distances, shows variations in the spectrum peculiar to each one.

It is impossible for the human imagination to visualize even dimly the interactions of innumerable streams of light emitted by billions upon billions of stars crossing and recrossing each other at countless points, filling the stupendous stretch of space at every spot from end to end. Similarly it is utterly impossible to picture or to depict even hazily the colossal world of prana, or life energy, as described by seers. Its unbounded extent is traversed by streams and cross-streams, currents and crosscurrents, radiating from innumerable stars and planets with motionless spots and storm centers, vortices and eddies, all throbbing with activity everywhere. The animate worlds rise out of this marvelously intelligent but subtle ocean of vital activity as foam appears on the surface of the perennially moving oceanic currents.

In order to explain the phenomenon of terrestrial life there is no alternative but to accept the existence of an intelligent vital medium which, using the elements and compounds of the material world as bricks and mortar, acts as the architect of organic structures. All show evidence of extraordinary intelligence and purpose, built with such amazing skill and produced in such profusion and in so many diverse forms as to falsify any idea of spontaneous generation or chance. The existence of this medium cannot be proved empirically; human ingenuity and skill have not yet attained the perfection where one can experiment with media of such subtlety.

Immense significance has been attached to the pranic radiations coming to earth from the sun and moon. In fact, some ancient authorities trace the origin of the human mind to the moon. The whole structure of yoga is based on the validity of prana as a cognizable superphysical stuff. For thousands of years, successive generations of yogis have verified the assertions of their precursors. The reality of prana as the chief agent leading to the superconscious condition known as samadhi has never been questioned by any school of yoga. Those who believe in yoga must first believe in prana.

Considering the fact that to attain success in yoga one must not only possess unusual mental and physical endowments but must also have all the attributes of saintly character—honesty, chastity, and rectitude—it would be nothing short of obstinacy to discredit the testimony of numerous renowned seers, who, in unequivocal terms, have testified to their own experience of the superconscious conditions resulting from systematic manipulation of prana as learnt by them from their own preceptors.

According to the religious beliefs in India dating back to prehistoric times, the existence of prana as a medium for the activity of thought and transference of sensations and impulses in living organisms, and as a normally imperceptible cosmic substance present in every formation of matter in terms of the classifications made by Hindu cosmologists in earth, water, air, fire, and ether, is an established fact, verifiable by the practice of yoga when undertaken by the right type of individual on proper lines. According to these beliefs, prana is not matter, nor is it mind or intelligence or consciousness, but rather an inseparable part of the cosmic energy or Shakti which resides in all of them. It is the driving force behind all cosmic phenomena, as force in matter and vitality in living organisms; in short, it is the medium by which the cosmic intelligence conducts the unimaginably vast activity of this stupendous world, by which it creates, maintains, and destroys the gigantic globular formations burning ceaselessly in space as well as the tiny bacteria, both malignant and beneficent, filling every part of the earth. In other words, Shakti, when applied to inorganic matter, is force, and when applied to the organic plane is life, the two being different aspects of the creative cosmic energy.

For the sake of convenience and to avoid confusion, the term prana or *prana-shakti* is generally applied to that aspect of the cosmic energy which operates in the organic sphere as nervous impulse and vitality, while the generic name Shakti is applied to every form of energy, animate and inanimate; in brief, to the creative and active aspect of the Reality. In dealing with kundalini we are concerned only with prana as *prana-shakti*.

Present-day science is being irresistibly led to the conclusion that energy is the basic substance of the physical world. The doubt about the existence of life as a deathless vital medium apart from the corporeal appendages is as old as civilization, and is occasioned mainly by the inexorable nature of physical laws operating on the body, the inevitability of decay and death, the extremely elusive nature of the vital principle, the utter impossibility of perceiving it apart from the organic frame, the finality of death as the end of the organism, and above all, the absence of demonstrable or incontrovertible proof of survival after bodily death.

According to the yogis, however, the existence of the life energy as a deathless entity becomes subjectively apparent in the superconscious state of samadhi, and its flow through the nerves can be experienced even before that as soon as certain measures of success are attained in meditation. When that happens, a greater demand for it is felt in the concentrated condition of the brain, and to meet this, prana, or vital energy, residing in other parts of the body, flows to the head, sometimes to such an extent that even vital organs like the heart, lungs, and the digestive system almost cease to function, the pulse and the breathing become imperceptible, and the whole body appears cold and lifeless.

With the additional fuel supplied by the enhanced flow of vital energy, the brain becomes more intensely alive; the surface consciousness rises above bodily sensations and its perceptive faculty is vastly enlarged, rendering it cognizant of superphysical existences. In this condition the first object of perception is prana, experienced as a lustrous, immaterial stuff, sentient and in a state of rapid vibration both within and outside the body, extending boundlessly on every side.

In yoga parlance, prana is life and life is prana. Life and vitality, in the sense used here, do not mean soul or the spark of the Divine in the human being. Prana is merely the life energy by which divinity brings into existence the organic kingdoms and acts on the organic structures, as it creates and acts on the universe by means of physical energy. It is not the reality, as sunshine is not the sun, and yet is essentially a part of it, assuming different shapes and appearances, entering into countless types of formations, building persistently the units or bricks to create the complicated organic structures in the same way that physical energy starts with electrons, protons, neutrons, and atoms to raise the mighty edifice of the universe, all its activity governed by eternal laws as rigid and universal as the laws which rule the physical world.

After creating the atoms, physical energy is transformed into countless kinds of molecules, resulting in the existence of innumerable compounds diverse in form, color, and taste, which again by combination and mixture, differences in temperature and pressure, create the amazingly diversified appearance of the physical world. Prana, starting with protoplasm and unicellular organisms, brings into existence the marvelous domain of life, endless in variety, exceedingly rich in shape and color, creating classes, genera, species, subspecies, and groups, using the materials furnished by the physical world and the environment to create diversity, acting intelligently and purposefully with full knowledge of the laws and properties of matter as well as of the multitudinous organic creations it has to bring into being.

While remaining constant and unaltered fundamentally, it enters into countless combinations, acting both as the architect and the object produced. It exists as a mighty universe, vaster and more wonderful than the cosmos perceived by our senses, with its own spheres and planes corresponding to the suns and earths of the latter, its own materials and bricks, its own movement and inertia, its own light and shadow, laws and properties, existing side by side with the universe we see, interwoven with our thoughts and actions, interpenetrating the atoms and molecules of matter, radiating with light, moving with wind and tide, marvelously subtle and agile, the stuff of our fancies and dreams, the life principle of creation, which is woven inextricably with the very texture of our being.

We do not realize what mysterious stuff animates the cells and organs of living bodies, causing marvelous physical and chemical reactions while the owners of the bodies, even the most intelligent and perceptive, know nothing of what is happening in them, know nothing of the intelligence which regulates the body machine, which builds it in the womb, preserves it in illness, sustains it in danger, heals it when injured, cares for it when asleep or delirious or unconscious, creates urges and tendencies which move and sway them as wind does a reed.

What is more astounding, after doing each and everything, even to the extent of drawing the breath and inducing the thoughts, because of its own marvelous and, for the human intelligence, absolutely incomprehensible nature, it keeps itself always behind the scenes, allowing the surface consciousness, which it maintains as oil does a flame, to think and act as the master, utterly unconscious of the invisible but amazing activity of the real mistress of the abode, the superphysical medium, *prana-shakti*, the life aspect of the cosmic energy.

The founders of the practice of kundalini yoga, accepting the existence of prana as a concrete reality, both in its individual and cosmic aspects, no doubt after experimentation carried out by many generations of savants, were led to the momentous discovery that it is possible to gain voluntary control over the nervous system to the extent of diverting a greater flow of prana into the brain, resulting naturally in an intensification of its activity, and hence devised all their methods of body control and mental discipline to achieve this end.

They succeeded admirably, as the main exercise, concentration, which is the cornerstone of every system of yoga, fits in with the methods prescribed by Nature for expediting human evolution. They found that on acquiring a certain degree of proficiency in mind control and concentration, they could, in favorable cases, draw up through the hollow backbone a vividly bright, fast-moving, powerful radiance into the brain for short periods of time in the beginning, then extending the duration with practice, which had a most amazing effect on the mind, enabling it to soar to regions of surpassing glory, beyond anything experienced in the crude material world.

They named the channel *sushumna*, and as the streaming radiance was distinctly felt mounting up from its base, they treated that spot as the seat of the Goddess, representing her as lying asleep there in the guise of a serpent, closing with her mouth the aperture leading to the spinal canal. The systems of nerves on the left and right of the *sushumna*, which contributed to the formation of the flaming radiance by yielding a part of the vital energy moving through them, were named *ida* and *pingala*.

Though lacking in the knowledge made available by modern science, it did not take the ancient teachers long in their heightened state of consciousness to postulate the existence of the subtle world of life, interpenetrating and existing side by side with the material cosmos. Consequently the ancient writings on hatha yoga abounded in cryptic references to *prana-shakti* or vital energy and its conducting network of systems in the body, which are not infrequently a source of confusion for beginners.

ELEVEN

Perennially Conscious of an Inner Luminosity

I QUITE REALIZE THAT it is impossible for me to convey accurately or for the average reader to understand clearly what I mean by the expressions "widening" and "contraction" of consciousness, which I use frequently to denote the fluctuations in my mental condition. However, it is only by employing these phrases that I can describe even vaguely a purely subjective experience that seldom falls to the lot of the average person. To the best of my knowledge, the weird phenomena following the awakening of kundalini have so far never been revealed in detail or made the subject of analytical study. The subject has remained shrouded in mystery, not only because of the extreme rarity and astounding nature of the manifestation, but also because certain essential features of the development are closely bound up with the intimate life and private parts of the individual who has the experiences. The disclosures made in this work are likely to appear startling, even incredible, because the subject is being discussed openly for the first time after centuries of a veiled existence.

We can more or less follow the meaning of words, however difficult they may be, which describe mental states common to us all, or discuss intellectual problems and abstract propositions based on common experience and knowledge. But the phenomenon which I have tried to explain in these pages is so rare and so removed from ordinary affairs that in all probability only a few of those who happen to read this account will have even heard of anything so extraordinary. Accomplished masters of kundalini yoga, always extremely rare in the past, are almost nonexistent nowadays, and the cases of a spontaneous type, where the awakening occurs suddenly at some period in life, more often than not end in mental disorder, which makes a coherent narration of the experience impossible. Under the circumstances it is no wonder that a detailed account of this strange experience is not available anywhere.

In spite of all this, the experience is not as singular or as unauthenticated as might at first appear. There is enough evidence available to suggest that from times immemorial, probably from the very birth of civilization and even before that, there have been cases, extremely rare indeed, of the awakening of kundalini spontaneously or by means of suitable exercises. In the few cases of the former type where the awakening proceeds towards a healthy culmination, the symptoms being usually mild and the development gradual, as in born mystics, the essential characteristics of the rebirth, which were startlingly apparent in my case, might conceivably escape notice or when noticed may be attributed to other causes.

In the large proportion of cases of the same class where the awakening is morbid, the frenzied expressions of the stricken, even when correct, would be utterly disregarded as the senseless rubbish of a delirious brain. In the case of awakening brought about by voluntary effort as, for example, in a monastic order, secluded yoga center, or solitary hermitage, the extraordinary phenomena attending it were most likely either not open to critical observation or, where they were observed, were treated as a necessary preternatural accompaniment to the adventure and hence not regarded seriously as something important to record and communicate. They may have been considered too sacred to be divulged and consequently were kept a closely guarded secret accessible to none save the initiates.

Accordingly, laboring under the difficulty of describing in this critical age of science a bizarre mental phenomenon never revealed in detail before, I am compelled, for reasons of prudence, to keep back certain details that should have found a place in this work and which, I am sure, will fall within the experience of many of those who, like me, chance to kindle the Serpent Fire accidentally without a preparatory period of training. In spite of many almost uncanny happenings which I witnessed within myself, during the succeeding months my mental condition continued to be the same as already described, but there was a perceptible improvement in my bodily health, and I found my former strength and vigor gradually returning.

The government offices usually moved from Jammu to Srinagar, the summer capital of the State, in the month of May, but being on leave and finding myself unable to withstand the deleterious effects of heat in the weakened state of my nerves, I left for Kashmir in early April, 1939. The change did me good. The valley was thick with blossoms and the crisp spring air filled with fragrance had an invigorating effect upon me.

There was absolutely no change in the constant movements of the radiant current or in the intensified behavior of the glow in my head. On the other hand, their activity was more intensified. But my mental strength, poise, and powers of endurance, which seemed to have been completely depleted, came back to me in part, and I found myself able to take a lively interest in conversation.

What was more precious to me, the deep feelings of love for my family, which had appeared to be dead, stirred in my heart again. Within a few weeks after arriving, I found myself able to take long walks and to attend to ordinary affairs not requiring too much exertion. Still, I could not read attentively for long and continued to have a fear of the supernatural. I persistently avoided thinking of or talking about the subject.

My former appetite returned and I could eat everything I used to previously without any fear of a few morsels more or less creating a storm in my interior. I could even prolong the interval between meals, but not too long without discomfort. By the time my office opened at Srinagar I had gained enough strength and endurance to be sure that I could again take up my official duties without the risk of aggravating my mental condition or making myself ridiculous by exhibiting a lack of efficiency in my work or any sign of abnormality in my behavior. When I went through the papers on my desk, I noticed that my memory was unimpaired and the awful experience I had undergone had in no way adversely affected my ability.

I was easily fatigued, however, and became restless after only a few hours of attentive application. After a prolonged spell of mental work, I invariably found, after closing my eyes and listening internally, that the luminous circle was more extended and the buzzing in the ears louder than usual. This served as an indication that I was still not capable of maintaining a sustained state of attention for lengthy periods and that I should proceed with caution to avoid a recrudescence of the previous symptoms. Accordingly, I decided to alternate spells of work with intervals of relaxation by chatting with my colleagues, by looking out of the window, or by moving from the office into the busy street outside, which offered a large variety of objects to divert my attention.

I do not know how it happened that, even in that extremely abnormal state of my mind, needing constantly the application of new measures to adapt it to changing circumstances, I often hit upon the right procedure to deal with unexpected and difficult situations arising in my day-to-day contacts. If I had even so much as hinted to colleagues a word about my abnormality and the bizarre manifestations which were now a regular feature of my life, I might have been labeled a lunatic and treated accordingly.

If I had tried to make capital out of the mysterious occurrence and pretended a knowledge of the occult, which I did not in reality possess, I might have been hailed as a saint and pestered day and night by people seeking a miraculous way of escape out of their difficulties. Beyond a few hints which I let drop to some of my relatives in the very beginning when I was taken completely aback by the strange malady, and beyond revealing my condition as well as I could to a few yoga experts for guidance, I maintained a strict reserve about my abnormal state and never referred to it in my conversation with intimate friends.

Even in my most sanguine moments, however, the fear of impending madness never left me completely. The magnitude of the risk that one has to run in the event of a powerful and sudden kundalini awakening can be gauged from the fact that simultaneously with the release of the new energy, profound functional and structural changes begin to occur with rapidity and violence in the delicate fabric of the nervous system. This can be sufficient to cause unhinging of the brain instantaneously if the organism as a whole does not possess enough power of adjustment to bear the tremendous strain, as actually happens in many cases. Among the inmates of mental hospitals there are often some who owe their malady to a prematurely active or morbidly functioning kundalini.

With the restoration of my faculties and the growing clarity of mind, I began to speculate about my condition. I read all that came my way pertaining to kundalini and yoga but did not find any detailed account of a similar phenomenon. The darting warm and cold currents, the effulgence in the head, the unearthly sounds in the ears, and the gripping fear were actually mentioned, but for me there was no sign of clairvoyance or ecstasy, or communication with disembodied spirits, or any other extraordinary psychic gift, all considered to be the distinctive characteristics of an awakened kundalini from the earliest times.

Often in the silence and darkness of my room at night I found myself looking with dread at horribly disfigured faces and distorted forms bending and twisting into shapes, appearing and disappearing rapidly in the shining medium, eddying and swirling in and around me. They left me trembling with fear, unable to account for their presence. At times, though such occurrences were rare, I could perceive within the luminous mist a brighter radiance emanating from a glowing, ethereal shape, with a hardly distinguishable face and figure, but nevertheless a presence, emitting a luster so soft, enchanting, and soothing that on such occasions my mind overflowed with happiness and an indescribable divine peace filled every fiber of my being.

Strangely enough, on every such occasion the memory of the

primary vision, which occurred on the first day of the awakening, came vividly to me as if to hearten me in the midst of despondency with a fleeting glimpse of a supercondition towards which I was being painfully and inexorably drawn.

I was not sure at that time whether the visions afforded actual glimpses of supermundane existence or were mere figments of my now highly excited and virtually glowing imagination. I did not know what was making me perennially conscious of luminosity, as if my own intangible mental stuff had been metamorphosed into a radiant substance and this metamorphosis of the mind substance was responsible for the radiancy in my thought images.

I continued to attend to my household and official duties, gaining more and more strength every day. After a few more weeks I was able to work attentively for hours with my now transformed mental equipment without feeling any distressing symptoms. But there was no perceptible change in my general outlook or efficiency, and barring the introduction of this mysterious and incomprehensible factor into my life, I was the same as before.

In the course of time the passage of the current through the scattered nerve threads became less perceptible and often I did not notice it at all. I could now devote myself attentively to any work for hours. Comparing my later stable mental condition with what it had been in the initial stages after the crisis, the realization came to me that I had escaped from the clutches of insanity by the narrowest margin, and that I owed my deliverance not to any effort of mine but to the benign disposition of the energy itself. In the primary stages, particularly before the crisis, for certain very cogent reasons, the vital current appeared to be acting erratically and blindly like the swollen waters of a flooded stream which, pouring out through a breach in the embankment, rushes madly here and there trying to scour out a new channel for its passage.

Years later I had an inkling of what had actually happened and could guess at the marvel lying hidden in the human body, unsuspected, waiting for the needed invocation from the owner and a favorable opportunity to leap into action, when, plowing its way through the flesh like a diverted stream in flood, it creates new channels in the nervous system and the brain to endow the fortunate individual with unbelievable mental and spiritual powers.

The six months of that summer spent in Kashmir passed without any remarkable event or noteworthy change in me. The stir caused by my strange indisposition gradually died down and most of the people who had any knowledge of it attributed my sudden breakdown to mental causes. A whisper had gone round in some quarters, however, that my strange distemper was the outcome of yoga practices, intimately connected with kundalini, and the curious came to see me on one pretext or another, trying to elicit further information to assure themselves, by the exhibition of some supernatural feat on my part, that I had really crossed the boundary which separates the human from the Divine. For many of them, the mere awakening of the Serpent Power meant a precipitate plunge into the supernatural.

They were not blameworthy. Many people seem to have the notion that it is but a step from human to cosmic consciousness, a step which one can take all at once with assistance from a teacher or with the aid of spiritual exercises as easily and safely as one crosses a threshold leading from a smaller to a larger room.

This fallacious idea is often bolstered by incompetent guides, trading on the credulity of some, who claim knowledge of yoga and ability to bring about positive results in their disciples, themselves utterly unaware of the fact that yoga as a progressive science has been dead for several hundred years and that beyond a few parrotlike recitations from the works of ancient masters they know no more about it than the uninformed whom they profess to teach. In olden days, however, the serious and difficult nature of the task was fully recognized and the aspirants who set about it took full care to divest themselves of all worldly responsibilities and to develop a stoical attitude of mind, prepared to meet all eventualities without flinching or yielding under stress.

To the frivolous inquiries directed to gathering more information about my experience, I usually turned a deaf ear, maintaining a reserve which has continued to this day. Failing to gain satisfaction for their curiosity and finding no remarkable change in me, the story of my spiritual adventure was treated as a myth, and to some I even became an object of ridicule for having mistaken a physical ailment for a divine dispensation.

At the end of summer I was almost as strong as before. Barring the luminous currents and the radiance in my head, I marked no other change in myself and felt none the worse for my awful adventure save that at certain times, usually in the afternoon, the passage of the current became disturbingly perceptible, accompanied by a slight uneasiness in the head. At such times I usually experienced difficulty in applying myself attentively to any task and often spent the interval talking or strolling in the open.

Sometimes on such occasions I noticed a greater pressure on the nerve centers in the cardiac and hepatic regions, especially the latter, as if a greater flow of the radiation was being forced into the organ to increase its activity. There was no other indication of anything remarkable or unusual in me. I slept well, ate heartily, and in order to overcome the effects on my body of several months of forced inactivity, took a little exercise, to which I had been accustomed since boyhood, avoiding undue strain and exhaustion. But after the hours spent in the office, I felt no inclination to read in the evening, as had been my habit in the past, or to do any mental work. Treating this as a hint from within not to tax the brain any further, I retired usually to my room for relaxation and rest soon after dinner.

Towards the end of October 1939, I made preparations for my departure to Jammu with the office. I felt myself so thoroughly fit for the journey and subsequent sojourn there for six months all by myself that for reasons of her health I left my wife, my one unfailing partner in all my vicissitudes, in Kashmir, confident of my own ability to look after myself. I did not realize at that time that I was taking a grave risk in not having her with me when away from home, that without my knowledge the stormy force released in my body was still as actively at work, and that though I was not acutely cognizant of its movements, the strain on my vital organs was no less heavy than it had been before.

The thought that I was in an abnormal state internally was, however, never entirely absent from my mind, for I was reminded of it constantly by the luminosity within. But as time wore on and the condition remained constant it lost for me much of its strangeness and unnaturalness, becoming, as it were, a part of my being, my usual and normal state.

In view of the immense significance of the regenerative and transformative processes at work in my body, especially during sleep, which ultimately resulted in the development of psychic gifts never possessed by me until I was over forty-six years old, it is necessary to dwell on this most important phase of my singular experience.

Not only the ancient treatises on yoga but numerous other spiritual texts of India contain references to the miraculous power of Shakti, or feminine cosmic energy, to bring about transformations in her devotees.

The famous *gayatri* mantra, which every Brahmin must recite daily after his morning ablutions, is an invocation to Kundalini to grant transcendence. The sacred thread worn by the Hindus, consisting generally of three or six separate threads held together by a knot, is symbolic of the three well-known channels of vital energy, *ida*, *pingala*, and *sushumna*, passing through the center and on either side of the spinal cord. The tuft of hair on the top of the head, usually worn by men, indicates the location of the inoperative conscious center in the brain which opens like a lotus in bloom when watered by the ambrosial current rising through *sushumna* and functions as the seat of the supersensible perception, the sixth sense or the third eye, in those divinely favored by Kundalini.

The obviously unambiguous references to her creative and transformative prowess contained in the hymns composed in praise of the Goddess by renowned sages and great spiritual teachers, venerated almost like gods and in most cases, if their own avowals are to be believed, themselves the beneficiaries of Her grace, cannot be dismissed lightly as mere poetic effusions devoid of any material foundation. Considering also the fact that the results attained by the masters formed subjects for experiment and verification by their disciples, who had, therefore, necessarily to gauge their correctness, the assertions cannot be treated either as mere metaphors, intended to convey some other meaning, or as crude exaggerations of trivial achievements.

In any case, it is on the universal acceptance of the truth of these ancient beliefs in India that all the systems of yoga and the massive structure of Vedic religion have been built, with a foundation so deeply laid that they have come to be an integral part of every religious act and ceremony of a Hindu. Consequently the average worshiper of Kali, Durga, Shiva, or Vishnu, when prostrate before the image of his deity with tearful eyes and lips quivering with emotion, implores the boon of not only worldly favors but also of superphysical attributes to enable him to look behind the veil of illusory appearances.

If the historic record extending to more than thirty centuries as embodied in the Vedas and other spiritual texts is to be relied upon, and credence lent to the unquestionable testimony of scores of clever investigators and shrewd observers, the ancient society of Indo-Aryans abounded with numerous genuine instances of transfiguration by means of spiritual strivings and yoga resulting in the complete metamorphosis of personality, as a result of which individuals of a common caliber were transformed into visionaries of extraordinary attainments by the touch of an invisible power which they recognized and worshiped with appropriate ceremony.

In fact, one of the basic tenets of Hindu religion and the archstone of the science of yoga is the belief, emphatically upheld by almost every scripture, that by properly directed effort it is possible for a person to complete the evolutionary cycle of human existence in one life and blossom into a transfigured adept in tune with the Infinite

Reality beyond the phenomenal world, forever released from the otherwise endless chain of births and deaths.

In addition to cases of spontaneous transformation brought about suddenly or by slow degrees in mystics and saints, ancient or modern, both in the East and West, and supported by unimpeachable evidence which confronts modern science with an enigma as insoluble now as it was in medieval times, there are also authentic instances where a definite alteration of personality has occurred as a result of yoga or other form of spiritual effort, undertaken deliberately and continued for some time, resulting ultimately in the sudden or slow development of abnormal psychic faculties and extraordinary mental attributes not visible before.

What is the mystery behind this oft-repeated and generally accepted phenomenon? What force, spiritual, psychical, or physical, is set into motion automatically or by voluntary striving, which, working mysteriously according to its own inscrutable laws, brings about a radical change in the organism, molding it into a distinct type with certain common characteristics that have distinguished mystics and seers of all ages and climes?

Not only in India, but in almost all the countries professing a revealed faith, the belief in the efficacy of worship, prayer, and other religious practices to induce a mental condition favorable to the dispensation of divine grace has been current from time immemorial, and the transformation occurring in consequence of such practices is, therefore, naturally attributed to divine favor. It must be remembered, however, that a hasty recourse to supernatural agencies to account for any obscure phenomenon not explicable by the intellect has also been a marked feature of human existence from the earliest stages of development as rational beings, and is almost as common now in the lower strata of any society as it was in prehistoric times. The habit is still there in the majority of human beings, though its operation has been somewhat restricted owing to the explanations furnished by science for many previously obscure phenomena of nature.

To bring in divinity for the explanation of isolated phenomena, when its perpetual suzerainty over the whole universe and its position as the primordial cause of all existence is recognized, is an inconsistency of which seasoned intellects should not be guilty. When viewed in the light of such recognition, neither a leaf can stir nor an atom move nor a raindrop descend nor any creature breath without divine providence; the inconsistency lies in furnishing rational explanations for some of the problems and invoking a supermundane agency for the rest. To the great sorrow of the human race, this has always been done in respect of matters temporal, on the one hand, and spiritual on the other. It has to be admitted that matter and spirit are radically different, perhaps diametrically opposite propositions, and that therefore, what is true of one may not be true of the other; but that can only serve as a sound reason for employing different methods of approach to the problems presented by each, and not for denying to one what we concede to the other, when the two owe their origin to the same eternal cause.

The existence of extraordinary intellectual talent or spiritual and psychic gifts in some people should not, therefore, be attributed to divine intervention; there can be no pampered favorites in the just hierarchy of heaven. However, as in the case of material phenomena, the variations from the rule, repeatedly observed, should act as a spur to goad us to investigate the problems presented by the extraordinary achievements of geniuses on the one hand and the amazing performances of visionaries on the other.

Working from this angle, the first effort of any investigator should be directed towards ascertaining the degree of relationship between the body and the mind, to determine whether the conditions and actions of the former invariably affect the latter and vice versa, or if each functions completely or partially as an independent unit. Only a moment's thought is enough to convince even the least intelligent that the body and mind are indissolubly bound to each other from birth to death, each exerting a tremendous influence over the other at every moment of their joint existence, to such an extent that many keen observers are sharply divided on the issue as to whether mind is the product of the biochemical reactions of the body or the latter is the result of the ideative processes of the mind. One is astounded at the depth of knowledge and the keenness of intellect displayed on either side, but neither group has been able to win the other completely to its view.

For the purpose of our point of view, it is enough to say that body and mind are mutually dependent and responsive to such an amazing extent that not an eyelid flickers nor does a muscle move nor an artery throb without the knowledge of the mind, and similarly not a memory stirs, nor does a thought strike, nor an idea occur without causing a reaction in the body. The effect of disease, of organic changes in the tissues, of exhaustion, of diet, of medicine, of intoxicants and narcotics on the mind, and of pleasure and pain, sorrow and suffering, emotion and passion, fear and anxiety on the body is too well known to need stressing. The close connection between body and mind may with justice be likened to that existing between a mirror and the object reflected in it. The least change in the object is instantaneously reflected by the mirror, and conversely any change in the reflection denotes a corresponding change in the object also.

In all temporal affairs, the correlationship and interdependence of the gross body and the ethereal mind is recognized and accepted without question; but strangely enough when dealing with spiritual matters, this obviously unalterable rule determining the relationship of the two in the physical world is inexplicably lost sight of. Even eminent scholars, when discussing psychic phenomena of the most extraordinary kind, argue as if the corporeal frame, which faithfully follows physical laws during its pilgrimage on this plane, has no place in the picture from the moment of entry into spiritual realms.

Even after making full allowance for the miracles performed by them, the life stories of known saints, mystics, and prophets make it undeniably clear that the inviolable biological laws affected them just the same as if they were ordinary human beings, and that they, too, were as prone to hunger, thirst, and fatigue and as easy a prey to disease, senescence and death as the others of their time. Not one of them survived for a remarkably longer span of time than that normally allotted to mortals—say a few dozen years—to demonstrate conclusively the victory of spirit over flesh, nor did any of them completely conquer hunger, thirst or sleep, nor radically alter the predisposition of the body to age, disease, and decay.

Most of them undoubtedly furnish unique examples of unparalleled courage and fortitude in adversity, extraordinary loftiness of character, unflinching adherence to truth, and other laudable virtues; but so far as this aspect of their existence is concerned, the histories of all nations contain numerous examples of normal men and women who exhibited in an almost equally outstanding manner some or many of the noble traits characterizing the visionaries, without ever attempting to trace their sterling qualities to any supernatural agency or exceptional divine favor.

One can easily cite countless instances of the dominance of spirit over the frailties of flesh true of any nation and relating to any period of history. They are encountered daily, particularly in the humbler sectors of society. Hence it would be a fallacy to assert that they are an exclusive feature of spirituality in the ordinary connotation of the term or that their occurrence in any way alters or nullifies the operation of the otherwise inviolable biological laws regulating the relation between the body and the mind. When we know that even the flicker of a thought or the momentary sway of passion has a perceptible reaction on the body, it is inconceivable that such abnormal and extraordinary states of mind associated with spiritual phenomena as are involved in the beholding of presences, hearing of unearthly voices, contemplation of enrapturing or awe-inspiring visions, entrancement and ecstasy, or any other form of psychical activity, should not exhibit a corresponding physiological reaction in the body.

It has been observed that at the time of psychic manifestations or physical phenomena in mystics or mediums, signs of faintness, partial or complete insensibility to surroundings, convulsive movements, and other symptoms of organic disturbance are frequently present. This fact alone should provide sufficient cause for questioning the attitude of those who accept their existence as a perfectly legitimate activity of the mind alone, beyond the pale of organic laws, as also of those who as readily and as complacently deny their occurrence. It has become a habit to treat such phenomena as freakish occurrences, not amenable to ordinary biological laws.

In all probability there is a basic misconception, owing to a wrong interpretation of religious doctrine or proceeding from superstitions, which allots to the cognitive faculty in human beings an entirely independent status utterly divorced from the body in relation to its supersensory and superphysical activity. It is under the influence of such erroneous premises that not infrequently even erudite people lend their support to dogmas crediting the human mind with unlimited powers, even to the extent of comprehending the ultimate reality behind the visible universe in its entirety or providing a suitable vehicle for its incarnation in human form.

Bearing in mind the stupendous extent of the universe, the reality of the Creator becomes so staggering that it is utterly beyond the conceptual capacity of the human brain. Even the developed consciousness of an ecstatic, though itself an indestructible universal substance risen above the sense-bound human intellect, is utterly incapable of apprehending the real nature of its immeasurable source.

Hence even in the highest condition of superconscious flight, the most which renowned mystics have been able to say is too fragmentary and vague to justify the conclusion that what they perceived through supersensory channels was the Reality in itself, and not merely a slightly brighter radiation from an extremely distant, unimaginable, conscious Sun. To come closer to this source would mean instantaneous destruction of a frail receptive instrument like the human body, incapable of sustaining at its present stage of evolution anything but the tiniest measure of vital energy streaming everywhere through the Universe in incalculable abundance from that inexhaustible source.

Speaking more clearly, the transcendental state may be nothing more than a fleeting glimpse of a tiny fragment of the superconscious world illumined by the rays of a stupendous unvisualizable Sun in the same manner as with our normal vision we see but a tiny portion of the gigantic physical universe around us. Since body is the vehicle and mind the product of the radiation filtering through it, animating its countless cells like a living electric current, vivifying the sensitive brain matter to a far greater pitch of vital activity than any other region, the whole machine can exhibit only a limited range of consciousness depending on the capacity of the brain and the efficiency of the various organs and parts composing it.

Because of the drastic restrictions imposed on our sensory equipment and the extremely narrow bounds of our mental orbit, the average person, never brought into contact with a state of consciousness distinctly superior to their own, is utterly unable to even dimly form a conception of a deathless, incorporeal conscious Energy of infinite volume, penetrative power, and mobility, able to act simultaneously in millions upon millions of living objects all over the earth, to say nothing of the unimaginably vast creation in other parts of the universe, to whose invisible activity we owe our own existence.

The main stumbling block in the visualization of even a slightly higher plane of consciousness is the normally unalterable and limited capacity of the human brain, which in each individual is able to utilize only a specific quantity of life energy for the activity of the body and the mind. There is no known method by which the brain of a normal individual can be made to overstep the boundaries set to it by nature, though it can be improved and sharpened with application and study and made to accommodate more information and assimilate more facts, assisted by interface with computers, but with the exception of gifted individuals fashioned in a slightly different form, it cannot be made to transcend the limits of its native state of consciousness, and to step into the next higher stratum, able to perceive what was imperceptible and to know what was unknowable before the transition.

The question to be answered is whether the basic transition from one sphere of consciousness to a higher one can be effected, and whether there are any authentic instances of it during recent times. The answer to the first part of the question is an emphatic yes. The whole armory of every system of yoga, of every occult creed and of every esoteric religious doctrine is directed to this end. The only shortcoming, which makes the claim appear absurd and fantastic to a strictly scientific mind, is that the biological process by which the change can be brought about has not been explained, or probably even thought of, under the false notion, already discussed, that the human mind can win entry to supersensory realms without affecting the body in any way.

Almost all the methods in use from time immemorial for gaining visionary experience or supersensory perception—concentration, breathing exercises, postures, prayer, fasting, asceticism, and the like—affect both the organic frame and the mind. It is therefore reasonable to suppose that any changes brought about by any of these methods in the sphere of thought must also be preceded by alterations in the chemistry of the body.

The ancient authorities on yoga, though aware of the important role played by the physical organism in developing supersensory channels of cognition, and fully conversant with the methods for diverting its energies in this direction, were far more interested in the spiritual than in the physical side of the science. They attached little significance to the biological changes occurring in the flesh as compared to the resulting momentous developments in the realm of mind. The general level of knowledge in those days and the tendencies of the time also precluded the possibility of such an investigation. Even the advocates of kundalini yoga, starting with the discipline and purification of internal organs, failed to give the corporeal frame the status it deserved as the sole channel for achieving a transcendent state in yoga practice.

From the very nature of the exercises and the discipline enjoined, it should be obvious that the pivot round which the whole system revolved was the living organism, and it was to bring it to the required degree of fitness that the initiates devoted precious years of their lives in acquiring proficiency in maintaining difficult postures. They also had to master the art of cleaning the colon, the stomach, the nasal passages and the throat, holding the breath almost to the point of asphyxiation, and other extremely difficult, even dangerous, practices.

In the light of the facts mentioned in this present book, it is not difficult to see that they are all indicative of a sustained endeavor to purify and regulate the system in order to adjust it to the heightened state of perception. They also indicate a preliminary arduous preparation of the body to bear safely a possible shock or excessive strain consequent on the bursting of the vital storm in it, released to effect drastic organic changes extending over years, and ending in death or immortality, or only bitter disappointment at the close of a life spent in ceaseless striving and self-denial.

It is abundantly clear that all the exercises were directed towards the manipulation of a definite organic control system in the body, capable of bringing about the earnestly desired consummation by mysterious means even less understood now than they were in olden days.

TWELVE

The Transformative Power
of the Divine Energy

DURING 1939, I RETURNED to Jammu in a cheerful frame of mind, restored almost to my normal physical and mental health. The fear of the supernatural and antipathy towards religion that had been constantly present during the first few months had partially disappeared. For a long time I could not account for this sudden revulsion of what had been a deep-rooted feeling in me, and even during the days of acute disturbance was surprised at this change in myself. It was not only because my irrepressible desire for religious experience had landed me in an awful predicament that I felt the fear and the aversion, but there seemed to have actually occurred an inexplicable alteration in the very depths of my personality, for which I was at a loss to assign a reason.

Devout and God-fearing until my abnormal condition, I had lost all feelings of love and veneration for the divine, all respect for the sacred and the holy, and all interest in the scriptural and sacramental. The very idea of the supernatural had become hateful and I did not allow my thoughts to dwell on it even for a moment. From a devotee, I had become an inveterate enemy of faith and felt seething resentment against those whom I saw going to or coming from places of worship. I had changed entirely, devoid completely of every religious sentiment, turned into a rank atheist, a violent heretic, the very antithesis of the religious and the spiritual.

In the early stages, desperately engaged in a neck-and-neck race, with death on one side and insanity on the other, I had neither the time nor the mental disposition to think seriously about this sudden disappearance of a powerful impulse which had dominated my thought from a very early age. As my mind grew clearer I wondered more and more at this quite unexpected alteration. When on the restoration of my general health, particularly the feelings of love, the distaste for the supernatural still persisted and I found myself still empty of religious desire, as if washed clean of it, I became uneasy at the thought that, after all, it might not be kundalini (considered to be the inexhaustible fount of divine love and the perennial source of spirituality which was active in me) but some evil force of darkness dragging me towards the depths of irreligiosity and impiety.

At such times the words of the Brahmin sadhu whom I had consulted during the preceding winter in a state of desperation always came back with an ominous significance. He had said slowly, emphasizing every word to make it sink deep into my terribly agitated mind, that the symptoms I had mentioned could in no way be attributed to Kundalini, the ocean of bliss, as She could never be associated with anything in the nature of pain or disturbance, and that my malady was most probably due to the vicious influence of some evilly disposed elemental spirit. I had been horrified at the words, which, spoken with certainty to a man fighting desperately with madness, spelled death for any spark of hope left in him. They often came back to me in the darkest moments to shut out the last glimmer of reason still struggling for existence. With sanity restored, but still strangely altered by a strongly marked characteristic, the idea recurred with overwhelming force to harass me when I failed to find a satisfactory explanation for the change.

However, shortly before returning to Jammu I had begun to feel vaguely the dim stirrings of the apparently dead impulse of religion. This happened usually in the early hours of morning, immediately on awakening from sleep, as if the refreshed state of the brain afforded an opportunity to the vanished urge to make a shadowy appearance for a brief interval.

At such moments my thoughts usually dwelt on the life stories of certain mystics whose utterances had once made a powerful appeal to me. I had wholly forgotten them during the preceding months, and when recalled by accident the remembrance failed to evoke any warmth. I usually turned my thoughts to other things to avoid thinking of them. Now their memory returned as of old for a moment, the sweetness tinctured with a certain bitterness, for they had said nothing clearly of the dread ordeal which they too must have gone through in one form or another, nothing about the dangers and pitfalls of the path which they too must have traveled and which must be common to reach a goal open to all.

But if they had suffered as much as I did or even a fraction of it and come out of the tribulation to compose inspiring verses which had captivated my heart at the very first hearing, they were indeed worthy of the greatest homage, far above and beyond a man like me, shaken and shattered by the same ordeal.

A few weeks after my arrival in Jammu I noticed that the gap was quickly filling and that my religious ideas, sentiments, and memories were all reviving rapidly. I felt again the same deep urge for religious experience and the same all-absorbing interest in the supernatural and the mystical. I could again sit all by myself brooding on the yet unanswered problem of being and the riddle of my own existence, or listen to devotional songs and mystical poetry with undiminished rapture from start to finish without the least sign of disturbance or any symptoms of haunting terror. When this religious mood came, the overhanging cloud of a malevolent spirit leading me towards degradation disappeared and my heart expanded in gratitude to the mysterious power working in me. It was only now that I really began to recognize myself, the being who about a year or so before had sat cross-legged in his ignorance that the average human frame of today, emasculated by a faulty civilization and enervated by uncontrolled ambitions and desires, is not strong enough to bear the splendor of the mighty vision without long preparatory training, austerity and discipline.

Slowly it began to dawn upon me that the torture I suffered in the beginning was caused by the unexpected release of the powerful vital energy through the wrong nerve, *pingala*, and that the hot blast coursing through my nerve and brain cells would have undoubtedly led to death but for miraculous intervention at the last minute. Later on, my suffering was probably due, firstly, to the damage already sustained by my nervous system; secondly, to the fact that I was entirely uninitiated into the mystery; and thirdly and mainly, to the circumstance that my body, though above the average in muscular strength, was not sufficiently developed internally to withstand the sudden onrush of a much more dynamic and potent life energy than that to which the average human body is normally accustomed.

I had experienced enough to realize that this powerful vital force, once let loose even by accident, cannot be restrained from carrying one onward and upward towards a higher and more penetrating consciousness for which it is the one and only instrument. The awakening of kundalini, it seemed to me, implied the introduction into the human body of a higher form of nerve force by the constant sublimation of the human seed, leading ultimately to the radiant transcendental consciousness aglow ever after in the transformed brain of successful initiates.

I speculated in this manner without being sure about the correctness of my surmises. I had undergone a singular experience, but how could I be sure that I was not the victim of an abnormal pathological condition, peculiar to me alone? How could I be sure that I was not suffering from a continuous hallucinatory affliction in this particular respect while normal in other ways, the unexpected result of prolonged concentration and too much absorption in the occult? If I had within reach a recorded experience even distantly similar to mine, or a really competent teacher to guide me, my doubts would have been resolved then and there, by which the whole course of my life might have been different and I might have been saved another equally long and equally awful period of agony, as the one I had just come through.

As I still failed to notice the development of any extraordinary talent or supernormal faculty, I continued to be tormented by serious doubts about the actual nature of the abnormality of which I was the victim. The ever-present radiation, bathing my head with luster and glowing along the path of countless nerves in the body, streaming here and there in a most wonderful and sometimes awe-inspiring manner, had little in common with the effulgent visions described by yogis and mystics. Beyond the spectacle of a luminous circle around the head, which was now constant in me, and an extended consciousness, I felt and saw nothing extraordinary in the least approaching the supernatural or divine, but for all practical purposes was the same man that I had always been.

The only difference was that I now saw the world reflected in a larger mental mirror. It is extremely difficult for me to express adequately this change in my cognitive apparatus. The best I can do is to say that it appeared as if an enlarged picture of the world was now being formed in my mind, not enlarged in the sense of magnification by a microscope, but as if the world image was now presented by a wider conscious surface than before. In other words, the knowing self appeared to have acquired distinctly extended proportions.

It was at an early stage that I had become conscious of this inexplicable alteration. At that time I was not in a condition to give it serious thought and took it for granted that the change was brought about by the luminous vapor streaming into my brain. As already mentioned, the dimensions of the shining mist in my head varied constantly, causing a widening and shrinking of consciousness. This rapid alteration in the perceptive mirror, accompanied by an ever-present sense of deadening fear, had been the first acutely distressing and completely bewildering feature of my uncanny experience.

As time wore on, the extension became more and more apparent, with less frequent contractions, but even in the narrowest state of perception my consciousness was wider than before. I could not fail to mark this startling alteration in myself as it occurred abruptly, carrying me from one conscious state to another almost overnight.

If the transition had taken place gradually, without the other accompanying factors like the radiating spinal currents and the extraordinary sensations that made the whole phenomenon so striking and bizarre, I might not have noticed the extension at all, as one does not notice the extremely slight daily changes in one's own face which immediately strike a friend after a long separation.

As the alteration in the state of my consciousness is the most important feature of my experience to which I wish to draw attention, having far-reaching results, it is necessary to say more about this extraordinary development, which for a long time I considered to be an abnormality or delusion. The state of exalted and extended consciousness, permeated with an inexpressible, supermundane happiness which I experienced on the first appearance of the Serpent Fire in me, was an internal phenomenon, subjective in nature, indicating an expansion of the field of awareness, or the cognitive self, formless, invisible, and infinitely subtle, the observer in the body, always beyond scrutiny, impossible to delineate or depict.

From a unit of consciousness, dominated by the ego, to which I was habituated from childhood, I had expanded all at once into a glowing conscious circle, growing larger and larger, until a maximum was reached, the "I" remaining as it was, but instead of a confining unit, now itself encompassed by a shining conscious globe of vast dimensions. For want of a better simile, I should say that from a tiny glow the awareness in me became a large radiating pool of light, the "I" immersed in it yet fully cognizant of the radiantly blissful volume of consciousness all around, both near and far. Speaking more precisely, there was ego consciousness as well as a vastly extended field of awareness, existing side by side, both distinct yet one.

This remarkable phenomenon, indelibly imprinted upon my memory, as vivid when recalled today as at the time of occurrence, was not repeated in all its original splendor until long afterwards. During the succeeding agonizing weeks and months there was absolutely no resemblance between my initial experience and the subsequent extremely disquieting mental condition, beyond the fact that I was painfully aware that an expansion had somehow taken place in the original area of my consciousness, subject frequently to partial contractions.

By the time I returned to Jammu, I had regained my equilibrium of mind and soon after was restored fully to myself, with all my individual traits and peculiarities. But the unmistakable alteration in my cognitive faculty, which I had noticed for some time and of which I was constantly reminded when contemplating an external object or an internal mental image, underwent no modification except that with the passage of time the luminous circle in my head grew larger and larger by imperceptible degrees, with a corresponding increase in the area of consciousness. It was certain that I was now looking at the universe with a perceptibly enlarged mental surface and that, in consequence, the world image which I perceived was reflected by a larger surface than that provided by my mind during all the years from my childhood to the time of the ecstatic vision. The area of my peripheral consciousness had undeniably increased, for I could not be mistaken about a fact continually in front of me during waking hours.

The phenomenon was so strange and so out of the ordinary that I felt convinced that it would be useless on my part to look for a parallel case, even if the weird transformation was because of the action of an awakened kundalini and not a unique abnormality affecting me only. Realizing also the futility of revealing this unheard-of development to others, I kept my secret strictly to myself, saying nothing of it even to those most intimately connected with me. As my physical and mental condition gave me no cause for uneasiness in any other respect, I gradually ceased to trouble myself about it.

As already mentioned in an earlier chapter, in the initial stages of my experience it appeared as if I were viewing the world through a mental haze, or to be more clear, as if a thin layer of extremely fine dust hung between me and the objects perceived. It was not an optical defect, as my eyesight was as sharp as ever and the haze seemed to envelop not the sensory but the perceptive organ. The dust was on the conscious mirror which reflected the image of the objects.

It seemed as if the objects seen were being viewed through a whitish medium that made them look as if an extremely fine and uniform coat of chalk dust were laid on them without in the least blurring the outline or the normal color peculiar to each. This coat hung between me and the sky, the branches and leaves of trees, the green grass, the houses, the paved streets, the dress and faces of people, lending to all a chalky appearance, precisely as if the conscious center in me, which interpreted sensory impressions, was now operating through a white medium, needing further refinement and cleaning to make it perfectly transparent.

As in the case of enlargement of the visual image, I was entirely at a loss to explain this phenomenon. Any change of time, place, or weather had absolutely no effect on the transformation. It was as apparent under lamplight as in sunlight, as noticeable in the clear light of morning as at dusk. Obviously the change was internal and not the result of alteration by changed external influences.

Surprised, yet keeping my own counsel, I continued to pass my days and nights at Jammu attending to my duties and minding my tasks as others were doing. The only plausible reason for the change in my cognitive faculty which I could think of was that the animating principle inhabiting the body was now operating the mechanism through an altered vital medium. This led to an alteration in the quality and behavior of the nerve currents regulating the functions of the organs as well as in the quality of the sensory impressions and their interpretations by the observing mind. But all that had happened and was still happening was so unprecedented and incredible that I felt easier in treating it all as an abnormality rather than as a natural growth governed by regular biological laws, which ultimately it proved to be.

In this manner, a prey to doubts and uneasiness, I continued to pass my time until one sunny day, when on my way to the office, I happened to look at the front block of the Rajgarh Palace, in which the government offices were located, taking in my glance the sky as well as the roof and the upper part of the building. I looked casually at first, then, struck by something strange in their appearance, more attentively, unable to withdraw my gaze, and finally rooted to the spot I stared in amazement at the spectacle, unable to believe the testimony of my eyes.

I was looking at a scene familiar to me in one way before the experience and in another during the last few months, but what I now saw was so extraordinary as to render me motionless with surprise. I was looking at a scene belonging not to the earth but to some fairyland, for the ancient, weather-stained front of the building, unadorned and commonplace, and the arch of the sky above it, bathed in the clear light of the sun, were both lit with a brilliant silvery luster that lent a beauty and a glory to both and created a marvelous light-and-shade effect impossible to describe. Wonderstruck, I turned my eyes in other directions, fascinated by the silvery shine which glorified everything. Clearly I was witnessing a new phase in my development; the luster which I perceived on every side and in all objects did not emanate from them but was undoubtedly a projection of my own internal radiance.

Entirely absorbed in the contemplation of the enchanting view, I lost all touch with my surroundings, completely forgetting that I was standing like a statue in the middle of a road thronged at that time of day with crowds of employees going to the Secretariat. Collecting my thoughts, like one suddenly awakened from a beatific vision, I looked around, withdrawing my gaze with difficulty from the delightful scene. Many pairs of eyes from the rapidly moving crowd on every side looked at me in surprise, unable to account for my abrupt halt and subsequent immobility.

Pulling myself together, I walked at a leisurely pace in the direction of the office, keeping my eyes on the building and the portion of the overhanging sky in front of me. Completely unprepared for such a development, I could not bring myself to believe that what I was gazing at was real and not a vision conjured up by my fancy stimulated to greater activity by the intriguing aureole, perceptible to me always around my head. I looked intently in front and around again and again, rubbing my eyes to assure myself that I was not dreaming. No, I was surely in the center of the Secretariat quadrangle, moving slowly in the midst of a bustling throng hastening in all directions, like them in all other respects except that I was looking at the world with a different vision.

On entering my room, instead of sitting at my desk I walked out onto the verandah at the back, where it was my habit to pass some time daily for a breath of fresh air while looking at the fine view open in front. There was a row of houses before me edged by a steep woody slope leading to the bank of the Tawi River, whose wide boulder-covered bed glistened in the sun with a thin stream of water running in the middle, bordered on the other side by another hillock with a small medieval fortress on top. I had looked at the same sight almost daily in winter for several years and the picture of it was vividly present in my memory. During the past few months, when gazing at it, I found that it too had assumed grander proportions and had the same chalky appearance I had noticed in all other objects.

On that memorable day, when my eyes swept across the riverbed to the hillock and from there to the sky, trying to take the whole panorama in one glance to make a comparison between what I was accustomed to seeing previously and what I perceived now, I was utterly amazed at the remarkable transformation. The magnified dimensions of the picture and the slightly chalky appearance of the objects were both present, but the dusty haze before my eyes had vanished and instead I was gazing fascinatedly at an extraordinarily rich blend of color and shade, shining with a silvery luster which lent an indescribable beauty to the scene.

Breathless with excitement, I turned my eyes in all directions, viewing each object attentively, eager to find whether the transformation was noticeable in all or whether it was an illusion caused by the particularly clear and sunny weather on that day. I looked and looked, allowing my gaze to linger for some time on each spot, convinced more firmly after each intent glance that far from being the victim of an optical illusion, I was seeing a brightly colored real scene before me, shining with a milky luster I had never before perceived.

A surge of emotion too deep for words filled my whole being, and tears gathered in my eyes in spite of myself at the significance of the new development in me. But even in that condition, looking through tears, I could perceive trembling beams of silvery light dancing before my vision, enhancing the radiant beauty of the scene. It was not difficult to understand that, without my being aware of it, an extraordinary change had taken place in the now luminous cognitive center in my brain and that the fascinating luster, which I perceived around every object, was not a figment of my fancy nor was it possessed by the objects, but was a projection of my own internal radiance.

Days and weeks passed without alteration in the lustrous new form of perception. A bright silvery sheen around every object, across the entire field of view, became a permanent feature of my vision. The azure dome of the sky, whenever I happened to glance at it, had a purity of color and a brightness impossible to describe. If I had possessed the same form of sight from my earliest childhood I should not have found anything striking in it, treating it as the usual endowment of every normal individual, but the alteration from the previous to the present state was so obvious, so remarkable, and so fascinating that I could not but be immensely moved and surprised by it.

Examining myself closely for any other change in my sensory perceptions, I became conscious of the fact that there also had occurred an amplification and refining of auditory sensations, as a result of which the sounds heard possessed now an exotic quality and a distinctiveness that lent to music and melody a greater sweetness and to noise and clamor a more disagreeable harshness. The alteration was not, however, so marked and striking as the change in visual impressions until a few years later. The olfactory, gustatory, and tactile centers as well exhibited a peculiar sensitivity and acuteness, clearly perceptible, but in point of magnitude nothing compared to what had happened with my sight.

The phenomenon was observable during darkness, too. At night, lamps glowed with a new brilliance, while illuminated objects glistened with a peculiar luster not wholly borrowed from the lamps.

In the course of a few weeks, the transformation ceased to cause me wonder or excitement, and gradually I came to treat it as an inseparable part of myself, a normal characteristic of my being. Wherever I went and whatever I did, I was conscious of myself in the new form, cognizant of the radiance within and the lustrous objectivity without. I was changing. The old self was yielding place to a new personality endowed with a brighter, more refined and artistic perceptive equipment, developed from the original one by a strange process of cellular and organic transformation.

Towards the middle of April that year, before leaving for Srinagar, I went to Hardwar with the sacred relics of my departed mother whom, to my sorrow, I had lost during the year preceding the experience. I had been to Hardwar once before on a similar errand after the death of my father. On this occasion, all through the journey by rail and during the few days of my stay at Hardwar, I was constantly reminded of the marvelous change in me. I traveled by the same route, saw the same stations, towns, and sights, until I reached my destination and there also saw the same quaint streets and buildings, the same Ganges with its swiftly flowing sapphire water, the same bathing places and ghats (terraced steps at sacred bathing places) thronged with pilgrims. They were all as I had seen them last but how different was the picture perceived by me on this occasion! Every object now formed a part of a greatly extended field of vision in striking contrast to the previous one; the whole assemblage lit with a glitter like that of freshly fallen snow when the sun shines upon it. After performing the sacred rites, I returned to Jammu, refreshed by the change, more firmly convinced about the new development in me. Soon after, I left for Srinagar with my office as usual.

Years passed. My health and vitality were completely restored. I could read continuously for long periods without fatigue and even indulge in my favorite pastime, chess, demanding close attention for hours. My diet became normal and the only article to remind me of my experience was a cup of milk in the morning and another in the afternoon with a slice of bread. I could not, however, stand a fast with impunity, but if obliged to keep one was not seriously affected by it either. In spite of all these signs of normality, it was easy to perceive that mentally I was not the same old self. The luster within and without became more and more perceptible with the passage of time.

With my inner vision I could distinctly perceive the flow of lucent currents of vital energy through the network of nerves in my body. A living silvery flame with a delicate golden tinge was clearly perceptible in the interior of my brain across the forehead. My thought images were vividly bright, and every object recalled to memory possessed radiance in the same manner as in the concrete form.

My reaction to infection and disease was not, however, normal. In every illness the characteristic symptoms of the ailment, though present, were distinctly milder in nature and usually there was an absence of temperature. The rapidity of the pulse was the main indication of an indisposition, but it was seldom, if ever, accompanied by a corresponding rise in the heat of the body as normally occurs with disease. This peculiarity is as observable now as it was in those days. The only explanation for it that I can think of is that my highly nervous organism does not permit the flow of heated blood to the brain, as a measure of safety to avoid injury to the now exceptionally sensitive cerebral matter, and adopts other devices to free the body from infection. I could not stand medication during illness or fasting and invariably resorted to dietetic remedies to get well.

I have said a good deal about the working of my mental equipment during waking hours without making any mention about its condition during sleep. The first time I became aware of an alteration in my dream consciousness was during the night in February 1938 when I passed the crisis, tasting sleep after several weeks of insomnia accompanied by a maddening mental condition. I fell asleep that night wrapped in a mantle of light perceptible in the dreams also.

From that day onwards, extraordinarily vivid dreams became habitual with me. The bright luster in my head, always present during wakefulness, continued undiminished during sleep; if anything, more clearly apparent and more active during the night than during the day. The moment I rested my head on the pillow and closed my eyes to invite sleep, the first object to draw my attention was the cranial glow, clearly distinguishable in darkness, not stationary and steady but spreading out and narrowing down like a whirlpool or swirling water in a shining sun. In the beginning and for many months after, it appeared as if a piston, working in the spinal tube at the bottom, was throwing up stream after stream of a very lustrous fluid, impalpable but distinctly visible, with such force that I actually felt my whole body shaking with the impact of the current to such an extent as made the bed creak at times.

The dreams were wonderful and always occurred against a shining background formed by the widespread luminous glow inside, which also lent a strange phosphorescence to the dream images. Every night during sleep I was transported to a glittering fairyland where, garbed in luster, I glided from place to place, as light as a feather. Scene after scene of inexpressible glory unfolded before my vision. The incidents were of the usual character common to dreams. They often lacked coherence and continuity, but although strange, fanciful and fantastic, they possessed a visionary character, surrounded by landscapes of a vastness and magnificence seldom seen in real life.

In my dreams I usually experienced a feeling of security and contentment, with the absence of anything in the least disturbing or disharmonious, all blended into a sense of peace and happiness, which gave my dream personality a character so unique and alluring that I never missed having ten hours of rest, and when distraught or dismayed during the day, invariably sought the sanctuary of sleep to rid myself of worry and fear. I had never dreamt such vivid dreams before. They naturally followed the pattern of my new personality and were woven of the same luminous stuff which formed the texture of my daytime thoughts and fancies. It was clear beyond a doubt that light not only pervaded my peripheral consciousness but had penetrated deep into the recesses of my subconscious being as well.

In course of time, the idea began to take root in my mind that the enhanced activity of the radiant current during sleep was an indication of the fact that in some incomprehensible way the opportunity afforded by the passive state of the brain was being utilized for immunizing it and the complicated nerve structures to the action of the newly released dynamic force in place of the former less potent vital energy.

But for years I was unable to guess what was happening inside me. I had come across vague statements in some of the ancient writings on kundalini yoga hinting at the transformative power of the divine energy. The hints were so obscure and so lacking in detail that I could not grasp how the human organism, with an unalterable legacy of innumerable hereditary factors stretching back for millions of years, possessing a certain strictly circumscribed brain power and intelligence, could be rebuilt from within to a far different or higher type of cerebral activity, enabling it to transcend the limits prescribed by Nature for it from birth. Taking into account the organic changes involved in a process of this kind, affecting simultaneously all constituents of the body and also the extremely delicate tissues of the brain and nervous system, the task of transformation envisaged in its true significance assumes such colossal proportions as to make it appear almost beyond the bounds of possibility.

But something wholly inexplicable was transpiring inside my

bodily frame, particularly during the long period devoted to sleep, when my inactive will was powerless to cause any interference in the new immensely accelerated anabolic and catabolic processes in the body. That my whole system was functioning in an altered manner, forced to a far higher pitch of metabolic activity under the compulsion of the lustrous vital energy racing through my nerves, I realized immediately after the crisis. It was impossible to mistake the increase in the pulse rate and the greater activity of the heart during the first part of the night, as well as the sudden undeniable alteration in my digestive and excretory functions.

I could not but believe the testimony of my own senses over months and years and the evidence of those who surrounded and looked after me, nor can I mistrust the proof furnished by my senses now, as the apparently abnormal metabolic activity which started more than twenty-five years ago continues undiminished to this hour and, from all indications, will continue to the end. It is not necessary for me to array proofs in support of the startling disclosure I am making. That would make this work too lengthy and specialized. But any trained observer who has the least knowledge of physiology can convince himself of the fact soon after kindling the Sacred Fire in himself.

The plan of this work does not permit me to describe in detail the constantly occurring physiological reactions and changes to which I was a daily witness, convincing me beyond doubt that my body was undergoing a process of purgation and rejuvenation side by side with some definite purpose entirely beyond my grasp. Otherwise there could be no other reasonable explanation for the feverish and sometimes even frantic activity continuously going on in my interior day and night, except that my whole organism was reacting to a new situation created inside by an altered activity of the vital organs to adjust itself to the changed environment within. Undoubtedly the disorder in my body was caused by the rapid passage of the luminous vital energy from cell to cell.

Under the action of a stronger current than that for which it was designed, any man-made mechanism, even a hundredth part as sensitive and intricate as the human frame, would be wrecked or damaged immediately, but because of certain inherent qualities developed by the human organism as a means of evolution, the sudden release of the Serpent Power, provided the blood is healthy and the organs sound, is not attended by fatal results in favorable cases because of safety devices already provided by Nature to meet a contingency of this kind in individuals ready for the experience.

Even in such cases it is essential that the energy be benignly disposed and that the subject take all necessary precautions to maintain the strength of the body and the balance of the mind during the subsequent period of inexpressibly severe trial. How far I was endowed with a constitution suited for the great ordeal I cannot say, but being an utter stranger to the science, taken unawares without the requisite preliminary course of physical and mental discipline, and prey to adversity, I was buffeted unceasingly for many years.

After the first most distressing period, I found in sleep the supreme healer for my physical and mental suffering during the day. There were unmistakable indications of abnormal activity in the region of kundalini from the moment of my retiring to sleep until the morning. It was obvious that by some mysterious process the precious secretion of the seminal glands was drawn up into the spinal tube and through the interlinking nerves, transferred into a subtle essence, then distributed to the brain and the vital organs, darting across the nerve filaments and the spinal cord to reach them. The suction was applied with such vigor as to be clearly apparent, and sometimes in the early stages with such violence as to cause actual pain to the delicate parts. At such times the ferment caused in the body resembled in effect the last minute frantic effort made for succor when a life is in imminent danger, and I, a dumb and helpless witness to the show, could not help but pass hours of agony thinking of this abnormal development in myself. It was easy to see that the aim of this entirely new and unexpected activity was to divert the seminal essence to the head and other vital organs, after sublimation, apparently to meet a contingency caused by a sudden disorder in any organ or a general discord inimical to the new development.

With the power of observation left to me even in the initial distraught condition of the mind, I could not fail to take notice of such a startling development in the sexual region which had functioned quite normally before. I could not fail to mark the agitated condition of the hitherto quiescent area, now in a state of feverish activity and ceaseless movement as if forced by an invisible but effective mechanism to produce the life fluid in superabundance without cessation in order to meet the unending demand of the cerebral lobes and the nervous system.

After only a few days of observation of this unmistakable organic phenomenon, the conviction dawned on me that I had unwittingly forced open a yet imperfectly developed center in the brain by the long-continued practice of concentration. This abnormal and apparently chaotic play of vital currents which I clearly felt was a natural effort of the organism to control the serious situation that was thus created. It was also apparent that in this grave emergency the body was making abundant use of the richest and most potent source of life energy in it, the vital essence, always available in the region commanded by kundalini.

I make but a simple statement of fact when I say that for years I was like one bound hand and foot to a log racing madly on a torrent, saved miraculously time after time from being dashed to death against the many boulders projecting out of the swirling water on every side by just a narrow margin, and in the nick of time turning and twisting this way and that, as if guided by a marvelously quick and dexterous hand, infallibly correct in its movement. Often at night for years, when lying awake in bed waiting for sleep to come, I felt the powerful new life energy sweep like a tempest in the abdominal and thoracic regions as well as the brain, with a roaring noise in the ears, a scintillating shower in the brain, and a feverish movement in the sexual region and its neighborhood around the base of the spine, both in front and behind, as if an all-out effort were being made to fight an emergency caused by some poison or obstruction in the organism threatening the supersensitive and extremely delicate condition of the cerebrospinal system.

At such times I felt instinctively that a life and death struggle was going on inside me in which I, the owner of the body, was entirely powerless to take part, forced to lie quietly and watch as a spectator the weird drama unfolded in my own flesh. Nothing can convey my condition more graphically than the representation of the God Shiva and his female power Shakti, pictured by an ancient master, in which the former is shown lying helpless and supine while the latter in an absolutely reckless mood dances gleefully on his prostrate frame.

The self-conscious observer in me, the self-styled possessor of the carnal frame, now completely subjugated and pushed into the background, found himself utterly at the mercy, literally under the feet of an awe-inspiring power indifferent to what he thought and felt, proceeding impassively to deal with the body as it chose, without even conceding to him the right to know what he had done to merit the indignity. I had every reason to believe the pictorial representation was designed to depict a condition exactly similar to mine by an initiate who had himself passed through the same ordeal.

The utter helplessness of the devotee and his entire dependence on the mercy and grace of the cosmic vital energy Shakti when kundalini is aroused is the constant theme of hymns addressed to the Goddess by eminent yogis of yore. As the supreme mistress of the body, She and She alone is considered to be competent to bestow on earnest aspirants (who worship Her with true devotion, centering their thoughts and actions in Her, resigning themselves entirely to Her will) the much coveted and hard-to-attain boon of transcendental knowledge and supernormal psychic powers. All these writings assign to Kundalini the supreme position of being the queen and architect of the living organism, having the power to mold it, transform it, or even to destroy it as She will.

But how She manages to do it, consistent with biological laws governing the organic world, no one has previously tried to state in explicit terms. Certainly it could not be done instantaneously, like a magical feat, setting at naught the law of causality in this one particular respect. It is more reasonable to assume that, even in those cases in which apparently a sudden spiritual development takes place, there must occur gradual changes in the cells and tissues of the body for a sufficiently long period, perhaps even from the embryonic stage or early childhood, without the individuals ever knowing what was happening in their own interior.

THIRTEEN

The Cause of All Genuine Spiritual Phenomena

VIEWED IN THE LIGHT of the physiological reactions for which unmistakable evidence was furnished by my body every day, I had ample ground for the supposition that some kind of transformative process was at work in me, but I could not tell with what object. The most I could imagine was that I was gradually being led towards a condition of the brain and the nervous system which would make it possible for me to attain occasionally the state of extended consciousness peculiar to yogis and mystics in trance conditions. I already had an enlarged consciousness from the time of my first experience of kundalini, which had caused me so much surprise and torture and of which I was constantly reminded whenever my thoughts rested on myself; but the extension I now had in mind was of a superior kind, signifying a complete negation of the ties that bind the spirit to the body, leaving it free to soar to superphysical heights and to return to the normal state refreshed and invigorated.

This was my idea of supersensible experience, gleaned from the scriptures, the stories of spiritual men and their own accounts of the ecstatic condition. Barring the blissful vision of extended personality which I perceived twice in succession in the very beginning, there was certainly no comparison between my now undeniably extended and luminous self, as securely bound to the body and the earth, as readily affected by physical needs and as strongly influenced by desire and passion, heat and cold, pleasure and pain, as the common one, and the exalted, full-of-happiness, free-from-fear, immune-from-pain, and indifferent-to-death superconsciousness of the ec-

240

static. I was still the same being mentally as I had been before; a man of common clay far below, intellectually and morally, the spiritual giants about whom I had read.

I missed no opportunity to study my symptoms critically and thoroughly. There was no other change save the unaccountable alteration in the nerve currents and the ever-present radiance inside and out. The lustrous visibility, which represented the latest phase in my strange development, had a heartening and uplifting effect upon me. This was indeed something that gave to my weird adventure a touch of sublimity. There could be no doubt now that I was undergoing a transformation, and although I had in no major respect risen above the average, I had at least the consolation that in this particular I was nearer to the hallowed hierarchy than to the people of common caliber whom I resembled in every other way.

But at the same time I could not shut my eyes to the glaring fact that the suffering I had undergone was out of all proportion to the results achieved, for which there was no explanation, save that either I had developed an abnormality or that the internal attempt at purification and transformation, which began with the awakening, had proved abortive in my case, and that consequently, perhaps as a result of inherent physical or mental deficiency, I had the unenviable position of being a rejected candidate—a yoga *brishta*—one who had been tried and then given up as utterly unfit for the supreme state of yoga.

As years passed and I perceived no other indication of spiritual unfolding or the growth of a higher personality endowed with superior intellectual and moral attributes, characterizing the blessed in whom kundalini kindles the sacred fire, I was more and more led towards the disheartening conclusion that I was not provided with the essential mental and physical equipment. But as there was no decrease in the activity of the radiant force, I did not altogether cease to hope that perhaps the attempt would not go wholly for nothing, and that one day I might unexpectedly find myself favored, if not to the maximum, at least to a noticeable extent.

Physically I became almost my old self again, hardy and tough, able to withstand hunger, the rigors of heat and cold, bodily and mental fatigue, disturbance and discomfort. The only thing I could not stand well was sleeplessness. It always caused haziness of mind and depression which lasted for several days and did not wear off until the deficiency was made good by a longer period of rest during the day or night following the sleepless night. I felt on such occasions as if my brain had been deprived of its usual dose of energy which enabled it to maintain the extensive dimension to which it had now grown gradually during the years.

But there was absolutely no diminution in the activity of the radiant vital currents during sleep. My dreams, which possessed a highly exotic and elusive quality, were so extraordinarily vivid and bright that in the dream condition I lived literally in a shining world in which every scene and every object glowed with luster against a marvelously luminous background, the whole presenting a picture of such resplendence and sublime beauty that, without implying the least exaggeration, I actually felt as if every night during slumber I roamed in enchanting empyrean regions of heavenly life.

The last thing I remembered on waking suddenly from sleep was usually a landscape or a figure enveloped in a bright blaze of light in such sharp contrast to the encircling gloom which met me on awakening that it seemed as if a celestial orb shining brilliantly in my interior was eclipsed all at once, leaving me to my fate in utter darkness. The vivid impressions left by a well-remembered happy dream during a night lingered for the whole day, a sweet memory of what appeared to be a supermundane existence of a few hours, to be followed by that of another seen on the succeeding night as sweet and vivid as that on the previous one.

The magnificently brilliant effect present in the dreams was noticeable, though in a considerably diminished form, in the waking state also, but the sense of exaltation felt in the former was entirely absent. I distinctly experienced a partial eclipse of personality, a descent from a higher to a lower plane of being during the interval separating the dream state from wakefulness and could clearly mark a narrowing down of the self, as if forced to shrink from a state of wide expansion to one of close confinement. There was undeniable evidence to show that the temporary transformation of personality apparent in the dreams was brought about by physiological processes which affected the whole organism, causing a heavy pressure on every part.

During sleep my pulse rate was often considerably higher than during the day. I verified the fact frequently by putting my fingers to the pulse immediately on awakening at any time during the night. On numerous occasions I found it so rapid as to cause anxiety. The full and rapid beats clearly pointed to an undoubtedly accelerated metabolic process, to a quickly racing blood stream, to countless formations and alterations in cellular tissues, all affected by the vital current which swept like a storm through the entire organism with the obvious aim of refashioning it to a higher pitch of efficiency.

Lack of sufficient knowledge of physiology made it difficult for the ancient adepts to correlate the psychic and physiological reactions caused by the activity of kundalini. I labored under the same disadvantage, but on account of the fact that a superficial knowledge of every branch of science is an easily acquired possession in these days of research and publicity, and that I had ample opportunity to study my condition day to day for many years, it became possible for me to observe critically the effects of the sudden development upon my system and to draw tentative inferences from it.

I was irresistibly led to the conclusion that this extraordinary activity of the nervous system and brain is present in varying degrees in all cases of supernormal spiritual and psychic development, in a lesser measure in all cases of genius, in a still diminished form in all men and women of exceptionally high intellectual caliber, and in a morbid manner, when too violent and sudden or operative through a wrong nerve, in many kinds of insanity, neurosis, and other obscure and difficult-to-cure nervous and mental afflictions.

Kundalini, as known to and described by the ancient authorities, signifies the development, sometimes spontaneous, and less frequently through special psychophysiological exercises, of extraordinary spiritual and mental powers associated with religion and the supernatural. There can be no doubt whatsoever that the incessant, easily perceptible, rapid movement at the base of my spine, affecting the nerves lining the whole area, was an indication of the fact that, controlled by an invisible mechanism, a hidden organ had begun to function all of a sudden in the hitherto innocent-looking region, converting the reproductive fluid into a radiant vital essence of high potency which, racing along the nerve fibers as well as the spinal canal, nourished the brain and the organs with a rejuvenating substance out of reach in any other way.

For a long time I labored under the belief that the glow in the head and the powerful nervous currents darting through my body were all simply occasioned by the sublimated seed itself, but as time wore on I was forced to alter my opinion. The activity in the reproductive region was not the only new development that had occurred.

A corresponding change in the brain and other nerve centers had also taken place which regulated the consumption and output of the new mechanism. After the crisis the luminous currents did not move chaotically but with definite aim and purpose, which was clearly evident from the fact that the whole organism overcame the initial resistance of recalcitrant and inferior parts and began gradually to adjust itself to the new development.

On the strength of these and other facts I gradually came to the conclusion, which it shall rest with future investigators to confirm or disprove, that by virtue of the evolutionary processes still going on in the human body, a high-powered conscious center is being evolved by nature in the human brain at a place near the crown of the head, built of exceptionally sensitive brain tissue. The location of the center allows it to command all parts of the brain and the entire nervous system with a direct connection with the reproductive organs through the spinal canal. In the ordinary person, the budding center draws its nourishment from the concentrated nerve food present in the seed in such extremely limited measure so as not to interfere with the normal reproductive function of the parts.

When completely modified, the center in evolved individuals is designed to function in place of the existing conscious center, using for its activity a more powerful vital fuel extracted by nerve fibers from the body tissues in extremely minute quantities, collected and rushed through the spinal tube into the brain.

When the center accidentally begins to function prematurely, before the nerve connections and links have been fully established and the delicate brain cells habituated to the flow of the powerful current, the result is likely to be disastrous. The delicate tissues of the body in that case are likely to be damaged irreparably, causing strange maladies, insanity, or death. In a grave emergency of this kind the only way open to nature to avoid a catastrophe is to use liberally the ambrosia contained in the human seed and to rush it in a sublimated form to the brain, the nervous network, and the main organs, in order to provide the injured and dying cells with the most powerful restorative and food available in the body to save life.

The whole organism now begins to function in a most amazing manner which cannot but strike terror into the stoutest heart. Tossed between the old and yet incomparably modified new conscious center, the subject, unprepared for such a startling development, sees himself losing control of his thoughts and actions. He finds himself confronted by a rebellious mind and unruly senses, and organs working in an inexplicable way, entirely foreign to him, as if the world, suddenly turned upside down, had dragged him to a topsy-turvy existence as weird and bizarre as the most fantastic dream.

It is for this reason that the ancient teachers of kundalini yoga, on the basis of experience extending for thousands of years, insisted on an exceptionally robust and hardy constitution, mastery over appetites and desires, voluntarily acquired control over vital functions and organs, and, above all, the possession of an inflexible will, as the essentially needed qualifications in those offering themselves for the supreme undertaking of rousing the Shakti. An excellent condition of both body and mind, difficult to achieve in the unfavorable environment of modern civilization, is absolutely necessary in an enterprise of this nature to prevent the brain from giving way completely under the unbearable strain. It is not surprising, therefore, that any one who set himself determinedly to the hazardous task of awakening Kundalini before Her time was acclaimed a *vira*, meaning a hero, and the practice itself designated as *vira sadhana*. or heroic undertaking, even by fearless ascetics themselves, indifferent to physical torture and death.

It should not be thought, even for an instant, that the alarming alteration in mental processes or the condition of the nervous system, tending to produce a most stupefying and bizarre effect on even the most daring yogi, persists for a short duration, only to be followed by a return to normality with a mastery over the newly developed powers. After the awakening, the devotee lives always at the mercy of kundalini, wafted to a new state of existence and introduced to a new world as far removed from this one of rapid change and decay as reality is from a dream.

The hypersensitive and critical condition of the nerves and the brain, caused by the unceasing effort of the marvelous invisible power to mold them to a higher and higher state of cognition, the possibility of injury and damage to the oversensitive tissues, the process of repair and rejuvenation with the administration of nerve tonics and restoratives present in the system, and the tremendous strain on the excessively worked reproductive organs, may continue undiminished for years. The only change is that with the lapse of time the individual becomes more and more accustomed to the play of the newly developed force in him and is able to regulate his habits and appetites according to the revised requirements of his system on the strength of the experience gained.

The time of sleep, when the body is at rest and the mind comparatively quiescent, provides the best occasion for the remodeling process to gather momentum, by using the surplus energy dissipated during the day in voluntary physical and mental activity for reconstructive purposes. This results in a greater flow of the radiant vital energy into the brain with a corresponding amplification of the dream personality and other contents of the dream. The entire matter of the brain is invigorated with a copious flow of the subtle essence, abundantly supplied by the organs of reproduction, which makes it possible for the delicate tissues to maintain their activity at the pitch to which they are raised by the powerful vital current streaming into the cephalic cavity in conformity with the needs of the newly opened center of higher consciousness. The self-regulating mechanism of the body, trying desperately to adjust itself to the sudden development, lets no opportunity escape to bring about the necessary changes in the organism on every favorable occasion, in spite of the resistance offered, particularly when awake, by the ego consciousness which, acting during the day and dreaming during the night, tossed up and down like a cork floating on the surface of a billowy sea, remains entirely in the dark about the wonders enacted in its mortal mold.

My dreams had, therefore, a peculiar significance, and from the time of the awakening to the present day they have been no less an active and remarkable feature of my existence than the busy hours of wakefulness.

Except for the fact that it is attended by psychic manifestations of an extraordinary nature, presenting an appearance of abnormality, the awakening of kundalini is a perfectly natural biological phenomenon of an uncommon kind, demonstrable by any healthy human body on the attainment of a certain state of evolutionary development. The only peculiarity which gives it a semblance of the bizarre and the uncanny is the biological process which, set afoot, leads to the emergence of a conscious personality so superior and possessing such astounding, almost superhuman, attributes as to make the whole phenomenon appear to be the performance of a supernatural agency rather than the outcome of the operation of natural, though as yet unknown, biological laws.

Those who possess an extensive knowledge of the animal kingdom know of numerous surprising instances of such extraordinary instinctive behavior in certain lower forms of life as can aptly be classed as marvelous and even uncanny, but when corresponding gifts of an amazing nature, developed by the operation of yet obscure biological laws, are consciously exercised by a human being with a more elaborately fashioned brain and nervous system, the phenomenon is often regarded with suspicion and disbelief by the same observers who would accept it unquestioningly in lower forms of life.

To deny that the human body is capable of exhibiting an organic activity that can sustain or lead to a consciousness of the supersensory type involves also the denial of some fundamental concepts of religion, of inspired prophethood, and of all kinds of spiritual phenomena. If the human system is incapable of developing a brain and nervous activity expressive of a higher form of consciousness than that which is common to all individuals, it is in that case equally incapable of exhibiting superordinary mental faculties and supernormal spiritual attributes, for the simple reason that in all forms of life existing on earth there is an unalterable relationship between the organism and the level of consciousness; and since it would be unscientific to suppose without demonstrable proof that, of all living creatures, the human being alone forms an exception to this rule, it will have to be admitted that an extraordinary development of the human mind, radically different from, or strikingly above its normal range of expression, must necessarily be attended by a corresponding change in or development of its biological equipment also.

The first pertinent question is likely to be how this alteration and development takes place in the face of the fact that for any such activity to be effective it must have existed as a continuous evolutionary process for ages, for which the human body, particularly the skull, provides no convincing proof, having exhibited no marked variation over past thousands of years conspicuous enough to furnish conclusive evidence for a radical change in the brain, the seat of its mental expression.

If the answer to this be that the alteration does not occur in the size or shape of the brain or any other vital organ or in the body as a whole but in the arrangement, quality, and composition of the constituents of the body in respect of the extremely subtle life element present in every cell and part of the organism, the point raised in the question would cease to have any weight. The obvious reluctance of many otherwise highly intelligent minds to accord recognition to the validity of spiritual experience and the reality of psychical phenomena is due mainly to the inability of empirical science to grasp or analyze the true nature of the life principle animating the cell, the ultimate unit of all organic structures.

At the present stage of our knowledge, the arousing of kundalini provides the only possible way to study the extraordinary behavior and possibilities of the life element and the subtle biochemical medium by means of which it manipulates the organism and is able to augment or reduce its efficacy and power, leading to bewildering diversity in intellectual acumen and spiritual insight of persons possessing approximately the same dimensions of the head and the same size and weight of the brain.

It is a great mistake to treat the human being as a completely finished and hermetically sealed product, entirely debarred from passing beyond the present limits imposed by his or her mental constitution. There is a big gap between the human and the most intelligent anthropoid apes, whose habits, it is said, we shared only a few thousand centuries ago, advancing in an inexplicable way beyond the mental boundary reached by the other members of that family. The cause of departure must have originated *within*, as external influences have no radically modifying effect on a mental compartment sealed by Nature.

According to the popular beliefs in India, Kundalini is possessed of marvelous attributes. She is Para-Shakti, the supreme energy, which, as illusive maya, inveigles the embodied jiva (individual soul) into the mesh of transitory appearances, bound helplessly to the ever-rotating wheel of life and death. She is the seductive female who lures him to the bed of enjoyment followed by procreation and pain, and She is also the compassionate mother who creates in him the thirst for knowledge and the desire for supersensible experience and endows him finally with spiritual insight to lead him towards the realization of his own celestial nature.

Amazing stories are current about the manner in which some very famous literary stars of India, whose names are household words, became the fortunate recipients of the grace of Kundalini and from being common men and women soared to unrivaled heights of poetic and literary genius almost overnight. They emerged as accomplished poets, rhetoricians, dramatists, and philosophers without the aid of teachers, without training, and sometimes without even the rudiments of education. There are also incredibly strange anecdotes of the marvelous psychic gifts showered by Kundalini on many exceptionally favored devotees almost on Her very first appearance before them in a vision, investing the hitherto unknown aspirants with such miraculous powers as enabled them apparently to defy at will some of the otherwise inviolable laws of Nature.

Yet try as I might, I could not at that time observe in myself the slightest sign of any such incredible development, and as year after year passed without bringing any major alteration in my mental or spiritual endowment, barring the luminosity and the widening of consciousness, I began to feel that the episode was over and the peculiarity in my mental makeup was probably all that I was destined to see of the supersensible in my life.

I was neither happy nor dejected at the idea. The awful experience I had undergone and the terror that had haunted me relentlessly for months had had a chastening and curbing effect on my previous desire for supernatural adventure. The boundary line dividing the natural from the supernatural was not, I thought, negotiable by all and sundry; and as subsequent events clearly revealed to me, this narrow strip is so well protected that the cleverest person is sure to blunder into one pitfall or another unless guided at every step by a higher self-illuminating intelligence, which ceases to shine at the slightest tinge of impurity in the heart.

The existence of a superintelligent internal monitor has been avowedly acknowledged by some very famous individuals, both past and present, the monitor being none other than the mystic personality developed by kundalini, imperceptibly active in them from birth.

After the incidents mentioned in the preceding chapters, I lived an almost normal life for years, similar to that of other men in all respects except for the ferment noticeable during the hours of sleep. The great increase in the metabolic activity of the body, resulting in more rapid heart action, followed by lassitude in the mornings, and the dynamic nature of my dreams, unmistakably pointed to the possibility that my system was being subjected to some kind of internal pressure which tended to accelerate the organic functions beyond the normal limit. On numerous occasions I was forcibly struck by the resemblance that I bore during those days to a growing baby, utterly unconscious of the great changes occurring in every part of the tiny frame, tending to bring it by imperceptible degrees nearer and nearer to the massive proportions of manhood. I also closely resembled a baby in the frequency of intake and more rapid digestion of food, quicker and more thorough elimination, longer periods of rest and sleep, and by an abnormal rapidity of the pulse, unaccompanied by fever or any other symptoms of illness. It was obvious that under the action of the transformed nervous energy my body functioned in a definitely altered manner in certain respects, forced to greater activity probably with some ultimate object in view which I could in no way guess at that time.

Apparently my body had become a target for invisible but super-intelligent living forces which, using the surplus energy provided by my considerably enhanced intake and better assimilation of food, temperate habits, and frequently long periods of strict continence, were hammering away at my interior, bending and twisting the cells and organs to the required shape or the required degree of functional activity in order to make the whole system fit for the operation of a more potent life energy. The consistency in the symptoms and the mechanical regularity with which my body functioned under the action of the new vital current made it evident that, even in its altered behavior, the organism was following a certain clearly marked rhythm, an essential characteristic of life in any form.

This was a matter of great consolation to a man like me whose every night was a witness to strange, incomprehensible activities in his interior, as it tended to provide proof for the fact that whatever transpired was taking place in accordance with certain biological laws to which the body was responding in an orderly, systematic manner. Such would not be the case if an unnatural and chaotic condition had overcome the organism.

In the beginning I mistook the normal mode of operation of the new vital energy for a sudden disorder of the nervous system attended by malformation and erratic behavior of the nervous currents. The descriptions contained in the ancient esoteric treatises on Kundalini represent the Goddess as a stream of radiant energy, ambrosial in effect, which, when roused by the power of concentration and *pranayama*, can be led gradually to Her supreme abode at the crown of the head, there to taste the ineffable bliss of an embrace with Her divine spouse, God Shiva, residing in the consciousness of the yogi.

In the course of Her ascent from Her seat at the base of the spine to the crown, it is averred that She waters with nectar the six lotuses flourishing at the six important nerve junctions on the cerebrospinal axis governing the vital and sensory organs, which bloom at Her approach, until She arrives at the thousand-petalled lotus at the top of the head and is absorbed in ecstatic union with Her heavenly consort. When released from the chains which bind it to earth, the embodied consciousness soars to sublime heights of self-realization, made aware for the first time after ages of bondage of its own ineffable, deathless nature.

It is said that at the time of Her descent She repasses the lotuses, which droop and close their petals at Her departure, until She assumes Her original dormant state at the base of the spine, bringing down with Her the temporarily liberated consciousness, adding link after link to the fetter which binds the attributeless eternal substance inexorably to the flesh until the chain is complete at the last stage, when the yogi, coming down gradually from a condition of unutterable beatitude, awakes again to the world as embodied spirit, dominated by the senses, retaining only a brief but striking memory of its flight into the Infinite.

The writings on hatha yoga contain graphic descriptions of these lotuses, their exact location, the number of petals on each, the name and form of the presiding deity, the letters of the Sanskrit alphabet associated with them, and the like. The students are enjoined to meditate on them in that form while practicing *pranayama*, beginning particularly with the lowest, or *muladhara*, chakra, close to the abode of the Goddess. The centers bearing the lotuses are called chakras. Five of them are considered to be the centers of vital energy distinguished by thick clusters of nerves situated at different points along the spinal cord, which some modern writers identify with the various plexuses. The sixth is said to be located in the brain at a spot corresponding to the point of junction of the two eyebrows and the root of the nose, and the seventh is in the cerebrum.

Biologically, a healthy human organism with an intelligent brain should provide at its present stage of evolution a fit abode for the manifestation of a higher form of consciousness than that which is the normal endowment of human beings in the present age. Its brain, nervous system, and the vital organs should have attained the state of perfection, according to the evolutionary standard, where a higher personality can step in without much commotion to take over control of the body.

But ages of incorrect living in obedience to the dictates of civilization have played havoc with this most intricate machine, marring the growth of the organs and the efficiency of the nerves and loading the system with nervous poisons too subtle to be eliminated by the administration of drugs or other therapeutic agents. This is the main reason why the present-day human organism, instead of expediting the process, offers a strong resistance to its investiture with a more potent form of vitality, an essential preliminary to the installation of a higher personality.

By no means known to science can this cleaning and remodeling of the body be done to make it fit for the transfer of power. All systems of yoga aim at achieving this by overcoming these deficiencies. Kundalini is the mechanism as well as the motive force by which this biological trimming and remodeling is accomplished in the most effective manner, provided the system is not too much deteriorated either by its own defective mode of life or because of a retrogressive heredity.

The kundalini awakening being a rare but natural biological phenomenon, it is futile to enter into a discussion of the reality of the lotuses, on which a good deal of emphasis has been laid by the ancient authorities. I did not come across any in the course of my own long adventure, not even a vestige of one in any part of the cerebrospinal system. To assume their existence even for an instant in these days of physiological knowledge and research would mean nothing short of an insult to intelligence. In all probability their existence was suggested graphically to the disciples with colorful detail as an aid to concentration and to signify the location of the more sensitive and easier-to-effect brain and nerve centers, as well as to symbolize chastity; the lotus flower, unaffected by the condition of water in which it grows, has always served as an emblem of purity.

By denying the tangible existence of the lotuses and other accessories associated with them, it is not intended in the least to undervalue or ridicule in any way the colossal work done by the ancient masters, whose achievement in this insecure and inaccessible domain has been nothing short of marvelous.

The idea of chakras and lotuses must have been suggested to the mind of the ancient teachers by the singular resemblance which, in the awakened state, the lustrous nerve centers bear to a luminous revolving disc, studded with lights, or to a lotus flower in full bloom glistening in the rays of the sun. The circle of glowing radiance round the head, tinged at times with rainbow colors and supported by the thin streak of light moving upward through the spinal duct, bears an unmistakable likeness to a blooming lotus with its thin stalk trailing downwards in the water, conveying to it the nutritive elements drawn by means of innumerable root fibers, exactly in the same manner as the living stalk of *sushumna* supplies the subtle organic essence drawn from every part of the corporeal frame by means of countless nerve filaments to feed the flame lit by kundalini. It resembles, in effect, a gorgeous lotus of extraordinary brilliance, having a thousand petals to denote its large dimensions.

In the absence of adequate physiological information the old savants probably could not seize hold of a better method, not only to indicate the position of the nerve clusters which had to become seats of intense activity simultaneously with the awakening but also to prepare the uninitiated disciples for their subsequent brightly illumined lotus-like appearance.

I have tried to make the point clear, as readers in the least familiar with the writings on kundalini are likely to be struck by the singular absence of any reference in this work to the reality of chakras and lotuses, so lavishly dealt with in other books that a whole literature has grown around them, detracting from the scientific value of the actual phenomenon. I never practiced yoga by Tantric methods of which *pranayama*, meditation on the nerve centers, and posture are essential features. If I had done so with a firm belief in the existence of the lotuses, I might well have mistaken the luminous formations and the glowing discs of light at the various nerve junctions along the spinal cord for lotuses, and in the excited state of my imagination might even have been led to perceive the letters and the presiding deities in vivid form, suggested by the pictures already present in my mind.

By the grace of the divine energy I was destined to witness a phenomenon of another kind, a unique phenomenon undoubtedly repeated many times during the past but in all probability seldom studied in detail and certainly never recorded in plain language free of unintelligible descriptions and metaphors. Astounding as it may appear, I am convinced that an emphasis was designedly laid on great suffering to me, particularly on such items of the experience as enabled me, though very imperfectly, to trace the biological processes responsible for the phenomenon.

It is mainly because of this that I am in a position to adduce certain hitherto inexplicable facts, fully confident that the indistinct track now pointed out, passing zig-zag through the thick undergrowth of superstition and ceremonial, will with the labor of competent investigators soon lead to surprising developments and momentous results.

I was destined to witness my own transformation, not comparable in any way to the great transfigurations in the past, nor similar in point of results to the marvelous achievements of genius; but though simple in nature and ordinary in effect, a transformation nevertheless attended all along by great physical and mental suffering. But what I witnessed and still witness within myself is so contrary to many accepted notions of science, at variance with many time-honored dogmas of faith, and so antagonistic to many of the universally followed dictums of civilization, that when what I have experienced is proved empirically there must occur a far-reaching, revolutionary change in every sphere of human activity and conduct.

What I realized beyond the least shadow of doubt is the fact, corroborated in part by ancient seers of many lands and more concretely by those in India, that in the human body there exists an extremely subtle and intricate mechanism located in the sexual region which, while active in the normal person in the naturally restricted form of intercourse and procreation, tends to develop the body generation after generation, subject of course to the vicissitudes of life, for the expression of a higher personality at the end; but when roused to rapid activity, it reacts strongly on the parent organism, effecting in course of time, subject again to numerous factors, a marvelous transformation of the nervous system and the brain, resulting in the manifestation of a superior type of consciousness, which will be the common inheritance of human beings in the distant future.

This mechanism, known as kundalini, is the real cause of all genuine spiritual and psychic phenomena, the biological basis of evolution and development of personality, the secret origin of all esoteric and occult doctrines, the master key to the unsolved mystery of creation, the inexhaustible source of philosophy, art, and science, and the fountainhead of all religious faiths, past, present, and future.

FOURTEEN

Losing Hope, I Prepared for Death

IT WAS MY GOOD FORTUNE to have relatives and friends whose affection, loyalty, and help contributed to make the risky path I was traversing safe and smooth for me. My two sisters, their husbands, the father and brothers of my wife, and also my friends, few but sincere, surrounded me with affection and loyalty. My mother had died more than one and a half years before the occurrence and yet it was no less to her excellent upbringing than to the great devotion of my wife that I owed my survival. Among all my benefactors they stand out like two ministering angels, and the debt of gratitude for the unbounded love they bore me and the invaluable service they rendered I can never hope to repay in this world. It was my great good luck to have a mother whose kindness of heart, nobility of character, sense of duty, and purity were exemplary, and whose boundless love molded my childhood and youth, exercising the greatest influence for good on my whole life.

Looking back now at the years which followed the awakening, I can affirm unhesitatingly that but for the robust constitution bequeathed to me by my parents and certain good traits of character inherited or learned from them I could never have survived the ordeal and lived to relate it. Although for many years of my altered life I never breathed freely like a man sure of himself and of what he had to do, and I was at no time entirely without doubt about my condition, I managed by adopting an attitude of calm resignation to the inevitable and indifference to death, partly the effect of parental influence and partly cultivation, to keep my mind undisturbed even in grave situations. Often my difficulties were caused by my own neglect of the conditions regulating my peculiar existence, unavoidable in the storm and stress of life, and sometimes by attacks of common ailments, for each of which I had to discover and apply the right treatment by trial and error suited to the changed reactions of my body.

An ordinary man in a humble walk of life, burdened with responsibilities, as I always have been and think myself to be, I never allowed any false idea about myself to take root in my mind after the new development. On the other hand, my absolute helplessness before the lately manifest power in me had the effect of humbling what little remnant of pride I still possessed. I attended to all my affairs in the same manner as I had always done before the change. The only thing to remind me of the internal upheaval was rigid regularity in diet and an adherence to certain other austere ways of conduct, which experience taught me to adopt in order to minimize resistance to the activity of the mighty energy at work inside me.

Outwardly I lived a strictly normal life, permitting no one, save my devoted wife, to have the least glimpse into the mysterious happenings in my interior. Every year I moved to Jammu in winter with my office and to Kashmir in summer, in this manner to escape the rigor of heat and cold which might have proved injurious to the growth of the supersensitive tissues then in a state of development within. Gradually, in the course of a few years my body attained a degree of hardiness and strength sufficient to withstand the effect of fasts, discomforts of travel, rigors of climate, irregularities in diet, overstrain, worries, and adverse circumstances which form an inevitable corollary to the struggle for existence.

I became almost my old self again, humbled and chastened by the experience, with a good deal less of ego and a great deal more of faith in the Unseen Arbitrator of human destiny. The main thing I was aware of was a progressively expanding field of consciousness and a slowly increasing brightness of the external and internal objects of perception, which, in course of time, brought the idea irresistibly home to me that though outwardly one with the restlessly active mass of humanity, I was a different being inside, living in a lustrous world of brilliant color of which others had no knowledge whatsoever.

In mentioning apparently minor details I am influenced by the consideration that I should not omit any relevant facts. Transformation of personality is fraught with risks, needing attention to every phase of conduct and careful regulation of activity. If all I have to relate had been known but a few centuries earlier, the knowledge properly systematized and applied might have helped physicians to save many persons from the clutches of insanity.

It was my ill luck not to have understood for many years what I have learned now after repeated bitter struggles. Side by side with the suffering, however, I have also tasted moments of incomparable happiness, supreme moments which liberally compensated me for long periods of pain and anguish, as the mere act of waking to reality instantaneously compensates a sleeper for the awful agony suffered in a prolonged nightmare.

About three years after the incidents narrated in the preceding chapters, I began to feel an irresistible desire for a more nourishing and substantial diet than that to which I had accustomed myself from the time of the awakening. The desire was more in evidence in winter when I was in Jammu than in the months of summer spent in Kashmir. Those were the closing years of the Second World War, and the prices of commodities had risen enormously. Unable to assign any reasons for the sudden excess in a now otherwise normal appetite, I restrained the inclination because I considered it improper to give way to a desire which had something of the gourmand in it and also because our extremely limited means did not allow me the additional expenditure. Despite meager resources our diet was sufficiently nutritious and balanced, including certain varieties of animal food, against which Kashmiri Brahmins as a community do not have any scruple. But the urge in me was not without good reason, and I had to pay bitterly for my shortsighted resistance to an impulse intended to expedite the process still going on as strongly as ever in my interior.

Soon after our annual move to Jammu in the month of November 1943 I received an invitation from my relatives in Multan to spend a few days with them during the ensuing winter. As it afforded me an opportunity to meet my cousins whom I had not seen for many years, I determined to accept the invitation to go there during the Christmas holidays, extending the period by a few more days if necessary. That year, feeling particularly fit and strong, I left my wife at Srinagar and came alone to Jammu to stay with her brother, the municipal engineer of the town. He hired a building in an open locality on the outskirts of the town where, having a room all to myself and finding all my simple needs well provided for, I felt entirely at home, happy at the change and harboring not the slightest suspicion that all my cheer would vanish in the horror of another awful trial.

I was happy to find myself in full possession of my normal health with a surplus amount of energy demanding an outlet. From early November I started taking easy physical exercises, beginning with the first gray streaks of dawn and ending with the sun just near the horizon, after which I had a cold bath and retired to my room for rest and study until office time. I do not know how it happened, but after only a few weeks of the program the urge to take exercise partially disappeared, yielding place to a strong, almost irresistible desire for meditation. The glow of vibrant health resulting from systematic exertion made me feel reckless, and looking for an avenue to make the best use of my superb physical condition, I felt half inclined to yield to the impulse and try my luck again, swayed by the thought that with the experience gained and the immunity acquired by the organism I might succeed without encountering the mishap I had suffered last time. I had escaped by a miracle to pass years of uncertainty and suspense before I found myself again on firm ground. What an imbecile I was, I sternly told myself, not to profit by my previous extremely bitter experience and to expose myself again to the same ghastly battle, the wounds of which were still fresh in my heart.

In spite of my sober reflections, in spite of myself, in spite of the suffering I had borne in consequence of it, I again felt an urge to meditate and yielded to this urge with disastrous results, which kept me in anguish, pain and suspense for a long time afterwards. Viewed from the knowledge gained in subsequent years, the details of the amazing experience I underwent are of tremendous importance. I believe the condition of my nervous system had become more stabilized by this time. The production of the gross pranic substance, its conversion into high-grade radiation which irradiated my brain day and night had now become an habitual function of my system. The nerves, the fleshy tissues, the visceral organs and the brain had become fully accustomed to the new activity and there were no ups and downs in my mind to keep me in fear and suspense. In other words, the alluring expanded state of consciousness with its glowing luster and blissful nature had now become the native state of my being.

During these days, we lived in a building on the outskirts of the city. On stepping up to the roof one could obtain a clear view of the city and the distant hills covered with trees. The spectacle was always fascinating for me. It was not only from this particular place that the panorama seen appeared so bewitching to my eyes, but wherever and whenever I happened to look from an elevated spot at a vast landscape in front, the effect was almost always the same. I had looked at some of these sights from the same spots once or several times before and had a clear recollection of the view they presented. But now there was a marvelous transformation. It seemed as if I was looking at the landscape of a master artist painted with brilliant crystalline colors that held me spellbound by their transparency and loveliness.

It was obvious that I was now looking at the world with a new instrument of perception. It mellowed and beautified even an ugly or sordid scene. A panorama, charming to the normal eye, appeared like a fairyland. How this change had occurred I did not know. The observer in me was invested with a new power of brightening and beautifying all the objects which I saw.

Could it be possible, I often debated within myself, that the great poets, the great musicians and the great artists have an element of the same perceptive quality ingrained in their cognitive faculty? They see a light, a harmony or a beauty which is not perceptible to the average human being. But they do not know that they alone possess this particular type of perception and not the others. The world is in ignorance of a momentous secret relating to our minds. Enlightenment, genius, high intelligence and the aesthetic sense are not gifts added to a uniform texture of our minds, but a part of the spectrum which makes up what we are.

When we compare one human being to another and say that A is more intelligent or more aesthetic or more artistic or more enlightened than B, we nearly always invest both of them with the same quality of consciousness, based on a picture of our mind, believing that one of them has more of certain talents or faculties than the other. This is not entirely correct. It is the very texture of the mind or consciousness which has a difference in quality, distinguishing one from the other. We cannot detect this variation in the texture of the mind because we can never fully perceive the personality of another, even those nearest and dearest to us. I could clearly observe this variation in the pattern of my consciousness before the awakening and the form it assumed years after, when a bright, alluring state of my vision became a permanent feature of the "knower" in me. I was definitely not the same personality which I had been before the memorable experience in December 1937.

This fact is of tremendous importance. The human mind or soul is not a uniform or untamable element, and all human beings are not alike in the fabric of their mind. It is a variable stuff. The enormous gulf that exists between the mind of an imbecile and an intellectual is not so much due to the difference in the pattern of the brain as in the texture of consciousness. This is what the empiricists fail to realize when they look into the fabric of the brain to account for the extraordinary ability of genius. They have to look into the mind and the source behind it, namely the pranic radiation which, for its subtle organic fuel, depends on a still-unknown activity of the nerves. I believe what I am asserting can be demonstrated experimentally. Observation of a few cases of a powerfully awakened kundalini would be sufficient to gain preliminary knowledge of the processes that occur to enhance the potency of the pranic radiation in order to install a new form of consciousness in the brain.

I felt almost stabilized in my new state of consciousness when I started to meditate again in December of the year 1943. The urge to meditate was irresistible. It overpowered me to such an extent that I ceased to remember the awful ordeals I had to face in yielding to the same urge in December of the year 1937. It seemed to me that some kind of a rhythm was operating in my system which began a new cycle in or about the month of December. I became more aware of this rhythm in the later years when I started to compose spontaneously in verse. An irresistible impulse to write occurred in December or a little earlier every year. The two or three following months served as my most productive period. It was only when an unfavorable state of the body or uncongenial circumstances occurred to prevent the desire from taking shape that I sometimes lost this period of productivity. The loss was then made up at some other time during the year.

I began to meditate again from the first week in December, starting from the early hours of dawn, losing myself in the contemplation of the wonderful lustrous glow within, until the sun, risen high above the horizon, shone full in my room, indicating the nearness of the office hour. For a number of days, in addition to the marvelous extension of personality and absorption in the enrapturing conscious glow that I had experienced on the first day of the awakening, differing only in the color of the radiance, I felt a sense of elation and power impossible to describe. It persisted through the day and in my dreams to the hour of practice, and was replenished again the next morning to last for another day.

During these spells of meditation I could distinctly perceive an effulgent aureole around my body stretching to some distance beyond it. This was now the area of my expanded consciousness. When I closed my eyes in meditation I felt a vast glowing circle of awareness round me. As usual, I focused my attention on the crown of my head and concentrated on the light which I perceived there. After only a few days this bore fruit and I became witness to a blissful experience which, if it had not been repeated in me several times, I could never have believed possible when described by another.

Astounded at the result of my effort, I increased the period of meditation by beginning earlier, completely overpowered by the wonder and glory of the vision which, luring away my senses from the harsh world of mingled joy and pain, carried me to a supersensory plane where, caressed by lustrous waves of indescribable rapture, I found myself immersed in the boundless ocean of unconditioned being.

It was indeed a marvelous experience, and I felt my hair literally stand on end when the stupendous vision wore its most majestic aspect. It seemed on every such occasion as if I or the invisible cognitive self in me, leaving its safe anchorage in the flesh, was carried by the strong outgoing tide of a lustrous consciousness towards an existence of such immensity and power as made everything I could conceive of on earth tame and trite in comparison: an existence where, untroubled by any idea of bondage or limitation, I found myself lost in an amazing immaterial universe so stupendous in extent, so sublime and marvelous in nature, that the human element still left in me, even when at the highest point of the experience, stared in amazement and trembled with awe at the mighty spectacle present before my internal eye.

To the best of my knowledge, this picture of kundalini arousal has never been described in plain language before. It has been metaphorically or obliquely mentioned, probably in order to prevent the uninitiated, attracted by its fascination and delight, from doing irretrievable harm to themselves by dabbling in its mysteries.

The symptoms attending a sudden powerful arousal of kundalini are so marked and characteristic that those who experience them seldom fail to take note of their real nature. The votaries of Shakti, the Taoists of China, the Buddhist followers of the Tantric path, and the hatha yogis of India have all borne witness in veiled language and metaphor to their involvement with the procreative kundalini. The medieval saints of India, the Christian mystics, and the Sufis, too, have not been remiss in noticing the resemblance between the rapture experienced in ecstasy and the transport of the conjugal union.

In fact, the intensity of love expressed for the deity by mystics of all ages and climes, both men and women, in many cases has clearly an overtone of the erotic in it. Even the great mystics have been misunderstood and misrepresented, vilified and criticized because the real nature of their experience and the somatic factors that gave rise to their passion of ecstatic love for the Divine have never been clearly understood.

I was overjoyed at the glorious possibility within my reach now. There could be absolutely no doubt that I was the exceedingly fortunate possessor of an awakened kundalini. It was only now that I could grasp the reason why in ancient times success in this undertaking was thought to be the highest achievement possible to a human being and why the followers of this path considered no sacrifice too much and no effort too great for the supreme prize attainable at the end. I now understood why accomplished yogis were always treated with the highest respect in India and how adepts, who had lived long ago, even now commanded an homage and a reverence which have not fallen to the share of any other class of people, including mighty rulers and potentates. There was certainly no honor more signal or fortune more precious than that which, without my asking for it, had been bestowed on me.

But, alas, my good luck was to be exceedingly short-lived, although this was not immediately apparent. After only a couple of weeks I found that the ferment caused in my mind by the breathtaking experience was so great that I could hardly sleep for excitement and was awake hours before the time of meditation, impatient to induce the blissful condition again as soon as possible. The impressions of the last three days terminating this extraordinary period of excursions into the normally forbidden domain of the supersensible are indelibly imprinted upon my memory.

Before losing myself entirely in the contemplation of an unbounded, glowing, conscious void, I had distinctly felt an incomparably blissful sensation in all my nerves, moving from the tips of fingers and toes and other parts of the trunk and limbs towards the spine, where, concentrated and intensified, it mounted upwards with a still more exquisitely pleasant feeling to pour into the upper region of the brain a rapturous and exhilarating stream of a rare radiating nerve secretion. In the absence of a more suitable appellation, I call it nectar, a name given to it by the ancient savants.

All the authorities on kundalini yoga are agreed about the reality of the ambrosial current, which irrigates the seventh center in the brain at the moment of the union of Shakti with Shiva, the superconscious principle behind the embodied self, and it is said that the flow of the nectar into it or into one of the lower centers on the spinal axis is always accompanied by a most exquisite rapture impossible to describe, exceeding many times in intensity that most pleasurable of bodily sensations, the orgasm, which marks the climax of sexual union.

On the last day of this unique experience I had no sleep during the night. My mind was in a state of excitement and turmoil with joy and exhilaration at this most unexpected and unbelievable stroke of luck. I rose up at my usual time in a hurry and after feasting my mental eye on the elevating beauty and grandeur that was now a reality for me, went to the market to make some purchases. I returned at nearly one o'clock in the afternoon in an unusual state of exhaustion, which surprised me. I had not taken my breakfast that day and accordingly attributed my weakness to an empty stomach. The next day, the twenty-fifth of December, I had to leave for Multan by the morning train to see my cousins. I remained busy until evening, making preparations for the journey, and after dining at the usual hour retired early to bed.

Only a few minutes after lying down, the stark realization came to me that I had woefully blundered again. My head reeled, my ears buzzed with a harsh, discordant noise, and in place of the usual resplendent glow in my head a wide column of fire was mounting up, shooting out forked tongues of flame in every direction. Trembling with fear, I watched the awful display. Too late I understood what had happened. I had overdone the practice of meditation and strained my already overstimulated nervous system to a dangerous limit.

It is needless for me to recapitulate all the incidents and details of the torture that I suffered again on this occasion for more than three months. Suffice it to say that after passing a terribly restless night I did not feel fit to undertake the long journey to Multan in the morning and was compelled to abandon the journey. Discarding meditation, I again took all care to regulate my diet as I had done the last time. In a few days I noticed a slight relief in the tension in my head, but the insomnia grew worse and I became weaker every day.

Alarmed at my condition, my brother-in-law expressed his intention of writing to my wife to come to Jammu. It was the middle of January now and the winding mountainous roads from Srinagar were covered with snow, making travel extremely uncomfortable and even risky. Anxious to avoid inconvenience to my wife as well as a shock, I dissuaded him from doing so, hoping that the disturbance would cease after some time.

One day, finding that I was unable to rise from bed without assistance and losing all hope of survival, I yielded to the exhortations of my brother-in-law to send a telegram to my wife. She arrived in all haste, half dead with anxiety, accompanied by her father and my younger son.

Day and night, without an hour's undisturbed rest for herself, my wife waited on me, attending to my every need, trying to soothe by her presence the internal agony I was suffering, which she could not visualize in all its horror but the external indications of which she could see every moment without difficulty. My father-in-law, whose parental love and solicitude for me had impelled him to undertake the arduous journey to Jammu despite his age, was beside himself with grief and anxiety at my precarious condition, but restrained by a feeling of awe, which all those who surrounded me at the time felt in spite of themselves, he made no attempt to offer any suggestions or advice.

Alarmed by the seriousness of my condition and unable to think of any other way, as a last resort, and without my knowledge, they decided to take experienced sadhus and fakirs into their confidence. But all those who were brought to treat me expressed their inability to do anything. One of them, a venerable saint hoary with age, then on a visit to Jammu, whom thousands flocked to see every day, after listening to me attentively shook his head, saying that he had not heard of anything like it in his life and suggested that I should seek directions from the same teacher who had prescribed the practice responsible for the disturbance.

Growing more desperate with my progressively worsening condition, they ultimately approached a Kashmiri sadhu staying at Lahore in those days and persuaded him to come to Jammu to see me. He stayed with us for some days studying my condition attentively. I had now grown extremely weak, almost exhausted, with spindle legs and emaciated arms, a skeleton with gleaming eyes, which made my wife wince every time she looked at me. For more than a month I had starved myself, subsisting on barely half a cup of boiled rice and a cup of milk two or three times a day. The poisoned condition of my nerves caused by acute digestive disturbances had translated itself into an ungovernable fear of eating because of a constant threat of dreadful consequence. I should have preferred not to eat anything at all, but knowing well that a completely empty stomach meant a dreadful death, in spite of the nausea and the revolt of my stomach I used all my willpower to perform the extremely unpleasant task of eating a little.

Unable to penetrate the cause of my distemper, the learned sadhu, imputing my dislike for food to a whim, asked me to eat in his presence, directing that the full quantity I was accustomed to take be served to me. On his insistence I swallowed with great difficulty a few morsels more than my usual intake, washing them down with water to overcome the resistance offered by my throat. The moment I did so a sudden unbearable stab of pain shot across my abdomen and the area around the sacral plexus, attaining such an intensity that I fell prostrate, writhing and twisting, casting a reproachful look at the sadhu for thus subjecting me to torture by his ill-timed advice.

Pale with mortification, he rose hurriedly and left the room. That evening he was attacked by a sudden sickness which kept him on his feet for the entire night without sleep, and he left the house in the early hours of the morning, attributing his own malady to the terrible power possessing me.

I recovered from the pain in a few hours without any serious aftereffects, but the incident exposed the helplessness of my condition as being entirely beyond human aid and added immensely to the worry of my wife.

Some days after this episode my son came into my room accidentally with a small plate of food in his chubby little hands. It was about noon. As usual I had taken a few spoonfuls of rice, my principal meal of the day, an hour before. The boy squatted down in front of me and began to eat, licking his lips and enjoying each mouthful in the manner of children.

Unlike other times, the sight of food caused no revulsion, and as I watched the child eating with delight I felt the dim stirrings of hunger for the first time in weeks. In place of the usual bitterness I noticed a reawakened sense of taste in my mouth. I could have eaten a few morsels with appetite at that time, but the fear of the awful consequences which followed the slightest error in diet in that hypertensed condition restrained me, and I could not gather strength enough to take the risk and ask for something to eat. After only a few minutes the feeling disappeared and the old chaotic condition overcame me again.

Puzzled at the occurrence, which could not fail to strike me forcibly even in that distraught condition, I racked my brain to find a satisfactory explanation for the apparently trifling incident, full of the greatest import for me. Could it be, I asked myself, that the interval between the meals set by me was too long in my present debilitated condition?

The next day I paid scrupulous attention to time, taking a few mouthfuls with a cup of milk every three hours, each time unwillingly and with fear gripping my heart. But I managed to carry out my purpose without noticing any adverse consequences, though there was no perceptible improvement either.

I continued in this matter for a few days, but the condition of my brain was deteriorating, and the convulsive movements of my limbs, coupled with intensely painful sensations along the path of nerves, especially in the back and abdomen, signified a serious disorder of the nervous system. I felt myself sinking and even the will to live, which had sustained me so far, appeared ready to give up the struggle as hopeless and to let the body drift to its doom.

After some days I noticed with a shock that I was slightly delirious at times. I had still enough sense to realize that if the condition worsened I was doomed. I had tried all expedients, used all my intelligence and exhausted all my resources, but had failed miserably to find a way out.

Finally, losing every hope of recovery and apprehending the worst in a mood of utter depression, I prepared myself for death, resolved to end my life before the delirium of madness rendered the task impossible. Overwhelmed by the horror which surrounded me, I had now almost lost the power to think rationally or to exert my will to resist the dread impulse. Before going to bed that night I embraced my wife with enfeebled, palsied arms for a long time, noting with anguish her pinched face, and with burning tears in my eyes I resigned her to God, in pain at the idea of the inevitable separation ahead, leaving me no opportunity now to repay her with redoubled love for her unparalleled loyalty and sacrifice.

Calling both my sons to me by name, I embraced them fondly, clasping each to my breast, entrusting them also to God's care for ever and ever. With a wrench at the heart I remembered that I could not have a last look at my dear daughter, who was at Srinagar looking after the house. Resigning her also to God, and looking for the last time at her image in my mind, I recovered my breath and stretching my aching body on the bed, closed my eyes, unable to stifle the great sobs that shook my breast.

It took me some time to grow a little composed after what I had thought was my last adieu to my wife and children, believing death to be inevitable. Then I began to think seriously about my resolve. It was foolish to expect, I told myself, that if the malady was allowed to run its course I would have a peaceful end. Death would definitely be preceded by a raging madness which I had to avoid at any cost. Arguing in this manner, I revolved in my mind the various methods within my reach to end my life, trying to select the one which was the easiest and the least painful, or possible of execution by one in an extremely weak condition. I weighed the possibilities, passing now and again into a delirious condition, all the while tossing from side to side in the relentless grip of unconquerable insomnia. Hours passed and my agitated brain refused to come to a decision, passing from one hazy chain of thought to another, without the power to complete any. I cannot say how it happened that towards the early hours of dawn I passed into a sleeplike condition, the first in weeks, and for a brief interval dreamed a vivid dream in which I saw myself seated at a meal with a half-filled plate in front of me containing boiled rice and a meat preparation common in Kashmir, which I ate with enjoyment.

I awoke immediately, the luster noticed in the dream persisting during wakefulness for some time. A sudden idea darted across my now almost delirious mind, and calling my wife to my side, in a weak voice I asked her to serve me nourishment every two hours that day, beginning early, each serving to include in addition to milk a few ounces of well-cooked, easy-to-digest meat.

Following my muttered instructions to the letter, my wife with her own hands cooked and served the food to me at the specified intervals, punctual to the minute. I ate mechanically, my arms and hands shaking while carrying the food to my mouth, a clear indication of a delirious condition. I found it even more difficult that day to chew the food and swallow it, but managed to gulp it down with milk.

After finishing the last meal at nine that evening, I felt a slight relief. The tension grew less, yielding to a feeling of extreme exhaustion followed by a soothing wave of drowsiness until, with an inexpressible transport of joy, which made tears stream from my eyes, I felt blissful sleep steal upon me. I slept soundly until morning, enveloped in a glowing sheet of light as usual.

The next day I reduced the interval to one hour, raising it to one and a half hours after a week, and adding in the course of this period fruits and a little curd to my diet. Gradually the signs of delirium vanished and the insomnia gave way to an excessive desire for sleep. I submitted willingly to the beneficial soporific influence day and night, awaking only at the time of eating in obedience to the gentle and cautious touch of my wife, who stayed in the kitchen all day preparing meal after meal and serving hot, appetizing dishes with a love and care which only a devoted wife can display. Thanks to her ministrations, stringent regard to time, and the excellence of the food, I began to grow in strength and in about two weeks was able to move from one room to another. After this period I prolonged the interval to two hours, thereby reducing to some extent the intake of food in a day.

Refreshed by sleep, my mind grew clearer, escaping by degrees the horror; in spite of the fact that the vital radiation had now assumed a colossal appearance, I began to feel a growing sense of confidence in myself and to hope that if nothing untoward happened I might pass the crisis with safety after all.

As if guided by a newly developed sense of taste, I selected the constituents of every meal, rejecting this article and taking more of that, choosing a combination of acids and alkalis, sugars and salts, fruits and vegetables, in a manner that helped my stomach to digest the enormously increased mass under the stimulation of the new, more powerful radiant current, without any undesirable reaction. I was now passing through an experience as amazing and weird as any I had passed so far, utterly bewildered by the new direction taken by my singularly functioning organism.

No one in their senses would believe such an abnormal performance of the digestive organs possible all of a sudden, turning me from a moderate eater into a voracious one; my stomach, working under the stimulation of a fiery vapor, consumed incredible quantities without causing the slightest adverse effect, as if licked up by fire. I had heard and read of yogis said to have commanded incredible powers of digestion, who could consume without ill effects prodigious loads of food with the aid of the luminous energy, but I had never lent credence to such stories. What I had disbelieved I now witnessed in myself, all the time overwhelmed with wonder at the powers and possibilities lying hidden in the body.

I was not so much alarmed by the voracity of my appetite as I was amazed at the capacity of my stomach. At the lowest computation I was consuming at least four times the amount of food I was used to before the occurrence. During the first week the quantity devoured must have been six times the normal amount. It was atrocious. The food disappeared in my stomach as if it had evaporated, no doubt sucked up greedily by the hungry cells of the body.

A disregard of time in eating was always visited with a sudden cessation of the desire for food and an absence of taste, aggravated at times to a feeling of nausea and utter dislike for any kind of nourishment. Experience had taught me that such symptoms indicated a poisoned state of nerves, an inevitable result of the awakening in the first stages, for which there is no known antidote except proper feeding, in spite of the aversion, done in a manner as may be indicated by the habits and the condition of the system. One should take care to use only the best, most easily digestible, complete natural foods in such a quantity as can be readily tolerated at regular intervals, normally of not more than three hours. The availability of a nutritious diet in the stomach is essential in all normal cases and has, therefore, to be arranged with due care to enable the nervous system to rid itself of impurities.

At the present moment we are entirely in the dark about the nature of the subtle organic essence in the body which serves as nourishment for the ever-active nerves and the constantly fleeting nervous and thought energy. In the first stages of the awakening and until the system grows accustomed to the flow of the radiant current, the one and the only preservative of life and sanity is diet in right measure, correct combination, and at proper intervals. The whole science of kundalini is fundamentally based on the assumption that it is possible for one to rouse to activity a mighty dormant power in the human body in order to gain freedom from sense domination for the embodied spirit, enabling it to soar unfettered to its celestial estate. The idea of stirring to activity a dormant vital force in the body, examined in the light of modern knowledge, can only signify the development or generation of a new type of vitality or life energy which clearly involves a recasting of the nervous system not possible without a biological evolution.

In the initial stages and later as well, nourishment suited to their appetite and constitution is taken by initiates of hatha yoga in surprising quantities as an offering to the power within. Aversion for food is a common feature in cases of a sudden awakening of kundalini; the abrupt release of the new force and its stormy dash through the nerves causes acute disturbances in the digestive and excretory systems. The constant presence of the teacher for guidance at this critical juncture has, for this reason, always been considered essential, and not infrequently forced feeding is resorted to in order to preserve life when the disciple, completely unnerved by the weird developments in his interior, loses command over himself and is unable to muster enough strength of will to perform the act of eating in spite of the nausea and the chaos prevailing within.

To avert disaster in acute conditions and to guard against the utterly unpredictable behavior of the digestive and excretory organs after the awakening, the students of hatha yoga have to devote many years of their life to acquire the ability to empty the stomach and colon at will to prepare for emergencies almost certain to arise sooner or later.

Except for this interpretation, there can be no other meaning or utility, barring a cheap demonstrative or gymnastical value, in the elaborate and extremely difficult system of physical discipline and body control enjoined by all the exponents of this form of yoga as an essential prerequisite for those initiated into the final esoteric practices of the cult. The would-be aspirants have necessarily to attain proficiency in all preliminary exercises and methods of body control before embarking on the supreme but hazardous course of awakening the Serpent Power.

We traveled to Srinagar in the beginning of April 1944. Owing to the joint efforts of my wife and her father and the pains taken by them to make every kind of provision for the two-day hilly journey, I reached Srinagar in my then extremely weak condition without mishap. There, surrounded by relatives and friends, and nursed with assiduous care by my wife and daughter, I made rapid progress, gaining enough strength in a few months to resume my duties in the office.

In the course of a year I grew hardy and strong, able to bear strain and fatigue, exertion and pressure, but I could not overcome the susceptibility of my system to digestive disorders in the event of unusual delay or irregularity in diet. I resumed my old habit of two meals a day, with a cup of milk and a slice of bread in the mornings and afternoons. By the end of the year my appetite became normal and the amount of food moderate, with a small measure of meat as a necessary ingredient.

The lustrous appearance of external objects as well as of thought forms and the brilliance of dream images was intensified during the worst period of the last disorder, and grew in brightness to such an extent that, when gazing at a beautiful sunlit landscape, I always felt as if I were looking at a heavenly scene transported to the earth from a distant Elysium, illuminated by dancing beams of molten silver. This astounding feature of my consciousness, purely subjective, of course, never exhibited any alteration, save that it gained in transparency, brilliance, and penetrative power with the passage of time and continues to clothe me and all I perceive in inexpressible luster today.

Years passed without bringing any new development in me to the surface. Whatever was happening was transpiring within, beyond my knowledge and away from the reach of my eyes. Failing to notice any other change in me except for the sea of luster in which I lived, and sternly warned by the last awful episode to desist from invoking the supernatural again, I occupied myself fully with the world and its affairs in an attempt to lead a normal life.

It was the summer of the year 1946. We had just come from Jammu to Srinagar with the annual move of our offices. I was in a fine state of health with a constant urge in my interior to do more healthy, constructive work in the time I could spare from my other duties. The high increase in the intake of my food, after the traumatic experience I had in Jammu years before, had made my body somewhat obese, but this increase in weight did not in any way interfere with the amazing transformation which was now a constant feature of my experience. The silvery luster that now pervaded the whole field of my vision had become brighter and more alluring than before. Whenever I turned my eyes to the sky or let them rest on a landscape or any objects in front of me, I was invariably fascinated by the change in perception that had occurred. The sight of a beautiful panorama or a fine row of buildings, a glistening lake, a flowing broad-bosomed river or a surging multitude of people, was so intensely alluring that my senses were almost ravished by the spectacle. I racked my brains for a solution to the problem created by this extraordinary perceptual change in me but could find no answer to it.

My dream experiences were no less striking. Sleep was my great mother and comforter. I did not remember all my dreams, but the fragments that came to my mind on awakening during the night or in the morning had a romantic and idyllic flavor in them. In the dream state I saw myself roaming over vast spaces, brightly lit up with the luster that I experienced during the day. Sometimes summit after summit of a vast mountain covered with greenery opened to my view as I climbed its steep slope to reach the top. On other occasions the boundless expanse of a lovely meadow, decked with beautiful flowers, surrounded me in the dream, delighting my senses with the loveliness and the grandeur that I beheld. At other times I saw myself sailing on fast-flowing, mighty rivers or billowing oceans, always attended by the fascinating light. These mighty feasts of transporting visionary experiences served as a continuation of the alluring mantle of glory in which the objects I observed were wrapped during the day. Every day I looked forward to the romantic peregrinations in the dream state with fond anticipation. When the night was over I looked forward with even greater anticipation to the panorama that would meet my view during the day.

A very remarkable feature in my dream life in those days was the prophetic nature of some of the dreams, especially those dreamed towards the morning. The reenaction of the dream scene or the fulfillment of the presage that very day, or during the course of the next few days, was so remarkable that I never ceased to wonder at the occurrences.

There was no question of a casual coincidence or paramnesia. There could be no false memory of a scene that I had witnessed only a few hours before and of which the details were fresh in my memory. For instance, one dream scene showed me reading a letter from a friend whom I had not met in years and about whose whereabouts I was not even aware at the time. The same day when the postman came I found a letter from him amongst the others delivered to me.

I saw a relative in my dream whom I had not met for months and he called on the same day.

One of the most remarkable of these dreams occurred on the night when China made an attack on India as the result of a boundary dispute. I saw at a distance a whole contingent of soldiers who looked Chinese, shooting with their rifles at another body of soldiers whose faces I could not distinguish. They were all around me, though some distance away, and I awoke with a slight throb of fear at my heart. Only three days later the invasion was announced in the newspapers and on the radio.

Fortunately I did not attach too much importance to this phenomenon. I took it as in some way connected with the transformation I was undergoing. I felt no sense of elation at the thought that my dreams were coming true or that I had developed the powers of prophecy and clairvoyance. On the contrary, the very fact that some of my dreams were premonitory or prophetic filled me with a vague sense of uneasiness. I could never know for certain which of the dream scenes I witnessed would be reenacted and if so, when, or which of the events would come true during the course of the next few days or weeks. This uncertainty kept me in a state of mental unrest which I did not at all relish. The materialization of the dreams became so common that at last I felt really disturbed in my mind. It was not good for me, I thought, for my mind to remain in a constant state of suspense, reviewing the dreams I had the previous night again and again to find out which of them had the likelihood of coming true in the near future.

Finally I decided to end the suspense. On awakening each morning I resolutely avoided dwelling in my mind on the scenes I had dreamed and made no attempt to recall them to my memory. The method worked very well. After a few days the rather unhealthy habit I had contracted of letting my mind revert again and again to the dreams I had seen began to lose its grip on my mind. I kept myself busy on the public tasks I had taken upon myself and firmly avoided relapsing into the old habit again. Whenever the thought arose or the memory of a dream came back to me, I determinedly brushed it aside and continued to concentrate on the work I had in hand.

In the course of time I realized that I had acted wisely. The knowledge that was dawning and the talents which were developing in me would have been seriously interfered with had I continued to attach exaggerated importance to my dream experiences and make my mind a slave to a habit that could never grant me the profound insight for which I longed.

In 1946, in collaboration with a few friends and colleagues, I started a movement for economic reform in all obligatory social functions in our community. I had become acutely conscious of the crushing load of misery and even infamy which a low-income family had to carry all its life, almost to the funeral pyre, for the transitory pleasure of excelling its neighbors in pomp and show, in the grandeur of a feast, in the richness of a dowry, or in other such items of social ceremonial. The child marriage was now no longer in vogue, but brides often had to endure hardships and injustices that made their life a bed of thorns with no hope of alleviation until they grew old.

The idea of introducing some measure of reform into the social customs of our society, especially those imposing certain disabilities on our womanhood, occurred to me time after time with a persistence that finally obliged me to translate it into action. I became more and more conscious of the inhumanity involved in the current practices.

As I was then working in the Education Department of the State and was on good relations not only with my colleagues in the office of the Director but also with most of the teachers and professors in colleges in all parts of the state, my burning desire to see justice done in every case, as far as lay in my power, had won me many friends and also a few enemies. The latter consisted of those who occupied privileged positions and were accustomed to gaining favor at the cost of less resourceful colleagues. But somehow I was allowed a free hand in carrying out my designs to set right the injustices suffered by teachers who had no powerful support in the Department or were too artless or poor to gain the favor they needed to gain their promotion or secure transfer in their turn.

My plan succeeded. A number of friends, both from the Department and also outside of it, expressed their agreement with my views and consented to form a body to start a campaign against the social evils in our community. A few of them showed enthusiasm, which created high hopes in my mind. We met a few times in small groups and finally decided upon a large meeting in which about fifty friends participated. Curiously enough this meeting was held in the large premises of the cremation site, which invested our enterprise with a solemn overtone from the beginning. A small organization designated as Samaj Sudhar Samiti was formed and our work began.

Our first act was to make the purpose of our movement known to the community in the form of a small brochure. This was followed by flyers and handbills. We formulated a reform scheme, prescribing a limit to the size of dowry and the number of guests to be invited to a marriage function, and even to other important religious functions, as for instance the sacred thread ceremony, and circulated our views widely with a fervent appeal for cooperation.

When looking at the whole idea subjectively, I saw no reason why the public should not respond to our efforts, since our aim was to save them from considerable extravagant expenditure of time, energy, and money. But when we tried to carry our plan in actual effect, we met a resistance as stiff as if we were out to do the gravest harm to them.

It was no easy task for our small, dedicated group of missionaries to achieve their purpose. Except in a few cases, they met resistance everywhere. Some people became our enemies simply out of jealousy, others out of spite, still others out of a fear that our effort was directed to snatching leadership out of their hands. The marriage parties listened patiently to our volunteers who went to persuade them to follow the reform scheme to save themselves and others from extravagance and misery, but seldom acted according to their advice. We then decided upon a program of public speeches in different parts of the city, and even in rural areas, to make our ideas widely known to the people.

It is a paradox of the human mind that, in the grip of habit, human beings submit readily and sometimes even gladly to ruthless exploitation by religious and political leaders, racketeers and impostors. They bleed themselves white to contribute munificently to the whims and fancies of pseudo-religious teachers who are ultimately proven to have been unworthy of the homage paid to them. They are ready to face hardships, police batons, bullets, and imprisonment in their loyalty to a political leader who, when raised to a position of power through their sacrifice and efforts, turns his back upon them and acts in the very opposite way promised at the start of his career. They fall easy victims to profiteers, racketeers, and impostors. But when an honest-hearted man who bleeds for their sorrows tries his utmost to lift them up from the mire of bloodsucking customs into which they have fallen, they turn upon him angrily and shower abuse or blows upon him to deter him from his task.

Although I knew it would not be easy to effect a change in customs that had been in vogue for many centuries, the urge was irresistible. I felt new ideas and new impulses surging in my head. Only a few years ago I had not even imagined that I could speak in an assembly of hundreds, even thousands of people. But I had now done so and with success. Only a few years ago I had been a passive spectator and observer of the very social customs which had now become abhorrent to me. I never tried to find an explanation for this change in my thinking and behavior. The transition was so imperceptible that it never impinged upon my mind as something new or remarkable. If I had thought over the issue at that stage the idea might never have occurred to me that a shift had occurred in the very roots of my being.

It is only now, when other changes have occurred and are still occurring, that I feel confident in asserting that this change from a passive observer of the customs prevailing in my society to that of an active reformer was the first result of the transformative process set afoot by my experience in the year 1937. Without knowing it, my personality had undergone a minor change which, but for the experience and its continued effects, I could easily have ascribed to the maturity of judgment at a more advanced age when I could view the issues with a greater insight than before.

There are countless instances in which conversions have occurred and continue to occur in all parts of the world, confirmed skeptics turning into religious-minded believers, evildoers transformed into pious men and women, and infidels converted into saints. There are also stories of the process working in the reverse direction, turning good souls into evil ways. The phenomenon of conversion from an irreligious to a pious mode of life is so clearly marked in the history of religion that there can be no doubt about it. But there has been no explanation how the transformation occurs overnight with suddenness or gradually in course of time. The answer lies in the operation of kundalini.

Intellectual and moral evolution of human beings involves a constant process of purification and regeneration of the nervous system and the brain. These processes are not discernible to scientists, because they have as yet no knowledge of the pranic energy which maintains and vivifies the organism. This intelligent "electricity"—the basis of all life in the universe—is yet an unknown entity to science since it is not normally perceptible to any of the senses known to us. It is not easy for human imagination to form a picture of the storm of activity raging in every living organism, from the lowest to the highest, or the intelligence displayed in the regulation of this activity. The play of electric currents darting through the network of wires in a telephone system serving a huge metropolis is a child's toy compared to it. We never realize when we arise in the morning the pranic activity through the billions of neurons in our system, more intricate than all the electrical lighting systems in the world, that has occurred to clean and repair our brains and to awaken us in the morning as fresh as ever. ˙

It is not possible for science to understand or evaluate fully the phenomenon of life without an understanding of prana. Scientists of the nineteenth century, carried away by the ideas of Darwin, failed to assess the profundity of life. Since then, science has become materialistic. It is only when subtle intelligent energies of the cosmos become the target of scientific observation that the complexity of the phenomenon of life and the bewildering nature of the cosmos will be realized. The Indian adepts used the term *maya* to describe creation, implying an illusory appearance, beyond the reach of the intellect alone.

In the summer of 1947, my daughter was married in an unostentatious manner in conformity with our reform scheme, the credit for which went not to us but to her husband, a struggling young lawyer, orphaned at an early age and left without resources, who refused tempting offers of rich dowries to marry the dowryless daughter of a poor man. The alliance was proposed to his elder brother by a friend while I was at Jammu, and all I had to do was signify my assent to it. In this way, in my peculiar mental condition, Nature spared me the ordeal of having to hunt indefinitely for a match for one who out of filial loyalty was as keen as I was myself to ensure that my principles in regard to dowry were not violated in any way.

In the autumn of the same year, the peaceful valley of Kashmir was thrown into convulsions by a sudden raid from marauding hordes of frontier tribesmen, who, organized and led by trained martial talent, came down upon the defenseless Kashmiris, pillaging, raping, and killing indiscriminately until almost the whole northern side of the valley shook with the lamentations of the bereaved and cries of the plundered and ravished. When the carnage was over and the invaders had retired after several scuffles with Indian forces, the members of our small band of enthusiasts, ready to devote their energies to a noble cause, threw themselves into the arduous task of providing relief to a large section of the ravaged victims.

That winter, because of stormy conditions in many of the border districts of the state, attended by wholesale massacres and rape, the offices did not move to Jammu, and I therefore continued to attend my duties at Srinagar, oblivious to the horror of the situation in the all-absorbing mission of service to which we had devoted ourselves. Entirely preoccupied with the task, I could not leave Kashmir during the winter of 1948 either and had to apply for leave of absence to complete the enterprise undertaken at a time when our own fate hung in the balance. During this interval momentous changes occurred in the political framework of the State. The hereditary ruler had to abdicate to make room for a people's government. This great upheaval brought in its wake countless smaller upheavals, bringing new values in place of the old and new ways of thought and action. The old order changed, as has always happened, often without effecting side by side the needed change for the better in human nature which, forgetting soon the lesson taught by a revolution, acts again in a manner that makes another upheaval inevitable after a time.

FIFTEEN ═══════════════════════════

Stretching Out
Immeasurably in
All Directions

IN NOVEMBER 1949, I AGAIN went to Jammu with the office. On this occasion my wife chose to stay at Srinagar to look after the house and children. She had grown confident of my health and ability to look after myself in view of the endurance displayed by me during the past two years. My system had functioned so regularly that there had occurred not the slightest cause for any perturbation. On the contrary, I had found myself fully equal to and in fact took pleasure in the strenuous task of relieving the distress of hundreds of families taken by us upon ourselves, a mere handful of men and women without resources or influence, at a time of extreme tension and under rigorous conditions.

I stayed at Jammu with an old friend who was good enough to place a room at my disposal. I was glad to accept his hospitality, offered with great cordiality and love, as it afforded me several facilities, especially the opportunity to be all to myself, absorbed in the contemplation of the luminous glow within, which had begun to assume to some extent the enrapturing character of the vision perceived on the first day of the awakening.

Profiting by the awful experience I had undergone previously, I made absolutely no attempt to meditate as before. What I did now was quite different. Without any effort and sometimes even without my knowing it, I sank deeper and deeper within myself, engulfed more and more by the lustrous waves of consciousness, which appeared to grow in size and extent the more I allowed myself to sink without resistance into the sea of consciousness in which I often

found myself immersed. After about twelve years, a curious transformation had occurred in the glowing circle of awareness around
my head which made me constantly conscious of a subtle world of
life stretching on all sides in which I breathed, walked, and acted
without in any way either affecting its all-pervasive homogeneous
character, or being affected by it in my day-to-day transactions in
the world.

Speaking more clearly, it seemed as if I were breathing, moving,
and acting surrounded by an extremely subtle, invisible, conscious
void, as we are surrounded by radio waves, with the difference that I
did not perceive or feel the existence of the waves but was compelled
to acknowledge their presence by the logic of certain facts. In this
case I was made aware of the invisible medium by internal conditions, as if my own confined consciousnss, transcending its limitations, was now in direct touch with its own substance on all sides,
like a sentient dewdrop floating intact in an ocean of pure being,
without mingling with the surrounding mass of water.

During the past months, on a few occasions I had noticed this
tendency of my mind to turn without encountering any barrier to its
expansion within itself, extending more like a drop of oil spreading
on the surface of water until, collecting myself with an effort, I came
back to my normal state, itself more extensive by far than the
original field of consciousness I had possessed before the awakening.
I had not attached much importance to this phase, believing it to be
an attempt of the mind to fall into reveries which, because of its
luminous spaciousness, created the impression of further internal
expansion without implying any additional change in my already
peculiar mental condition.

About a month after my arrival at Jammu, I noticed that not only
had this tendency become more marked and frequent, but the daily
plunge into the depths of my lucent being was maturing into a great
source of happiness and strength for me. The development was,
however, so gradual and the change so imperceptible that I was led
to believe that the whole occurrence was the outcome of the general

improvement in my health due to the salubrious climate rather than to any new factor operating within me.

Towards the third week of December, I noticed that when returning from these prolonged spells of absorption, which had now become a regular feature of my solitary hours, my mind usually dwelt on the lyrics of my favorite mystics. Without the least idea of trying my skill at poetic composition, I nevertheless found myself attempting this when not in an absorbed mood, keeping the mystical rhymes which I liked most as models before me. Beyond the fact that I had committed to memory a few dozen Sanskrit verses culled from the scriptures and a few dozen couplets picked up from the works of mystics, I knew nothing of poetry. After a few days of mere playful dabbling I became restless, and for the first time in my life I felt an urge to write verse. Not at all impressed seriously by what I thought was a passing impulse, I put to paper a few stanzas, devoting several hours every day to the task.

I wrote in Kashmiri, but after about a fortnight of daily endeavor I found I did not improve. The sterility of my efforts to write in verse, instead of dampening my spirits, urged me to greater efforts, however, and I devoted more and more time to what had now become a regular, fascinating hobby for me. The standard of the compositions did not improve in the least, and I had often to labor for hours to complete a line and then longer to find another to match it. I never associated the new tendency with the mysterious agency at work in my body. But these unsuccessful attempts I was making at verse formation were, in fact, a deliberately maneuvered prelude to a startling occurrence soon afterwards. I was being taught internally to exercise a newly developed talent in me, the existence of which I could have had no inkling otherwise; my crude attempts were the first indication of the schooling.

During those days, an ardent member of our small band of zealous workers in Kashmir was on a visit to Jammu. She often came to my place, usually to have news of our work at Srinagar, about which I received regular reports from our treasurer or our secretary. One day I offered to accompany her home when she rose to depart, intending by the long stroll to rid myself of a slight depression I felt at the time.

We walked leisurely, discussing our work, when suddenly while crossing the Tawi Bridge I felt a mood of deep absorption settling upon me until I almost lost touch with my surroundings. I no longer heard the voice of my companion; she seemed to have receded into the distance, though walking by my side. Near me, in a blaze of brilliant light, I suddenly felt what seemed to be a mighty conscious presence, sprung from nowhere, encompassing me and overshadowing all the objects around, from which two lines of a beautiful verse in Kashmiri poured out to float before my vision, like luminous writing in the air, disappearing as suddenly as they had come.

When I came to myself, I found the girl looking at me in blank amazement, bewildered by my abrupt silence and the expression of utter detachment on my face. Without revealing to her all that had happened, I repeated the verse, saying that it had all of a sudden taken form in my mind in spite of myself, and that it accounted for the break in our conversation.

She listened in surprise, struck by the beauty of the rhyme, weighing every word, and then said that it was indeed nothing short of miraculous for one who had never been favored by the muse before to compose so exquisite a verse on the very first attempt with such lightning rapidity. I heard her in silence, carried away by the profundity of the experience I had just gone through. Until that hour, all I had experienced of the superconscious was purely subjective, neither demonstrable to nor verifiable by others. But now for the first time I had before me a tangible proof of the change that had occurred in me, unintelligible to and independently of my surface consciousness.

After escorting my companion to her destination I returned to my residence in time for dinner. All the way back, in the stillness of a pleasant evening and the welcome solitude of an unfrequented path, I remained deeply engrossed in the enigma presented by the vision and the sudden leap taken by my mind in a new direction. The more intently I examined the problem the more surprised I became at the deep meaning of the production, the exquisite formation, and the highly appealing language of the lines. On no account could I claim the artistic composition as mine, the voluntary creation of my own deliberate thought.

I reached my place while still deeply absorbed in the same train of thought and, still engrossed, sat down for dinner. I took the first few morsels mechanically, in silence, oblivious to my surroundings and unappreciative of the food in front of me, unable to bring myself out of the state of intense absorption into which I had fallen, retaining only a slender link with my environment, like a sleepwalker instinctively restrained from colliding with the objects in his path without consciously being aware of them.

In the middle of the meal, while still in the same condition of semi-entrancement, I stopped abruptly, contemplating with awe and amazement, which made the hair on my skin stand on end, a marvelous phenomenon in progress in the depths of my being. Without any effort on my part, and while seated comfortably on a chair, I had gradually passed off, without becoming aware of it, into a condition of exaltation and self-expansion similar to that which I had experienced on the very first occasion, in December 1937, with the modification that in place of a roaring noise in my ears there was now a cadence like the humming of a swarm of bees, enchanting and melodious, and the encircling glow was replaced by a penetrating silvery radiance, already a feature of my being within and without.

The marvelous aspect of the condition lay in the sudden realization that, although linked to the body and surroundings, I had expanded in an indescribable manner into a titanic personality, conscious from within of an immediate and direct contact with an intensely conscious universe, a wonderful inexpressible immanence all around me. My body, the chair I was sitting on, the table in front of me, the room enclosed by walls, the lawn outside and the space beyond, including the earth and sky, appeared to be most amazingly mere phantoms in this real, interpenetrating, and all-pervasive ocean of existence which, to explain the most incredible part of it as best I can, seemed to be simultaneously unbounded, stretching out immeasurably in all directions, and yet no bigger than an infinitely small point.

From this marvelous point the entire existence, of which my body and its surroundings were a part, poured out like radiation, as if a reflection as vast as my conception of the cosmos were thrown out upon infinity by a projector no bigger than a pinpoint, the entire intensely active and gigantic world picture dependent on the beams issuing from it. The shoreless ocean of consciousness in which I was now immersed appeared infinitely large and infinitely small at the same time—large when considered in relation to the world picture floating in it and small when considered in itself, measureless, without form or size—nothing and yet everything.

It was an amazing and staggering experience for which I can cite no parallel and no simile, an experience beyond all and everything belonging to this world conceivable by the mind or perceptible to the senses. I was intensely aware internally of a marvelous being so concentratedly and massively conscious as to outluster and outstature infinitely the cosmic image present before me, not only in point of extent and brightness, but in point of reality and substance as well. The phenomenal world, ceaselessly in motion, characterized by creation, incessant change, and dissolution, receded into the background and assumed the appearance of an extremely thin, rapidly melting layer of foam upon a substantial rolling ocean of life, a veil of exceedingly fine vapor before an infinitely large conscious sun, constituting a complete reversal of the relationship between the world and the limited human consiousness. It showed the previously all-dominating cosmos reduced to the state of a transitory appearance, and the formerly care-ridden point of awareness, circumscribed by the body, grown to the spacious dimensions of a mighty universe and the exalted stature of a majestic immanence before which the material cosmos shrank to the subordinate position of an evanescent and illusive appendage.

I awoke from the semi-trance condition after about half an hour, affected to the roots of my being by the majesty and marvel of the vision, entirely oblivious to the passage of time, having in the intensity of the experience lived a life of ordinary existence. During this period, probably due to fluctuations in the state of my body and mind caused by internal and external stimuli, there were intervals of deeper and lesser penetration not distinguishable by the flow of time but by the state of immanence, which, at the point of the deepest penetration, assumed such an awe-inspiring, almighty, all-knowing, blissful, and at the same time absolutely motionless, intangible, and formless character that the invisible line demarcating the material world and the boundless, all-conscious Reality ceased to exist, the two fusing into one; the mighty ocean sucked up by a drop, the enormous three-dimensional universe swallowed by a grain of sand, the entire creation, the knower and the known, the seer and the seen, reduced to an inexpressible sizeless void which no ordinary mind could conceive nor any language describe.

Before coming out completely from this condition and before the glory in which I found myself had completely faded, I found, floating in the luminous glow of my mind, the rhymes following the couplet that had suddenly taken shape in me near the Tawi Bridge that day. The lines occurred one after the other, as if dropped into the three-dimensional field of my consciousness by another source of condensed knowledge within me. They started from the glowing recesses of my being, developing suddenly into fully formed couplets like falling snowflakes which, from tiny specks high up, become clear-cut, regularly shaped crystals when nearing the eye, and vanished so suddenly as to leave me hardly any time to retain them in my memory. They came fully formed, complete with language, rhyme, and meter, finished products originating, as it seemed, from the surrounding intelligence, to pass before my internal eye for expression.

I was still in an elevated state when I rose from the table and went to my room. The first thing I did was to write down the lines as far as I could remember them. It was not an easy task. I found that during the short interval that had elapsed I had forgotten not only the order in which the rhymes had occurred but also whole portions of the matter, which it was extremely difficult for me to recollect or supply. It took me more than two hours to supply the omissions.

I went to bed that night in an excited and happy frame of mind. After years of acute suffering I had at last been given a glimpse into the supersensible and at the same time made the fortunate recipient of divine grace, which all fitted admirably with the traditional concepts of kundalini. I could not believe in my good luck; I felt it was too astounding to be true. But when I looked within myself to find out what I had done to deserve it, I felt extremely humbled. I had to my credit no achievement remarkable enough to entitle me to the honor bestowed on me. I had lived an ordinary life, never done anything exceptionally meritorious and never achieved a complete subdual of desires and appetites.

I reviewed all the noteworthy incidents of the last twelve years in my mind, studying them in the light of the latest development, and found that much of what had been dark and obscure so far was now assuming a deep and startling significance. In the intensity of joy which I felt at the revelation I forgot the terrible ordeal I had passed through, as also the grueling suspense and anxiety that had been my companions for all that period. I had drunk the cup of suffering to the dregs to come upon a resplendent, never-ending source of unutterable joy and peace lying hidden in my interior, waiting for a favorable opportunity to reveal itself, affording me in one instant a deeper insight into the essence of things than a whole life devoted to study could do.

Thinking such thoughts I fell asleep at last, waking again in the luminous realm of dreams in which I had my abode every night. When I awoke in the morning the first recollection that came to my mind was of the transcendental experience of the previous evening.

Even the fleeting memory of a superconscious flight into the wonderland of Infinity is transporting, surpassing anything we can think of or encounter in the physical world. Considering the stupendous nature of the vision it is no wonder that the ancient seers of India, in constant communion with the transcendental reality, regarded the world as no more than an inexplicable shadow, an impermanent, illusory appearance before an eternal resplendent sun of indescribable grandeur and sublimity.

Every day during the next two weeks I wrote a few stanzas in Kashmiri that, without exception, dealt with some aspect of the unknown; some of them were definitely apocalyptic in nature. The verses occurred suddenly at odd times in the day or night, preceded by a voluntary pause on my part in the normal process of thinking. This preliminary cessation of mental activity was soon followed by a state of deep absorption, as if I were diving within myself to reach a certain depth where I could catch the vibrations of the message always expressed in poetry. The lines developed from an extremely subtle form, an invisible seed, and instantaneously passed before my mind as fully formed verses, following each other in rapid succession until the whole passage was completed, when I suddenly experienced a desire to withdraw myself from the state of semi-entrancement and return to normality.

On one more occasion during that fortnight I had the same transcendental experience as on the first day, tallying in almost all respects with the original one. I was sitting on a chair reading a piece written on the preceding day when, noticing the command, I leaned back in the chair and closed my eyes in a mood of relaxation, waiting for the results. The moment I did so I felt myself expanding in all directions, oblivious to the surroundings, and enveloped in an immense sea of glowing radiance, entertained by a sweet internal cadence unlike any symphony heard on earth, drawing nearer to the supreme condition, until with a plunge I found myself detached from all belonging to the causal world, lost in the inexpressible void, a marvelous state of being absolutely devoid of spatial and temporal distinctions. I returned to my normal state after more than half an hour and during the few moments of transition found a beautiful composition waiting for cognizance by my mind, staggered by the extraordinary experience that it had just gone through.

After a fortnight, the language changed and instead of rhymes in Kashmiri they occurred in English. The slight knowledge of English verse which I possessed was confined to the study of a few selected poems forming a part of my school and college texts. Beyond that, having no inherent taste for poetry, I had never cared to read it. But I could easily perceive that the passage before me was similar to the poems I had read, but having no knowledge of the rhyme and meter of English poetry, I could not form any judgment about its merit.

A few days afterwards, the poems appeared in Urdu instead of in English. Having a workable knowledge of the former, I did not feel any difficulty in writing down the lines, but all the same many blanks were left which were filled only months later. Urdu was succeeded by Punjabi in a few days. I had not read any book in Punjabi but had learned the language by constant contact with Punjabi-speaking friends and associates during my several years stay in Lahore as a school and college student.

My surprise, however, knew no bounds when a few days later the direction came that I should prepare to receive verses in Persian. I had never read the language, nor could I in the least understand or speak it. I waited in breathless expectancy and immediately after the signal a few Persian verses flashed before my mind in the same manner as the compositions in other languages. I had no difficulty in recognizing many Persian words and even the verse form of the lines. Kashmiri being rich in Persian words, it was easy for me to understand words already used in my mother tongue. After a great deal of exertion and straining, I at last succeeded in penning down the lines, but there were many blanks and mistakes which could not be filled in or set right until long after.

The few short poems in Persian that I was able to jot down involved such a strenuous effort that after some days I was obliged to desist from the onerous task. I felt entirely exhausted and what was more serious, the unhealthy effect of the exertion and excitement elicited was becoming seriously apparent in the prolonged spells of restlessness preceding my sleep. Consequently I gave myself complete rest for more than a week.

After a short time, feeling somewhat restored to health, I no longer felt it necessary to resist the impulse and submitted to the elevating moods at opportune moments. One day when I had obeyed the unspoken direction for relaxing my mind to prepare myself for reception, and had sunk deeply enough to reach the subtle emanations from the amazing conscious source within, yet tantalizingly out of my reach, I felt a thrill of deep excitement not unmixed with fear pass through every fiber of my being when the signal flashed across my own quiescent mind to make myself ready for taking down a piece in German. I came back from the semi-trance condition with a ferment in my mind, unable to reconcile myself to the idea that such a weird performance could ever be possible. I had never learned German, nor seen a book written in that language, nor to the best of my knowledge ever heard it spoken in my presence, and yet I was expected to write down a poem in it, which in plain terms meant a complete negation of the time-honored truth that language is an acquired and not inherited possession.

German was followed by French and Italian. Then came a few verses in Sanskrit, followed by Arabic. Surely there could be nothing more convincing than the phenomena I had witnessed during the previous few weeks to bring the idea irresistibly home to me that I was in occasional contact with an inexpressible fount of all knowledge and that, but for my inability to understand and transcribe, I could take down poetic pieces in most of the well-known languages of the earth. I felt wave after wave of conscious electricity pass through me, replete with knowledge to which, because of the poor capacity of my brain, I could not have full access.

Language fails me when I attempt to describe the experience which off and on has all along since then been the most sublime and the most elevating feature of my existence. On every such occasion I am made to feel as if the observer in me, or speaking more precisely, my lustrous conscious self, is floating, with but an extremely dim idea of the corporeal frame, in a vividly bright conscious plane, every fragment of which represents a boundless world of knowledge, embracing the present, past, and future, commanding all the sciences, philosophies, and arts ever known or that will be known in the ages to come, all concentrated and contained in a point existing here and everywhere, now and always, a formless, measureless ocean of wisdom from which, drop by drop, knowledge has filtered and will continue to filter into the human brain.

On every visit to the supersensible realm I am so overwhelmed by the mystery and the wonder of it that everything else of this world, everything conceived by us of the next, every fact and incident of my life save this, every momentous event of history, every ambition and desire, and above all even my own existence, life and death, appear to be trite and trivial before the indescribable glory, the unfathomable mystery, and the unimaginable extent of the marvelous ocean of life, of which I am at times permitted to approach the shore.

The daily dive into the conscious ocean to which I had now unexpectedly found access had a most exhilarating effect on my mind. I was overwhelmed with wonder at the incalculable wealth I had found within myself. The distracting anxiety I had felt previously and the grave doubts I had entertained about my condition vanished altogether, yielding place to a feeling of inexpressible thankfulness to the Divine Power, which in spite of my ignorance, constant resistance, many faults, frailties, and mistakes, had wrought with matchless skill a new channel of perception in me, a new and more penetrating sight in order to introduce me to a stupendous existence.

In spite of all my efforts, the news of the strange psychic manifestations in me leaked out. My host, friends, and colleagues at the office were struck by my altered behavior and my constant mood of deep absorption. Even if I had tried, I could not have shaken it off, being myself entirely carried away by the wonder of an occurrence beyond anything I could have imagined. I certainly could not hide from my close associates a development that had the effect of startling me out of my equilibrium.

My host, uneasy at my constant perambulations in a state of deep abstraction, almost to the point of being totally oblivious at times, grew positively alarmed at seeing my lights on at odd hours in the night and finding me awake, writing in a mood of utter preoccupation. Knowing of my mystical tendencies, he remonstrated with me gently under the misapprehension that my constant absorption and nocturnal exertions were a prelude to a complete renunciation of the world in order to take up a monastic life.

In the course of a few weeks, unable to resist the fascination of the newly found subliminal existence, I found myself powerless to come out of my contemplative moods. Except for a few hours of irregular sleep at night they were continuously upon me for the whole day, making it almost impossible for me to apply my mind to anything. I ate mechanically, almost as a child does in sleep, and when obliged to speak talked and heard like a man who is engrossed in watching a most fascinating drama enacted before him and returns laconic answers to the comments of those seated beside him, often without comprehending and remembering fully what is said.

I went to the office more by force of habit than by choice or inclination. My whole being rose in revolt when I attempted to climb down from the ethereal heights of transcendence to the dry files lying unattended on my table. After some days the mere act of sitting in the cramped atmosphere of the room for hours became so unpleasant and oppressive that I proceeded on long leave, never to enter the premises again. I realized that the severance of my connection with the office would reduce my income to a great extent, but the urge in me to liberate myself from the bonds of servitude was too stong to be suppressed by monetary or worldly considerations.

In the meantime the strange news traveled through the town, and crowds of people called at my residence, attracted by the rumors of the miraculous development in me. Most of them came merely to satisfy their curiosity and to verify what they had heard, much as they would have gone to look at a freak or to watch the astounding performance of a conjurer. But few of them evinced any interest in the genesis of the change or the reason for the sudden manifestation.

In a few days the rush of people became so great and continuous that from early morning to the hour of darkness I had not a moment to myself. Feeling that it would be discourteous to refuse interviews and laboring under the notion that such an attitude on my part would be misconstrued as pride, I bore the daily rush patiently at the cost of my mental peace, which ought to have been my primary concern in the initial states of the new development. I was usually in an exalted state of mind throughout, and in the same condition talked to the people gathered round me, frequently passing into deeper moods under their gaze from which I was often recalled to my surroundings by the entry of other groups. I greeted the eager crowds mechanically, barely mindful of what I said or of those who arrived and left during the day.

After a few days the strain became unbearable, and I began to feel its adverse effects on my health. The first indication of the trouble was a growing restlessness during nights, which soon assumed the state of partial insomnia. Instead of feeling alarmed at the reappearance of an enemy that had caused me so much agony in the past, I interpreted it as the first sign of a liberated existence, of freedom from the domination of the flesh, considered to be an essential feature of true spiritual growth.

Lacking the care of my wife, who, with a woman's true instinct always exercised a strict supervision of my diet, I also grew indifferent to food, reveling in the thought that I had at last overcome a weakness which had compelled me to be too attentive to my nutrition and a slave to regularity. Gradually a feeling of detachment from the world began to take hold of me, accompanied by an increasing desire to break the chains that bound me to my family and to lead the live of a *sannyasi* (renunciate), untroubled by desire and unfettered by customs and conventions.

I had passed through a most strange experience which had culminated in a development entirely beyond my expectations and one which it was necessary to make known to others. It was therefore my duty, I argued with myself, to lead a life entirely free of the fret and fever of a worldly existence, devoted exclusively to the service of mankind, with the object of making known the great truth I had found. The only obstacle to the execution of this resolve, I thought, would be presented by the strong ties of affection which bound me to my family and friends and which, judging from my own past experience and inherent tendencies, would be very hard to break. But when I pondered more deeply on the issue and searched my heart for the answer, I found to my great surprise that the amazing experience I had now undergone had purged me clean of worldly love also, and that I could part from my family and friends forever without so much as a single look behind, to perform unhampered by any thought of family obligations the sacred task I eagerly wished to take upon myself.

But though I was afforded a glimpse into the state of mind and the motive power behind it that drove the prophets and seers of old to unparalleled feats of renunciation and asceticism which appear beyond the capacity of the ordinary human being, I was not destined to follow in their footsteps, due to the extreme susceptibility of my system to disorder under the stress of unfavorable and harsh conditions. There was a weak spot in me somewhere which often gave way under the rigor imposed by an ascetic way of life or continued irregularity in the matter of diet and sleep. I believe it is because of this vulnerability that I was able to trace the close connection existing between the body and the mind, even in transcendental conditions of the brain, which might not have been so clearly apparent to me otherwise.

For more than a month I lived in a state of triumph and spiritual exaltation which is impossible to describe. During all this period my whole being was always pervaded by a distinct feeling that while moving, sitting or acting I was constantly encompassed by a stupendous silent presence from which I drew my individual existence. Frequently I had moods of deeper absorption when, speechless with wonder, I lost myself completely in the indescribable. These moods were attended occasionally by inspirational flashes towards the close.

After the end of this period, owing to insufficient sleep and irregularity in diet, the feeling of exaltation and happiness, which had been present continuously, diminished perceptibly, and I again began to feel signs of exhaustion and at times even of uneasiness in my mind. I was roughly shaken out of this short-lived state of heavenly joy when one morning, rising from bed after a restless night, I found myself in the grip of acute depression which continued for the whole day, acting like a dip in ice-cold water on one in a state of inebriation.

Startled out of my mistaken optimism and reprimanding myself sharply for the neglect, I forced myself to give immediate attention to my diet and after some days noticed signs of improvement in my condition.

But my immoderate indulgence in psychic enjoyment, excessive mental exertion, and neglect of organic needs had, without my detecting it, depleted my vitality to an alarming extent, creating a poisoned state of the nervous system which prevented me from noticing the extremely slow deterioration in time to take appropriate precautionary measures. I had heard stories of men who, intoxicated with joy to the point of madness on their first glimpse of the supersensory state of existence after the awakening, had been so entirely carried away from earthly life that they found it impossible to come down to the normal level of consciousness in order to attend to the needs of the body; their spirits in unbroken ecstatic contemplation of the fascinating supersensual realm from the beginning to the end had departed the starved body without even once descending back to earth.

I immediately refrained from exhibiting myself before the curious crowds that came and went in an unending stream. Instead of encouraging the moods of intense absorption, always ready to settle upon me the moment my mind turned inwards, I deliberately avoided introversion, devoting myself exclusively to worldly trifles in order to allow a period of rest to the already overstimulated brain.

It was about the middle of March, marking the beginning of spring in Kashmir, and I felt I should no longer delay returning to my home, my only asylum in times of distress, in order to submit myself to the affectionate care of my wife, my sole guardian during illness. Without losing a single day I journeyed to Srinagar by air, relinquishing forever the thought of roaming the earth in the traditional way of the renunciate to effect the regeneration of mankind, a fantasy born in my case from the desire for power and the yearning for mental conquest which often accompanies the activity of kundalini in the intellectual center, causing a slightly intoxicated condition of the brain too subtle to be noticed by the subject himself or by his uninformed companions, however erudite and intelligent they may be.

At home I entrusted myself completely to the care of my wife, who from the absence of color in my face and the look in my eyes at once concluded that I was in a state of exhaustion and stood in urgent need of rest and recuperation. The news of my strange feats had traveled to Srinagar before me, and it became a difficult problem to prevent the crowds which assembled at my house from gaining access to me.

After a few days I was able to devote several hours daily to meet the visitors without fatigue and kept myself lightly engaged for the rest of the time to avoid the influence of contemplative moods which even now exercised such a fascination over me that I had to exert my will to the utmost to resist the temptation completely for even a day. In the course of a few weeks the crowds began to thin and ultimately ceased, allowing me more respite which, coupled with the precautions taken in diet, helped me to overcome the deficiency caused by my own lack of restraint. But it took more than six months for me to be normal again and to attend to my duties without losing myself all of a sudden in the rapt contemplation of an unconditioned existence.

By the time my leave expired, I had made up my mind not to serve any longer. The way of escape from the sordidness and misery of the material world into the unutterable peace and tranquility of the effulgent internal universe was too narrow and too risky to allow me to make use of it with a heavy load of worldly responsibilities upon my shoulders. In order to taste the fruit of true spiritual liberation, it was necessary for me to free myself as far as possible from the chains that bound me to the material world. The secluded corner of a busy office room, throbbing with noiseless activity and tense with subdued excitement was not a place where a man now constantly preoccupied with the unseen could pass several hours at a stretch always at the call of others without running the risk of serious injury to his mental health.

There were other reasons, too, which precipitated my decision to sever my connections entirely with the office. The change of government had brought in its wake a host of burning problems, all demanding immediate solution. They had to be handled, and handled carefully, at a time when the whole country was in a state of ferment caused by a wild scramble for power and possessions on the one side and the efforts made to avert deprivation and dispossession on the other. Our office could not escape the general commotion visible everywhere, and soon its atmosphere grew charged with mutual suspicion to an extent that for a man in my condition it was positively dangerous. Accordingly I applied for premature retirement which, after the usual formalities, was ultimately sanctioned.

I was now free to pass my time as I pleased, untroubled by any thoughts of how to find my way out of the ever-present official dilemmas and the constant conflicts between my conscience and the wishes of my superiors. After an absence of many months, during which there had literally occurred a world of difference in me, I again joined the staunch group of friends who had kept our movement alive during the interval. I again participated in their activities, which were now directed towards providing amenities for the utterly destitute widows in our society or towards removing the barrier of public opinion against the remarriage of those who were agreeable to it, in this way mitigating to some extent the suffering of many subjected to inhuman treatment in the name of religion and caste by their own families.

In spite of the deep desire of every member of the little group to confine their activities to the mission of service, they were drawn unwillingly into the troubled waters of political rivalry and ambition by constant opposition, aimed at forcing their allegiance. In the course of a few years it was made difficult for them even to carry on the humanitarian work in which they were engaged. But determined to persist, they managed to continue their activities in a restricted form, always anxious to steer clear of rival political groups angling for their support.

SIXTEEN

A Triumph of Love

IT WAS ABOUT TEN O'CLOCK in the morning when a visitor was announced and ushered into my sitting room in Karan Nagar. He was a middle-aged man of about forty-five years, simply dressed and looking somewhat nervous as he sat before me. The preceding day had been a very busy one for me and I was sorting out some papers to put them in order.

I looked at the stranger and asked the reason for his visit. He was silent for a moment, trying to make up his mind how to begin and then said that he had heard that the Samiti was interested in arranging marriages of parties that were not in a position to arrange a normal wedding in the conventional manner.

"Please explain a little more clearly what you wish," I said.

"I have heard," he replied, "that the Samiti has arranged marriages of couples who loved each other and who did not wish to go to a court of law for a legal marriage and who wished to avoid the pomp and show, with all its heavy expenditure, of a conventional wedding ceremony."

"Who is the girl," I asked, "and what is her age?"

"She lives in my neighborhood," he answered, "and her age is about twenty years. She and I intensely love each other and all we wish is that your organization would solemnize our nuptials."

"Are the parents of the girl willing to agree to her marriage with you," I said, "and if so, have they agreed to the performance of the ceremony in the Samiti to avoid the expenses that an official ceremony would involve?"

He was silent for a while and then said slowly, "I have not consulted the parents and cannot say whether they would agree. But the girl and I are determined on the marriage. I have approached you as I know the Samiti is interested in preventing scandals in the society. We will live as man and wife in any case and no one can prevent us, as the girl is of an age to decide for herself. Only we do not wish to live as outcasts, ostracized by the community, and it is for this reason that I have come to seek your help."

I thought for a moment. As a rule we never solemnized a marriage, save in the case of widows, except with the consent of the parents or guardians of a girl. At the same time, experience had taught me that an outright rejection of the request could lead to elopement, with resultant agony to the parents and also a possible disaster for the girl, as she would have no one to protect her if the man turned out to be an imposter who would leave her to her fate as soon as he was satiated. In order to have some time to know the full details of the case, I asked the man to send an application in accordance with the prescribed procedure of the Samiti.

The man left and returned with his application in the afternoon. He and the girl lived at no great distance from Karan Nagar. The girl resided in his neighborhood in the house of her mother's brother and his wife. Her own father, a widower, lived in another locality. He was employed in a government concern and had let his daughter stay in the house of her maternal uncle for better protection. The suitor was a bus driver by profession, plying his vehicle between Srinagar and Jammu, separated from each other by a distance of about two hundred miles.

On receipt of the application, as was our custom, we started an independent investigation of the case. The members entrusted to this work lost no time in making the inquiries but came back with a startling report which made us extremely anxious about the whole issue.

The man and the girl, it was found, had an illicit connection and the girl was about eight months pregnant. So far the girl had not divulged the secret to her uncle and aunt or to her father. One of our lady workers who met her personally stated that she was in a desperate frame of mind and contemplated suicide as a last resort to save herself from disgrace, which was inevitable once the truth was known.

I felt deeply disturbed at this narrative and, together with my friends, spent long hours trying to find a solution to the problem. The next day we sent the same member again to the girl to reassure her that every possible help would be rendered to her in her misfortune and that we would solemnize her marriage with the father of the child, if she wished it, or find another suitable partner for her who would take responsibility for the unborn child. We also gave her the assurance that we would intervene with her father to save her from his anger and secure his consent to her marriage, which would be performed openly in such a way that no blemish would attach to her name.

With the other disabilities attending pregnancy, the fear and the agony that gripped the mind of the unfortunate girl must have inflicted a torture beyond words. We passed restless hours in our search for a remedy to alleviate her suffering. Every day, one of our lady workers went to console her and to give her the strength that she urgently needed. Slowly they gained her confidence with their assiduous care for her, and bit by bit she narrated the whole story of her fall.

Like a good neighbor, the man used to come to their house quite often and in this way became very friendly with the family. They exchanged presents and sacramental preparations on holy days. One day, when her uncle and aunt were away, he came with a plate filled with sweet cookies and met her alone in the house. That was her undoing. He took advantage of her loneliness to overcome her resistance and she succumbed. After that, he made use of every opportunity when the other relatives were absent to be with her and to indulge his passion without restraint. She soon became a willing accomplice in his designs without awareness of the danger she was in. It was after three or four months that the appalling truth dawned on her that she was with child, and she almost collapsed with the shock. There was no one in whom she could confide and no one could come to her succor in this calamity.

She broke the news to her paramour with tears streaming from her eyes and begged him to fetch her a medicine to cause an abortion so that she might be saved the horror of giving birth to an illegitimate child. She could not even bear the thought of it. The man, with loud protestations of his love for her and his wish to die in her service, promised to bring the most efficacious drug for her use. The medicine came, a pill that had to be swallowed daily for a couple of weeks until the abortion occurred. The girl obeyed the instructions implicitly. But nothing happened by the end of the period of two weeks. The empty phial, examined afterwards, was found to contain a tonic and not the drug for abortion which the girl had fervently sought.

Our female Samiti members were mystified at this story and could not understand why the man should have brought her a tonic instead of the medicine which the girl badly wanted and had begged for with streaming tears. The subsequent actions of the man clarified the mystery. He wanted to marry the girl. He knew that if an abortion occurred he would have no hold on her or her parents to marry her. The difference in their age, as also in their social status, made the marriage between the two extremely improbable. He had no illusions about it. Therefore, in order to leave no loophole for the girl to escape from his clutches, his effort was to keep her in the state of pregnancy until the fear of public disgrace forced her and her father to consummate her marriage with him. This was a villainous plan. The aim was to subject the poor victim of his lust to continued mental torture for months to force her into wedlock with him.

We were appalled at the betrayal involved in this inhuman plan of the treacherous lover. It was hard for me to reconcile myself to the truth that a man could be capable of such villainy towards a woman whom he professed to love. But there was more to come. When the girl finally understood the deceit practiced on her she was frantic with grief, and vowed never to see the man again. Whenever he entered the room where she was sitting with other members of the family, she abruptly left and refused to meet him or to talk to him. He tried his utmost to have a few minutes conversation with her. But in vain. She was adamant and would have nothing to do with the man who had so deeply wronged her.

The poor girl confessed that she had taken an oath not to marry the man even if she had to die to save herself from disgrace. With tears in her eyes she expressed her gratitude to our members for their solicitude and assurance of help. But at the same time she affirmed her determination not to marry the wicked father of her child under any circumstances whatsoever. The man had already learnt of this resolve on her part and went to further nefarious depths to gain his end. In a bid to prevent abortion of the child he made a report to the police, stating that the girl was with child by him and he feared that she would try to destroy it before birth. The police could act on the application under the antiabortion laws then in force. It is incredible that evil in the nature of man can sink to such abominable depths. I found it difficult to believe that a normal human being could act in this way with a girl whom he had betrayed. Meanwhile, the police could take no action until a crime was actually committed. The girl was not, therefore, harassed in any way.

These events took place shortly after the raid of Pakistani tribesmen on Kashmir in the autumn of the year 1949. The whole economic structure of the valley was in chaos. Lack of sufficient supplies of salt and sugar and other essential commodities had raised the price of some of them to an incredible degree. In his journeys between Jammu and Srinagar, this bus driver had the opportunity of bringing some of these articles, scarce in Srinagar at the time, and distributing them amongst those he wished to favor. Apart from informing the police, he took recourse to another abominable expedient to force his will upon the girl. He bribed a few ruffians in the locality to keep a watch on the girl's house from a distance, to prevent her going out to some other place. There was a state of tension prevailing in the city during those days which allowed such antisocial elements opportunities to do what they liked.

All these details made us aware of the intricacy of the position and the terrible situation in which the girl was placed. She could not destroy the child, nor even leave the house without creating an upheaval. In desperation the harassed creature decided that the only course open to her was suicide.

We racked our brains to find a solution. The girl frankly confessed to her friends, who now visited her daily on our behalf, that she was determined to kill herself and that her plan was to jump from the top floor of the house as soon as she could muster the courage to do so. She even admitted that she was going close to the window and looking down with the thought ever present in her mind that shortly she would take the jump to end her life and the mental torture that allowed her no rest day or night.

What could we do to prevent the tragedy? We thought and thought and, at last, hit upon a plan to save the girl and free her from the agony for all time to come.

I asked some of our friends to look out for a young man up to thirty years of age, healthy and good-looking, able to earn his own livelihood, who would be willing to marry the girl in her present condition and agree to act as father to the child. In a few days three candidates were selected, and we were asked to choose one of them. Our choice fell on a man about twenty-nine years of age, who had his own house and a large farm from which he derived an income sufficient for his needs. He was a handsome, well-built man and he solemnly assured us that he would take every care of the child if the girl was married to him. But how could the marriage take place? The girl was almost in a state of confinement. How could she be taken out of the house under the full gaze of the ruffians who were watching it at the instigation of her unscrupulous lover?

Our plan was to send one of our lady workers dressed as a nurse, covered with a *bougah* (veil worn by Muslim women). She was attended by a man who made it known deliberately to the loiterers close to the building that she was being brought to examine the girl. When the pair went up, they quietly put the *bougah* over the pregnant girl and after a short interval she came down with the man and they both passed into the street before the very eyes of the watchers, who thought that it was the nurse and her companion who were leaving. Close to the street where the river flowed by, a boat with another of our members in it was already waiting at the foot of the stone steps leading to the water.

The pair boarded the boat, which swiftly made for another landing place on the river a few hundred yards away. A tonga (horse cart) was waiting at the landing site for which the boat was bound. The tonga took all the three of them to a house in another part of the city where the marriage ceremony was performed during the night with many of our members and other friends participating. Soon after sunrise, the bride and the bridegroom went to their house. The girl looked at us with a beaming face, relieved for the first time of the terrible load that had weighed on her mind for months.

It was about nine o'clock in the evening. I had just finished my last meal of the day and was sitting in the kitchen, facing my wife who had been serving me with her usual tenderness. She sat perched on a small wooden board about six inches higher than the concrete floor of our cooking room in Karan Nagar.

The kitchen was her kingdom. In spite of my protests that she should have an occasional day off to relieve herself of monotony, she invariably seated herself at the accustomed place to make sure that the meals for the children and myself were ready on time. There was no holiday for her and no relief. If an illness intervened to keep her from her duty, the only lament she had was that it prevented her from doing the household work to keep things going for the family.

We are so accustomed to dwelling on the qualities of those who make a conspicuous success in life, in art, literature, politics, religion, or science, that we usually have no time to devote to those stratas of society which live in obscurity without ever appearing in the limelight of publicity. But, in actual fact, if our aim be to find the most noble, most perfect specimens of humanity, that is where we must look in order to find them.

For achieving noteworthy success in life, whether it be in politics or business, the individual needs must shed some of his principles and scruples to get the better of the other competitors in the field and to compromise with his conscience time after time to maintain his leading position. The ordinary men and women, who have no lofty and ambitious heights in view and who make the round of their duties in life without ever attempting to supersede others or snatch their rights in their own scramble for precedence, live more in harmony with their inner self than the ambitious celebrities whose names become household words in fields of human endeavor.

This is the reason why, in almost every revolution, it is the common men and women who rise to the seats of power, ousting the effete nobility, aristocracy, or the wealthy tycoons who had previously usurped all the seats of power and claimed all the attention of the masses exclusively for themselves. In my contacts with thousands of people in many parts of the world I have come across men and women who were models of truth, sacrifice and service and yet who never knew of their own greatness. They were unknown and unsought-after because too often the average human mind is not even able independently to assess the stature of a human being and must depend for its opinion on the views expressed in the books or other media or on the assessments made by other celebrities.

On that particular evening my wife and I were in a state of anxiety. Ragina, our daughter, was seriously ill in a hospital and we had had no news of her for the last two days. When my meal was finished I saw my wife looking pensively at me with anxiety writ large on her face. She made no attempt to serve the simple meal on her own plate as was her habit after serving the meal to me. I tried to break the silence with a few words of consolation, but at that very moment there was a loud knocking on the outer door leading into the compound. My wife gave a startled look and her face turned pale. Could it be a telegram from Delhi? Motioning her to remain seated I stood up and unlocked the door.

There were several people standing outside, indistinctly visible in the dim light shed by the street lamp. Looking attentively I saw three older members of the Samiti, one of them a senior police officer and another a lawyer, the elder brother of my son-in-law. For all three of them the mission of service we had undertaken was a sacred duty to which they had devoted themselves. They all trooped into my sitting room where I could see their faces clearly. Two other members with the party were a woman, tall and slim with a fair complexion, probably in her thirties, and a girl of about nine years of age. Both the mother and the daughter looked unkempt and disheveled, dressed in clothes that did not seem to belong to them and that were obviously borrowed and donned in haste.

"This lady and her daughter," explained Mr. Kaul, the lawyer, "have been entrusted to us by the police. She has eloped from her home in Khrew, a village about fourteen miles from Srinagar, with a stranger who worked as a blacksmith in the village. On the application of her husband the police have arrested them and handed them over to us for safe custody pending decision of the case in a court of law."

I understood the whole situation at once. The husband was over seventy years of age, and this was his second marriage. As we came to know later on, besides the disability of his age the man was an extremely closefisted miser who denied to his wife even the basic necessities of life. She had chosen escape from her home as the only way to free herself from a virtual prison house.

The time was not opportune for me to have a fugitive from justice and her daughter thrust into my care. It is true our home had provided an asylum for scores of such cases of fallen women, disowned and condemned by society, until it had been possible to rehabilitate them in the best way possible with the means at our disposal. But today my wife, who had to share the greater part of the responsibility, was in no mood to have two such suspicious-looking, disheveled strangers in the house.

I gently explained the position to my friends and asked them to keep the strangers with one of their families for a few days until we were free of anxiety, after which they could certainly bring them to us. But all my three friends declined to accept the responsibility on one excuse or the other. The main reason was that the woman was an apostate, since the man with whom she had eloped belonged to another faith. For this reason, they said, their ladies would not tolerate the presence of the woman and her daughter in their own homes, especially considering their dirty appearance and the dress they were wearing at the time. The scruples of orthodoxy, I knew, were too strong in the minds of the womenfolk to be brushed aside in a moment. There was no choice for me other than to accept the responsibility.

I went to my wife in the kitchen and told her the story of the unfortunate woman. She had never demurred whenever a victim was brought to my home for shelter and had always done her best to help. She thought for a moment and then said, "We cannot turn this poor creature out, so let us keep her, since there is no other place for her to go."

She came with me to the sitting room and, taking the woman by her hand, escorted her and the child into the kitchen and made them sit before her. She had not taken her meal yet. The disturbance caused by the knocking at the door and the entrance of the party had kept her from the meal. The mother and her daughter, she found, had not eaten anything for the whole day. The idea of eating alone while the other two continued to sit hungry was repellent to her. She instantly lit the fire and started to cook for the two.

The woman was wonderstruck by this kindness. After my friends had departed, I went to my wife to inquire where she had intended to lodge the mother and the daughter for the night. She at once replied, "They will sleep in my room."

The next morning, rising at her usual early hour, my wife also awoke the woman and escorted her to the bathroom, where the water had already been warmed up. She asked her to take her bath and offered her own freshly washed saree to her for a change of clothing. The woman protested at this change of dress, which would imply her reentry into her own caste. But my wife insisted, telling her that she was her sister and it would make her happy to take her to the temple. Overcome by her kindness, and with the memory of the previous evening still fresh in her mind, she obeyed, changed her dress and went to the temple and returned from there with my wife with the caste mark on her forehead.

The girl, too, took a bath and changed her dress. The mother and the daughter both now looked like presentable human beings. But the woman was adamant in respect of her relationship with her lover.

"I would never give him up," she said. She would stay with us as long as the case was in the court and, after that, join her lover to live with him. It was impossible to shake her from this position. For days on end we did all we could to persuade her to change her decision. But she was inflexible. She was a courageous woman. The police and the court had no terrors for her. Her argument was that her adherence to her own faith had played havoc with her life and happiness. How could she, therefore, retrace her steps to suffer the same torture she had endured before.

It was fruitless to argue with her. I felt that she now needed time to decide what was best for her own welfare. Meanwhile, after consultation with my friends, I had come to the conclusion that it would be sheer inhumanity to force the woman back to live with an eccentric and senile husband who had made her life a bed of thorns. If she agreed, we planned to marry her to a younger man, matching her in age. This course was not strictly lawful, as her marriage had not been dissolved and divorce granted. The old man would never have agreed to such a course. A dilemma faced us on every side. To force her into her former life of misery would be a sin, but it would be a greater crime if we allowed her to have her way and marry the man with whom she had eloped. He was a repulsive man, entirely unsuited to a woman of culture.

We also learnt from inquiries made that he intended to take the woman and her child to an unknown destination, probably to make the two over to a third party for a price. But the young woman was infatuated and all we said or did had no effect on her resolution. She understood that we were all doing our best to help her. She knew that my wife cooked, fed and served her as she would do to a member of the family. She was wearing the clothes which my wife freely gave to her. But all this did not suffice to convince her that her love for the man was misplaced and might lead her to a worse position very soon.

In order to give her more freedom, I placed a small kitchen at her disposal to cook what she liked and sanctioned a monthly allowance to meet her needs. The mother and the daughter had now a room all to themselves and a kitchen for their cooking. Weeks passed and still there was no change in her attitude. She often went for a walk with her daughter and returned after an hour or so to the house without ever making any attempt to escape. I allowed her every freedom of action and was happy that she took a walk daily to stretch her legs for a while. But soon we discovered that these walks had a secret purpose, of which we had known nothing.

One day, during the afternoon, Kashi Nath Chhattabali, one of our enthusiastic members, returning home from his office along the main road, a little distance from our house, saw the lady talking to a stranger with the daughter standing close by. On coming nearer he recognized the man as her paramour and, in a fit of rage at the betrayal on her part, he roared at them, threatening to hand them over to the police then and there. The man took to his heels and ran, but the lady, who knew Kashi Nath, stood unmoved without showing any signs of fear. Kashi Nath went in pursuit of the man and the woman and her daughter returned to the house.

In the evening, Kashi Nath came to tell me about the episode. The other members of our Samiti were also informed. We found that the little girl was serving as an intermediary between the two and it was through her that they could communicate with each other. The child had gone out often, we didn't know where, and returned soon after. In this way, the meeting place was fixed and the two lovers could meet now and then at some place chosen by the man and communicated by the girl for the information of her mother. Our members came to us one after the other, angry at the deception. Ramchand Nakshi, the retired police officer, even suggested that the woman no longer stay in my house, to avoid a public scandal. Some of the members talked to her in angry tones, pointing out the deception involved in her behavior and asked her to desist from meeting the man in the future. But all that was said made no serious impact upon her determination.

I felt greatly disturbed. We could not keep the lady as a prisoner. But, at the same time, to allow her freedom was to give her permission to meet her friend. For a long time that night sleep refused to come to my eyes. I had two precious lives in my care and was responsible to Heaven to see that they were fairly treated. Had I felt certain that the woman could be happy with the man we might have allowed her to live with him. But actually the position was very dubious and we could not adopt this course without serious misgivings in our hearts.

Next morning, when she had returned from the temple with my wife, I called her into my room and spoke to her gently on the happenings of the previous day.

"I have treated you as a sister or a daughter during all this period," I said, "and my wife has treated you as a dear member of the family. Do you not see what damage your conduct has done to our reputation? Did you notice how reproachful the members of the Samiti were and how they resented the freedom that we had allowed to you? I cannot understand what made you act in this way to cause me pain and to lower my image in the eyes of my friends."

She looked at my face for a moment and the blood mounted to her cheeks. But then, suddenly as if under the impact of another emotion, she lowered her eyes and burst into a paroxysm of tears and sobs as if her heart would break.

Something in my words had touched her and swayed her iron determination. For the first time I saw her like a woman in the grip of heartrending sorrow. In a voice broken with sobs she said, "I promise you never to repeat this incident again. Kindly do with me as you like. I entrust everything into your hands."

The struggle was over. Love and kindness had conquered her heart. She knew instinctively that I was trying to do my best for her and she yielded, to save me from further mental worry on her behalf.

I put my hand on her shoulders and consoled her until she ceased her tears. The next day in a meeting with my friends, we decided to marry her to a suitable young man about her own age who would also be prepared to take the responsibility for the daughter. Our members also met her husband and persuaded him to accept the reality of the situation. He acted on their advice and ceased to proceed with the case against his wife. We then started to look for a suitable young man to marry her. Soon there were several suitors for her hand. She saw them one by one and finally made her choice. It was a young man from a village some miles from Srinagar. He was in service with landed property and a small fruit garden, sufficient for the two to lead a happy life.

The marriage was performed in the Samiti premises without any ostentation. The woman soon proved herself to be a model house-wife and a good mother. Reports from the village showed that she had adjusted herself admirably to the new life. Her young daughter received all the attention she needed from her stepfather and grew into healthy womanhood. Years afterwards, she was married, and we participated in her marriage. For years her mother came to us at the time of Shivaratri, the annual spring holy festival, when young brides come to their parental home to receive the blessings of their parents. She treated our home as her parental house and acted in accordance with the custom.

The most important event in the lives of men and women of our community is marriage. There is no doubt that marriage is a major event in the lives of men and women all over the world. The thought of their life's partner is a constant feature in the imagination of adolescent boys and girls everywhere. The ideal image of their life's companion is a recurrent theme in the reveries and daydreams of men and women of marriageable age. But, apart from this common feature, the importance attached to wedlock in our community revolves around other weighty matters incidental to it.

The most important of these incidental matters is the dowry. As soon as the young men draw near to marriageable age, their parents dream of the wealth and the objects of luxury with which the bride would ornament the house. For the mother-in-law in particular, this is the most opportune time, when Goddess Lakshmi can bless the family. They dream of the delicacies that will start arriving from the bride's side after the marriage is celebrated.

There is a special class of men and women who act as intermediaries in the case of marriages. They are few in number, mostly males, and their services are eagerly sought, often years before the parents feel that their children are about to attain the age when they would like to marry them off. The intermediaries generally possess precise information about the men and maidens eligible for marriage in their clientele. They soon start coming to the parents who have asked for their help in the search for a suitable partner for the girl or boy. A horoscope showing the constellations that rule the future of the individual is prepared by the priest of the family. From this horoscope, a brief chart known as *tekni*, showing the time of birth of the boy and the position of the stars, is drawn up and a copy is supplied by the intermediary to the parents of the girl so that it can be compared with her chart. If the two horoscopes or the charts do not harmonize, marriage between the parties often becomes impossible. In some rare cases, the horoscopes are not tallied and the marriage is settled without adhering to this condition.

When the horoscopes accord with each other there is usually a hint from the bridegroom's side, demanding to know the dowry which the bride would bring from her family. This is a crucial issue and many otherwise appropriate marriage proposals break down on this account.

Before negotiations for the final settlement of the marriage take place, the parties are often in possession of all the particulars and data of the other side. This includes the family status, their financial position, their lineage, relationships, the character of the boy, his academic qualifications, his earning capacity, and his future prospects.

The bridegroom's side make similar inquiries about the other side. These include the appearance of the bride and her social graces. The particulars are supplied by the intermediary. But almost always the parents use other channels to gather the information.

In spite of all these precautions deceptions do occur sometimes, blasting the life of one of the partners with the selection of a life mate not at all suitable or with a physical or mental defect about which no hint had been divulged.

Several such cases came to my notice during the course of our social work. In one such case a deformed moron, whose face became twisted and distorted when he attempted to speak, was married to a healthy, handsome girl for whom every sight of her twitching and stammering husband was a torture all her life.

One of the prominent characteristics of parenthood in our society is the love lavished on the child. The ecstasy experienced on the birth of a male child is something to be remembered. The girls too, in spite of the burden they impose on their parents in this terrible, faulty social system, receive their due share of love. The parents stint and save, often to the point of denying themselves sufficient food and comfort, to ensure that their children have a proper education. The parents of a bright boy would gladly sell their heirlooms or mortgage their house to pay for the higher education of their child. There is no sacrifice they would not make to ensure a bright future for their offspring.

In addition to the expenses incurred on the education of a girl child, the thrifty parents must start to build up her dowry, bit by bit, while the child is still in her early teens. She must have a good husband, well-placed in life and a well-to-do family to take care of her. It does not matter if the girl has received a higher education than her husband or, because of her distinctions, is able to earn more than he does. She must bring in a dowry and, in addition to her service, attend to the household work to cook and wash for her lord.

The preparations for the marriage festival on the daughter's side have the semblance of an expedition to the top of Mount Everest or any other such Herculean project, involving a tremendous strain on the household. Months ahead, the family sits together to draw up the plan of the feast to be served to the bridegroom's party on the marriage day. Friends, neighbors, and relatives are dutybound to offer their assistance in the function. There is a good reason for this. Formerly there was no restriction on the number of guests that a bridegroom could bring with himself to feed at the house of the bride. Even now, in spite of the regulations limiting the number of invitees to fifty or less, the girl's side is never sure of the size of the marriage procession accompanying the bridegroom.

The practice is often to cook for at least five hundred people apart from the other guests which the girl's parents invite from their own side. Consultations, discussions, and confabulations continue for weeks and months to make sure that the procession has the best possible reception and the place where they are to be seated for their meal is lavishly decorated. The meal served is often vegetarian, but its richness and the number of dishes cooked make it expensive beyond the means of the average individual. I have seen as many as fifty and even more varieties of food prepared with meticulous care for hundreds, much of it only to be wasted and thrown into the gutter when the number actually sitting down to eat is too small.

The magnificent decorations and the sumptuous meal do not limit the responsibilities to be shouldered by the bride's family. Besides a number of gold ornaments, the dowry must include rich dresses for the bride and a choice set of clothes for the bridegroom. There is no limit to the goods, dresses, finery, furniture, bedding, television sets, silverware, radios, watches, motorcycles, cars, and other luxuries that the bride is expected to add to the household of her husband. She must have everything needed to run her own home.

For the first few years after the nuptials, tributes from the girl's family must reach her in-laws in cash or kind. There are specific occasions when the presents have to be sent and even conventional standards according to which they are to be calculated. The girl's parents often seek the advice of an elder in the neighborhood who is conversant with these customs.

It is incredible to what extent these practices have been elaborated to keep the parents of the girl in a constant state of fret and fever to satisfy usage. On at least four festive occasions in the year—on the birthday of the husband, his father, his brother-in-law or other honorable relatives, on every occasion of illness or death in the bridegroom's family, every time the girl comes to visit the parents and every time the parents accidentally meet their in-laws during the first year—a handsome tribute or present, in cash, fruit, cooked food, dresses, or in other ways must be delivered to the family of the bridegroom. It is unbelievable but even on the day when brinjals, a popular vegetable in Kashmir, are first eaten during the summer, a tribute must reach the husband's parents to keep them in good humor and to avoid constant reproaches to the young wife.

Except for some humane exceptions, these outrageous practices and exorbitant demands are enforced rigidly as a matter of right by the bridegroom's side. The torture they cause to the innocent brides—most of them models of decorum, modesty, and fidelity—is beyond description. I have known of numerous cases in which the bride, criticized and tormented day in and day out by her mother-in-law and sisters-in-law, never uttered a word of the torment she was enduring in order to spare her parents the agony of begging or borrowing heavy sums to appease the bridegroom's family. I have seen young brides wasting away and sinking slowly to death with the daily wounds inflicted on them by the sharp rebukes they have to listen to in silence without uttering a single word in reply.

I knew that these evil, inhuman customs and conventions were eating into the very vitals of our society within a few years after the marriage. I had seen beautiful, blooming maidens wither like flowers bitten by a frost, so different from what they had been before marriage that it was hard to recognize them. In a conservative, middle-class family the poor daughter-in-law has to be the first to be astir in the family at daybreak, to retire to her room at night last of all, to eat after the men have eaten, and to be at work some way or the other through all the hours of the day.

Ours is a cultured community, hardworking and thrifty, whose main profession has involved reading and writing from very ancient times. Vicissitudes have taught it to be tolerant and adaptable, God-fearing and religious-minded. Members of the community distinguished themselves in every sphere of knowledge and field of activity throughout the course of history. They are capable of blazing a trail for themselves and rising to elevated heights in any part of the world. But, by a strange perversity of the mind, the evil custom of dowry and the cruelty sometimes inflicted on young daughters-in-law to extort tributes from their parents is eroding the very foundation on which the community stands, and even government legislation has failed to remove abuses.

While our Samiti was still agitating for a raise in the salaries of the low-paid employees of the State, a sudden strange change in my thinking made me aware of the serious faults in our customs and conventions to which I had been an impassive spectator in the past. In fact, I had myself actively participated in the decorations and the feasts or the marriage celebrations of my close relatives and helped in the spectacular displays and enjoyed the delectable feasts. I had no remorse or prick of conscience on those occasions that I was helping in celebrations that were sucking the very blood of indigent parents who had several daughters to marry off. The thought had never previously even entered my mind that the society was adhering to inhuman customs that caused unbearable torture to and undermined the vitality of our womenfolk.

I was not conscious of it at the time, but it is clear that a change had occurred in my thinking. What had appeared to be a normal procedure before, to which it was necessary for us to conform, now seemed to be an atrocious custom against which every human being with a feeling heart must raise his voice. It is amazing how his own mind can deceive an individual. An egotist takes care that his interest is served first of all and thinks this is the right thing to do. The loss or pain caused another through his efforts are for him only natural and do not concern him at all.

On the contrary, the heart of a humanitarian bleeds when he sees another put to pain or loss on account of any action on his part and tries his utmost to recompense him for it, even at his own cost. The inherently honest and dishonest man look at the same deal from different angles, each believing in his own judgment. The mirror of our mind can become murky without our being aware of the change that has occurred. Our power of discrimination and judgement is not of our own making but comes from the spark of the Divine within us.

SEVENTEEN

More and More, I Returned Towards Normal Living

DURING THE CRITICAL YEARS that followed my first experience of the unseen, the work center of our group served for me the twofold purpose of providing congenial occupation without any curtailment of my freedom and also a fruitful and healthy hobby for my leisure. I had for the first time tasted the joy of a new existence and it maddened me to an extent I could not believe possible, creating a feeling of estrangement from the world and an aversion towards the things of life, as if I were a captive in an alien land, impatient to break away from prison but unable to do so.

I might have turned a recluse to assuage the fire of renunciation kindled in me but for the constant contact with suffering and misery and the slender chance I had of alleviating it. My active participation in the charitable endeavor, though extremely limited in scope, conduced to some extent to keep me normal with enough attachment to the world to combat the morbid escapist tendencies that had developed in me. The rest was accomplished by my wife, whose immense love, unremitting attention to my smallest need and constant care made me so dependent on her that the idea of residing in solitude, away from her even for a short time, appeared too formidable to be possible of execution by one in such an extremely delicate and peculiar state of health as I was.

From the very beginning of the new development, many persons, prompted by desire or driven by necessity, came to see me with an ulterior object in view. They waited for hours, seeking an opportunity to talk to me alone about the purpose of their visit. During the earlier period, when the crowds showed no sign of diminution and I was generally in an elevated and far-from-communicative mood, they came several times in succession until able to snatch a few minutes of private conversation with me.

For most of them I had attained a state of authority, of command over the subtle forces of nature, able to do and undo things, competent to alter circumstances, to change the destiny and modify the effect of other people's actions and conduct. They allotted to me a position of suzerainty, of close intimacy with the Almighty, with powers to defy the laws of nature and to interrupt the march of events by merely a gesture or an effort of my will.

I heard their stories in silence, touched at the scenes of human misery and tales of harrowing grief which they narrated. Some were destitute, some unemployed, some childless, some involved in litigation, some hopeless invalids, some in the grip of reverses, some entangled in domestic troubles, and so on. They expected me to intercede with fate on their behalf to rid them of their sorrows and to free them from their difficulties against which they were powerless to battle, and were eager to catch at every passing chance, holding the slenderest ray of hope as a drowning man catches at a straw. They were all of them afflicted, frustrated, or disillusioned men and women for whom life was a bed of thorns.

The general belief among the masses about psychics and men of vision, stretching back to prehistoric times, credits them with amazing supernatural powers. The impression is that they possess a mysterious link with, or control over, subtle intelligent forces of nature and command over the elementals and spirits. I could not escape the consequences of this misconception, and no amount of denial and argument on my part was effective in carrying conviction to people not only deeply steeped in the superstition from early childhood but also forced by exceedingly painful situations to be eagerly on the lookout for a supernatural source to extricate them from their difficulties. Not a few of them, ascribing my honestly expressed inability to help them out of their afflictions to reluctance

on my part to do anything, behaved like children, imploring my
assistance with folded hands and tears in their eyes. The sight of
tears and manly voices husky with emotion left me powerfully
affected, as shaken with grief as they were.

Those afflicted men and women who came to me for a miraculous
escape from their ills were mostly the victims of social injustice, and
my heart went out to them in sympathy. In their position, I too might
have acted in the same manner. My utter inability to relieve their
distress added so greatly to my sorrow at their misery that, unable
to bear it, I sometimes had to seek the sanctuary of my deeper being
to gain assurance and strength to overcome it.

I consoled them as best as I could, and often they went away in a
more peaceful frame of mind than that in which they had come,
leaving me restless and unsatisfied, heavy with their grief, vividly
conscious of the fact that, forming as we do the tiny individual cells
of a mighty organism, we share alike the sorrows and misery existing
in the world; but, debarred from realizing this by the wall of ego
segregating each cell from the rest, we feel happy and proud at
acquisitions, often purchased at our own cost, which we mistakenly
believe have been paid for by others.

While there is a solid foundation for the venerable belief which
attributes transcendental powers to visionaries, the popular idea has
persisted through centuries that those possessing the power are in a
position to set aside the laws of nature and to change the ordained
course of events. This idea rests on an incorrect evaluation of the
position and also on an unhealthy attitude towards the problems of
life. The development of a supersensory channel of knowledge for
the perception of subtle realities beyond the reach of the senses and
reason is not intended to supplant but rather to aid the rational
faculty in the management of temporal affairs rigidly ruled by
temporal laws.

The psychic and even physical powers possessed by prophets and
seers are merely in the nature of a manifestation, an emblem of
sovereignty bestowed by nature. In the circumstance, the application

of the extremely rare spiritual endowments to the solution of the day-to-day problems of human physical existence, for which intellect is the proper instrument, would be no less irrational than the utilization of the quality of heaviness in gold for the purpose of crushing stones with it to provide material for roads. The curative and other powers sometimes exercised by mystics and saints never went beyond the sphere of individual application, and it was left for people of genius who brought vision to the aid of intellect to devise universally efficacious remedies for scourges like smallpox and to make other discoveries in the physical realm, a task which was neither accomplished by nor fell within the province of prophets and visionaries.

As time wore on and I firmly refused to be tempted into making a vulgar exhibition or impious use of the priceless gift which Heaven had bestowed on me, there occurred a perceptible thinning in the number of supplicants who came purely with the object of a miraculous redress, and ultimately they ceased altogether.

I scrupulously adhered to a normal mode of life, performing all the duties incumbent on me as the head of a family, and in my dress, manner, and behavior displayed not the slightest deviation from the pattern which I should have followed in the usual course of events. This made most of the people, who in the beginning had evinced the deepest interest in my astounding performance, revise their opinion and regard the development as either freakish, disappearing as mysteriously as it had come to pass, or as an abnormality that subsided of its own accord with the passage of time.

In the course of a few years these incidents, after existing as a nine-day wonder, were almost forgotten and are now seldom mentioned save by traducers, who refer to them as an incontestable proof of my eccentric disposition when they wish to find fault with me.

In view of this experience I wonder at the inability of the mass mind to move out even an inch beyond the accustomed rut. Barring not more than half a dozen people in all, the thousands who came to see me evinced not the least curiosity to know how the development had occurred and what the mystery was behind the surprising manifestation. If in the beginning, side by side with the manifestation, I had started to talk and whisper in a mysterious manner and edited recondite volumes for mystified readers to pore over, each at liberty to draw his own meaning from the vague expressions and obscure passages, instead of making a plain, unambiguous statement of facts, and had followed the same principle in my dress and behavior, the interest and curiosity created would have increased enormously, at least for a period, securing me not only popularity but money as well, at the cost of truth.

In the course of time I returned more and more towards normal living, while retaining the heightened state of consciousness inviolate, and descending from a state of mental intoxication to one of sobriety. I became more keenly conscious of the fact that, though my psychophysiological equipment had now attained a condition that made it possible for me on occasions to transcend the boundary rigidly confining the mental activity of my fellow beings, I was essentially in no way different from or superior to them.

Physically I was what I had been before, as susceptible to disease, decay, and age, as liable to accident and calamity, as prone to hunger and thirst, as I always had been, a normal man in every other way save the alteration in the mental and consciousness spheres, which, by bringing me on occasions nearer to sober metaphysical realities as astounding and remote from our ordinary conceptions as light is from darkness, had a curbing effect upon the frivolous and vain tendencies of my mind. I had in no way overcome the biological limitations of my body, in no manner exceeded the measure of its endurance and physical capacity, or attained any miraculous powers to defy the laws of nature.

On the contrary, my system had grown more delicate. I was the same man, now advanced in age, who had sat for meditation on that memorable day when I had my first experience of the superphysical, with the difference that since then my brain had been attuned to finer vibrations from the unimaginable conscious universe all around us, and had in consequence acquired a deeper and more penetrating inner vision. Except for the alteration in the vital current and certain peculiar biological changes, there was no distinctive external feature to mark me out from other human beings. The moods of deep absorption, leading to the indescribable supercondition, on occasions became a normal feature of my existence. I lost touch with it, however, during intervals of illness and in the debilitated condition of the system which followed in its wake.

The slightest disturbance in the system becomes highly enlarged in an expanded state of consciousness. Emotions and feelings become magnified and the imagination highly evocative, excitable, and vivid. In this, I believe, lies the reason for the emotional imbalance and eccentricity of genius and the exaggerated response of the mystic's mind. It is the change in the volume and the depth of consciousness which is at the root of the gulf of difference existing between the exuberance of genius, the unitive experience of the mystic, and the normal mind.

I knew instinctively that I was witness to an extraordinary phenomenon and was the subject of a rare experiment. Slowly, by a decree of Fate which I could not understand, I was being initiated into a secret that has defied all attempts made to unearth it so far. It was the secret of the still-persisting organic evolution of the human brain. Since I had practiced no austerities, denied no legitimate desire, and made no attempt to renounce family or the world, I felt safe in assuming that a healthy natural life was not an obstacle in the attainment of a more evolved consciousness. What proved of inestimable value in the ordeals I had to face was the habit of moderation I had cultivated and also the fair degree of control I could exercise over myself. Without these two acquisitions I could not have survived the tumult caused in my mind soon after the awakening.

To cite but one instance of the mastery I had gained over my nature, the following episode should suffice. A colleague in the office persistently invited me to lunch at his residence during our stay in

Jammu. On account of the regimen I followed, I usually refused invitations to eat at the houses of friends and even relatives. But he was so insistent and even importunate that I ultimately gave in, and a day was settled for my partaking lunch at his house. I arrived in time at the address given. In a short while, after a brief chat, the meal was served.

A richly prepared dish was placed in front of me. I put forth my hand to pick up the first morsel and then reeled back in horror. It had been stormy in the morning. It is usual on such days for the wind to drive swarms of flies inside the rooms, away from the surrounding areas where the strong current does not allow them to stay firmly on anything. This had happened on this day. It seems that a crowd of flies, forced by the wind, dashed against the chimney where the wife of my friend had cooked the viands. Unnoticed by her, the flies, in hundreds, must have dropped into the cooking pots simmering on the fire. The light in the kitchen must have been dim, made dimmer by the storm. The small blackish bodies swimming in the gravy must have therefore escaped the eye of the lady. I myself could not easily distinguish the black marks at first as the light, even in the sitting room where we sat for the meal, was dim. But when I touched a black thing with my forefinger, the sickening truth dawned on me at once.

What could I do? To point out the mess and refuse the meal would have brought down furious anger of the husband upon the head of the poor woman. She had a pallor on her face, which told me she was not healthy. She had been so kind and attentive to me since the time of my arrival that I could not find it in my heart to cause her the least distraction which was inevitable if I refused the food. With a strong effort of will, I overcame the nausea which I felt at the sight of the dirty flies. The dishes were cooked in boiling oil and water so, I consoled myself, there was little fear of infection. Without allowing it to be seen by the husband who was sitting a few feet away, I carefully picked up the flies and placed them on one side of the plate. Then I proceeded to put morsel after morsel into my mouth while my stomach and all my body revolted against the outrage. But I was compelled to leave a part of the meal uneaten as it was too much for me. After I had eaten enough, I mixed up the flies again with the leavings which, according to practice, have to be thrown away.

I have read of people who had the strength of will to hold their finger over a flame till the fat melted, who castrated themselves with red-hot irons, or those who stretched themselves naked upon scorching iron sheets, with a raging fire burning beneath, turning from side to side till they were roasted to death, or who endured the most excruciating torture without flinching or surrendering a principle or a secret entrusted to them. The mere hearing or reading of these incredible feats of human endurance made me shudder and wince, shrinking with horror at the mere thought of having to face a similar ordeal.

Compared to these exploits, the episode I have narrated dwindles to a mere trifle. It is nothing compared to the penances practiced by some classes of ascetics in India—holding the arm upward till it is withered to a stump, sleeping on a bed of nails, hanging face downwards from a tree over a burning fire giving out fumes of pungent smoke, standing on one leg for the whole day, sitting atop a tree for days, dwelling naked on snowy heights, and the like.

But I had no ambition to be acclaimed a champion for any spectacular feat of endurance. What I had striven for was to have a moderate amount of control over my feelings and my reflexes in the ordinary battle of life. In my exercises for physical fitness or in my efforts at self-control, I never went beyond the limit of moderation, beyond what others could also achieve with only a small amount of persistent effort. Glancing backward to my later twenties, when for a time I exercised hard to excel in wrestling, I remember distinctly that every effort on my part to overdo things was countered by my own body in various ways. Any overexertion was followed not only by exhaustion and fatigue, which are usual, but also adverse mental reactions which soon made me desist from a too strenuous course.

Could it be that I was instinctively obeying an inner mandate not to force my body too far beyond the limit of endurance prescribed for it by nature? Try as I might, I never succeeded in exercising control over some of my desires beyond a certain point. My attempt was not to attain Herculean results and to tame every ounce of feeling, passion, or desire in me. The aim was to moderate them and keep their temper under the exercise of my will. This too, involved a hard battle lasting several years.

I do not believe nature has prescribed complete suppression of our feelings, ambitions, passions, and desires to gain self-awareness or the Divine Vision. I do not believe that small lapses and errors are not allowed in those who are granted the boon. I also do not believe that a complete denial of the pleasures, thrills, and delights of life is even wholesome for those who set out on the path to higher consciousness.

The issue now arises whether the suppression of the erotic impulse or a monastic way of life does, in actual fact, confer purity or holiness on one who completely masters his carnal desire. Let us make this point a little clearer. Does the ability to live without food for a month or the power to survive without sleep for the same period make one able to perform these feats holier or purer than other people? Does the denial of any other demand of nature raise one to a higher or purer level than the ordinary run of mortals? If not, what perversity in thinking makes us believe that even the legitimate indulgence of carnal passion is polluting and those who rise above it are purer in comparison?

As a Punjabi mystic has put it, "If you call one who subsists on milk only a *siddha* (an accomplished saint), then babies and calves all belong to the category of *siddhas*. If you call one who takes a cleansing bath every day a *siddha*, then every frog and fish belongs to the class of *siddhas*. If you call one who has obliterated his carnal desire a *siddha*, then every hermaphrodite and eunuch is a *siddha*."

The effort at suppression often creates adverse reactions endangering both sanity and health. In the case of a born genius or a born saint the erotic urge can be innately absent in some cases or

334 LIVING WITH KUNDALINI

consciously sublimated. Celibacy in cases of continence can be healthy and fruitful, but emulation of the born celibate by one with a normal appetite for love can prove unhealthy and harmful.

The popular notion that celibacy is a mark of sainthood, like some other popular notions, is based on fallacy. No doubt this idea originated from a dim awareness of some connection between sexual energy and higher consciousness. Buddha stressed it for those who wished to attain nirvana. Since his time, monastic orders established a firm foothold in Buddhism, Hinduism, and later in Christianity. Modern study and investigation have unearthed the hidden cesspools of licentiousness, depravity, and vice which often vitiated the holy atmosphere of these houses of penitence and the worship of God. The suppression of the carnal desire did not prove as easy as its advocates had anticipated. The arrows of Cupid, denied entrance in one way, often penetrated through another.

The damage caused by the sense of guilt experienced by countless men and women in all walks of life when they indulged in the pleasures of love has been incalculable. The great disservice done to humanity by narrow-minded religious zealots who inculcated the idea that the procreative act was sinful is beyond expression. This false supposition has acted as a blight on the spiritual aspirations of innumerable human beings who were led to hate and condemn themselves because of their inability to uproot the urge. Those who believe that an individual cannot reach God as a whole but only as a mutilated wretch, half-crazed with loss of sleep, insufficiency of food, starvation of emotions, and denial of love, make of God a sadistic tyrant who draws pleasure from the pain, anguish, and tears of those He has created. Those who have drawn this picture of the Almighty have been guilty of grave disloyalty to Him and of grave offense against humanity.

Humanity has to reach the precious estate of Higher Consciousness intact and whole, not mutilated, not withered, not starved, not sleepless, not demented, not devoid of love or of the instincts of self-preservation and survival which Nature has wisely implanted in us.

The least departure from a balanced mode of life prescribed by Nature, if followed for a number of generations with constant aggravation, can prove disastrous for a family. This is what sometimes happens to aristocracy and affluence in the course of time, producing at the end an enfeebled or degenerate progeny which brings the ancestral greatness to dust. The suppression of any single basic urge, if practiced on a collective basis, can prove disastrous for the race. Those who inculcate false ideas of piety, purity, or holiness based on the starvation of feelings or negation of any instinct are guilty of seriously misguiding those who listen to them.

The desire for purity is inherent in the intelligent human mind. This is one of the main reasons why religion, with its emphasis on truth, chastity, virtue, and goodness has an instinctive appeal to the masses. Carnal passion with its restless state of the mind, enslavement of the faculties, recurrent desire soon after it is satisfied, unrequited hopeless love, perennial domination over the ego, and endless search for an ideal to adore, by its very urgency and intensity that brooks no interference, creates a revulsion in one tormented by the fire. The wish to control the domineering urge is, therefore, natural. But if this wish were totally fulfilled no one would like to miss the romance and the delight which it provides. It needs heroic control to keep the flame totally under one's will. The fact that this state of mastery is hard to achieve impels the average ranks of mortals to regard with reverence those who, they believe, are above the pangs of desire.

This is one reason why the crowds often evince an instinctive reverence for the holy man said to have renounced the demands of carnal passion. He seems to have achieved, in their eyes, what they vainly try to accomplish. They see in his calm demeanor the signs of victory denied to themselves. The object of their veneration may himself be seething with passion inside, a worse sinner than they are, an addict to vice or perversion, but the aura with which he is surrounded, the order which he represents, or the dress and manners he assumes are sufficient for ordinary people to treat him as one who has won where they themselves have been defeated.

A boyhood friend in Lahore, himself a medical doctor, took me one day to visit his guru, residing at a small distance from his house. This was the first time I returned to Lahore after my appointment in Kashmir that led to our emigration from the capital town where I had spent most of my studentship period.

The guru was seated on a small wooden settee about three feet square, raised about nine inches from the ground. The large room in which he sat was filled with devotees, many of them sitting with folded hands, their gaze fixed on the teacher. On entry into the room my friend motioned me to a vacant seat in the middle and himself went to make his obeisance to his spiritual instructor. He sat on his knees about two feet from the settee and locking both his hands together at the back bent low, touching the carpeted floor with his forehead. It was like the posture of a conquered enemy of an ancient king, with his hands tied behind his back, kneeling before the victor to sue for pardon to save his neck. I stood transfixed with amazement at the spectacle.

The guru raised his right hand imperiously and brought it down with a "whack" on the back of my suppliant friend. During the period of about half an hour for which we sat there, several other well-dressed and intelligent-looking people entered the room and bowed in the same way to receive the blessing in the form of the heavy blow on the back. It seemed that the guru insisted on this form of obeisance as a precondition to gain his favor. He looked at me intently for a moment as if expecting a similar show of homage from me. But I saluted him from my own place with folded hands and bent head and this seemed to satisfy him as a sufficient mark of respect for my first visit. When my friend rose up from his recumbent position, the guru graciously presented him with a handful of dried fruit for himself and for me, indicating this favor with a gesture of his finger.

On my way back, mystified by such utter surrender on the part of my doctor friend, I asked him how he came to know the guru and what he thought about his spiritual prowess. My friend replied, "He is a wonderful man with amazing spiritual powers. On some occasions, when the room is full, sounds come out of the wooden settee which convey answers to the questions posed in their minds by members of the audience, without ever bringing them to their lips. During this interval the guru sits in a trancelike state with his face lit up by a glow that is not present at other times."

I was stunned by the credulity of my friend. How had the disciples been certain that some contrivance was not hidden below the surface of the settee or that it was not linked to a phonograph in another room of the house? Even admitting that the sounds might be genuine, the phenomenon could easily be ascribed to the ability of the guru as a psychic medium. Where then was the occasion for this humiliating salutation, resembling the posture of a slave cringing at the feet of his master to beg the boon of his life for some offense he had committed? Why even intelligent people forget their dignity and prostrate themselves at the feet of gurus or spiritual teachers in such an abject fashion, as if their very life rested in his hands, is an enigma which is hard to explain. The human mass-mind has been so saturated with stories of the supernatural powers exercised by the founders of faiths, enlightened sages, mystics, and saints that frequently the more susceptible and gullible feel a flutter in their hearts and a feeling of awe in their minds in the presence of those about whose miraculous powers rumors have already reached their ears.

The supernatural has a powerful grip on the human mind. The awe experienced in the presence of phenomena which appear magical or miraculous is one of the most common emotions felt by human beings. At times even the most stout-hearted sometimes quake in their shoes at the sight of an apparition conjured up by a medium, though it may be found afterwards that the phenomenon was a fake. A weird ghostlike figure crossing the path of a person suddenly at night, when unprepared for the sight, makes even the boldest heart miss a beat.

The false prophets, pseudo-yogis, and fake masters do not have to make much effort to create a powerful impression on many of those who come to visit them in response to an invitation or to satisfy the curiosity excited by their reputation. If, by a stroke of luck, the supposed holy man has a singular cast of countenance, an unfathomable expression, a flashing eye, an alluring smile or a fascinating look, the visitors, already expecting to see something remarkable, allow their minds to be captivated and hypnotize themselves into the belief that they are in the presence of an exceptional personality possessed of the powers peculiar to the enlightened. If, by even a greater stroke of luck, the guru has some mediumistic gift, as for instance mind reading or clairvoyance and the art to display it at the most opportune time, his fortune is assured and his fame spreads like wildfire. Peole fall over one another to touch the sandals on his feet or the hem of his robe or to catch the dust under his step to apply to their eyes.

Spiritual imposture has been common in India. *Pakhandis* (pretenders) have been more common than genuine yogis. The notorious "thugs" sometimes strangled their unsuspecting victims after approaching them in the garb of holy men. Sleight of hand, grotesque bodily postures and contortions, induction of a corpse-like condition of the body, mind reading, swallowing of poison, and other such wonder-exciting feats have been used to project a superhuman image of a guru on the minds of the people. These tricks have worked times without number.

It is human frailty which vitiated the teachings of the illumined founders of faiths from the very beginning and continues to do so even today. The revelations made by prophets and saviors were not intended to be accepted as the last word on the science of the soul or institutionalized to form the pivot of a mighty propaganda machine that will not allow the least encroachment on the sacred precincts from anyone born in succeeding ages. If the pioneers of modern science had not repudiated the prisonhouse of dogma erected by faith, humanity would still be dwelling in the frigid environment of the dark ages. Institutional religions prevented not only reason from exercising its native powers, but even the soul from attaining the stature destined for it.

In spite of the skeptical attitude of freethinking scholars and scientists, the habit of blind faith in spiritual knowledge continues to be as strong as ever. Science has not been able to liberate the masses from the thraldom of religious dogma because it has never investigated the phenomenon of faith.

With the discovery of certain elements, forces, and laws of Nature, modern science has transformed our lives and made the earth a far more felicitous abode for us to dwell in. With the painstaking discovery of potent medical remedies it has succeeded in eradicating some of the most virulent contagious diseases that took a heavy toll of life or incapacitated myriads of human beings, condemning them to a life of agony. With many discoveries and inventions science has succeeded in attaining a position of trust and honor which few dare to contend.

If material science, which now keeps itself strictly aloof from the polemics of religion, has been able to discover momentous laws of Nature and their application for the welfare of human beings, why could not faith, whose revelations are claimed to have emanated from the Lord God Himself, unearth the secrets of the soul that would have a universal value and application, like the other laws ruling the universe? Why is there chaos, confusion, and conflict of opinions in the science that deals with the soul and God which no one has been able to reconcile?

The world is divided into giant warring camps because there is no unanimity about the vital issues of life and death or agreement about the purpose of human existence. Two bloody global wars have already been fought and the third is in the offing because, at the present stage of its intellectual growth, the human species is still unaware of or indifferent to the spiritual laws that rule its destiny. The ideas of infallibility of the founders, the finality of their doctrines and the superiority of their own faith, assumed and propagated by the dignitaries and the servitors of the church, had no true sanction behind them, nor agreement of reason, but were merely the outgrowths of ego and pride. The custodians as well as the adherents of every major faith tend to believe in the infallibility and divine nature of their own revelation and its founders against the revelations of rival faiths. There are irreconcilable differences between the tenets of one faith and the others. Who can decide which of them is right in the light of the fact that each faith has millions of followers who contend that only the founder of their faith has been right and the others are wrong, or, at best, inferior?

The ideas I am presenting demand a radical change in the present religious thought of mankind. The idea of a God or Creator or Brahman or Allah, framed in the likeness of an Omnipotent or Omniscient human being, has to be discarded eventually. The Intelligence that rules the universe is entirely beyond the grasp of our intellect. The disproportion between human intellect and Divine Intelligence can be illustrated by the analogy of the brightly lit specks of dust floating in a state of motion in a shaft of sunlight entering a dark chamber, as compared to the blinding radiance on the surface of the sun.

Our incapacity to transcend the limits imposed by our senses prevents us from encountering other Intelligences in the universe. Humanity with all its technological achievements is like a colony of ants running hither and thither in search of food, and the human wars are like the sustained battles fought by ant colonies hostile to one another. Because of the sensory bondage on his perception, the average human being misses the glory, the majesty, and the Omnipotence of Cosmic Intelligence.

Yet the human race is slowly moving in the direction of a titanic consciousness. The process of evolution is not active in the brain alone but operates to bring the whole organism in line with the highly expanded state of the mind. The average human frame of our day is not yet sturdy enough to maintain the brightly burning flame of Cosmic Consciousness. It needs to be remodeled to make heightened spiritual activity possible. In numerous cases of psychosis the malady is due to the disproportion between the body and the mind. The former is not able to maintain a brighter light of consciousness on account of the inability to supply the subtle fuel or bioenergy at the rate, or of the standard, demanded by the brain. Future scientific investigation should show that many of the inmates of mental clinics consist of rejected models of evolution—the unfortunate creatures who, because of a physical or mental disability, lack of self-control, or adverse hereditary factors, were cursed with a malfunctioning evolutionary process either from birth or at some later stage in life.

There are large numbers of men and women in whom the process of this evolution becomes accelerated. The tendency to accelerated evolution is carried by genes and runs in families, transmitted from the parents to the children. A hundred constitutional peculiarities affect the evolutionary processes just as they affect the other characteristics of an individual. Where the process of accelerated evolution operates in an unhealthy body with constitutional faults or a genetically defective organ, it often terminates in some kind of mental aberration or psychosis which is not easily amenable to treatment. It is often individuals of this category who feel themselves irresistibly drawn towards the supernatural or the Divine.

The greatest blessing which was bestowed on me during my period of transition was that I instinctively followed a pattern of behavior for my body and my mind which conformed to the needs of the new activity and did not prove a serious hindrance in its path. There were periods when depression, disillusionment, a mild show of anger, failure, or defeat in an honest effort agitated my mind or caused spells of pain and sorrow. But these occasions were rare.

On the whole, the circumstances befriended me, and the Power working within me remained benign throughout. The result was that, by an act of providence which I have never been able to understand so far, I advanced step by step on the narrow and risky path which can lead an average mind into the fantastic world of the awakened self.

EIGHTEEN =======

The Marvelous
Ingenuity of Nature

WARNED BY THE ILL EFFECTS that followed my excessive absorption in the superconscious at Jammu, I tried and gradually succeeded in exercising restraint and moderation on the supersensory activity of my mind by keeping myself engaged in healthy temporal pursuits and the social work of the Samiti organization.

A sufficient amount of sleep and the fascinating adventures I had in my dreams were absolutely necessary for my well-being. I slept for at least ten hours every day. This is my habit even now.

The exhausting mental effort needed for the reception of compositions in languages other than those known to me was too high a price to be paid for a performance which, at best, had only a sensational or surprise value for others. I found in the course of time that only a slight knowledge of a language was sufficient to enable me to receive passages in verse without straining the memory or causing a harmful fatigue of the sensitive brain.

Perhaps because of the possibility of injury due to the strenuous mental exertion required in the reception of unknown languages, this phase of the newly developed psychic activity ceased after a while. Passages in the known languages continued to come on and off, especially during the three months of winter when, probably owing to a greater adaptability to cold than to heat, my system could sustain the higher moods more easily than in summer. But whether summer or winter, it became essential for the supersensual play of my mind that the body be in normal health, entirely free of sickness and infection.

The luminous glow in the head and cadence in the ears continues undiminished. There is a light variation in the luster as well as in the quality of the sounds during bodily or mental disturbance, which clearly indicates at least as close a relationship between the now highly extended consciousness and organism as existed between the two before the awakening.

My reaction to infection and disease is slightly different; first, an utter absence of or only a slight rise in temperature during illness, with an abnormal rapidity of pulse; secondly, my inability to undergo a fast with safety. It appears that the drain on the vital fuel in my system to feed the ever-burning flame across the forehead is too excessive and the reserve of energy too small to allow it to carry on the highly increased vital activity for lengthy periods without replenishment.

This susceptibility of the organism might be because of the tremendous strain borne, or even slight damage sustained by my nervous system on more than one occasion, owing to my unconscious violation of the conditions governing my new existence, or to the inherent weakness of some vital organ, or to both. For this reason, in any disorder of the system I have to be extremely careful about diet and regularity.

Apart from the crises I had to face in the spiritual domain, fate had destined me for no less severe trials in the temporal sphere as well. The severance of my connection with the office resulted in the reduction of my income by one half, on which I had to maintain myself and my family. I was in too delicate and precarious a condition both mentally and physically for years to allow me to augment my resources by taking up any other occupation requiring sustained attention and labor. I needed freedom and rest to save myself from a mental disaster in that extremely sensitive condition of the brain. During this very period the prices of commodities soared, making it difficult for us with our small income to make ends meet. Far from stretching my hand to anyone for help, I did not even allow the least indication of our crushing poverty to leak out. I had no brother or uncle from whom to expect assistance.

My poor father-in-law, always solicitous for my welfare, was shot dead by the raiders at the time of their incursion in 1947, and his eldest son was held captive at Bunji, where he underwent great hardships for more than a year before securing his freedom. His younger brothers had their own hands full trying to retrieve the ruined fortunes of the plundered and ravaged family. My two sisters, both extremely kind and affectionate to me, were themselves caught in economic distress and for years could not extricate themselves sufficiently to plant their feet on firm ground again.

The chilling wave of penury which submerged us swept over almost all the families closely bound to us in ties of kinship, and there could be no possibility of support from any side. Even if there had been, I should have been the last person to avail myself of it. Although we suffered terribly, not the least gesture was made to anyone for help. Compared to prewar prices, the cost of food had risen many times as the result of inflation apparent everywhere. The whole salary I received from the office before my retirement, even if doubled, could not have enabled us to meet the needs of our small family in the face of the high rise in prices, and even in the normal course would have entailed financial difficulties. But with the income halved, the cost of living at least fourfold, and the unavoidable demand for a more nutritious and hence more costly diet for me, with absolutely no other source of income and no possibility of one, I was placed in an indescribable predicament at a time when I was mentally in a precarious condition.

The struggle lasted for nearly seven years. Only the heroism of my wife saved my life. She sold her ornaments and denied herself to the limit to provide the indispensable articles of food needed for my use. I was utterly powerless to prevent her from doing so and had to continue as an impotent witness to her sacrifice. She was the only person who knew all about my condition, and, without in the least understanding the real significance of the development, tortured herself to save me from the pain of violent bodily disorders which invariably followed in the wake of a marked irregularity or deficiency in diet.

On no less than three occasions during this period I came near to the jaws of death, not because of any caprice of the mighty energy now inhabiting my body, or owing to any deliberate omission on my part, but because of grinding poverty, lack of amenities, insufficient and unsuitable diet which, in spite of the heroism of my wife and the sacrifice of my two young sons, who often insisted on surrendering a part of their own share to me, could not be what it should have been because of the utter inadequacy of our finances. On such occasions, lying in a state of utter exhaustion on the sickbed, I wondered at the stupendous mystery of fate which allowed one destined to reveal a mighty secret to be distressed and tortured for the lack of a few coins which flowed in streams on every side and were scattered right and left by many on trifles every day.

But even in the most gloomy conditions, an unshakable conviction always persisted in my mind like a solitary star, gleaming faintly in an otherwise darkly threatening sky, that I would somehow survive the crisis and live to place in the hands of other human beings the great secret on which depended the future safety of the race. It was mainly because of this inward strength, which no external source could infuse in me, that I was able to put up a strong resistance, even in the most desperate situation with no possibility of help from any earthly source.

The evil effects of these serious breakdowns in health, the unavoidable result of destitution, lasted for several months each time and once for nearly two years. During such periods, until the body regained the depleted store of vital energy, I lost the sublime moods and for part of the time even suffered from disquieting mental symptoms. But there was no diminution in the vital current or in the radiant halo around the head even in the weakest conditions. The violent reaction of my system to any default on my part which impeded in any way the action of the processes going on inside,

especially any laxity in the matter of nutrition, was clearly understandable.

It is necessary for any natural transformative tendency to be
effective that it should be attended by a biological activity directed
to that end, and for any biological activity to be operative, food in
sufficient quantity and wholesome form is an indispensable and
primary requirement.

If it is obligatory for an athlete to adhere to certain rigid rules of
conduct, to have regular hours of rest and a balanced diet, how
much more necessary it is for one whose entire organism is in a state
of feverish activity, akin to the exertions of an athlete during
intensive training, to be cautious in all these and other respects in
order to save his system from irreparable harm. The process at work
in him is not merely aimed at building the arm, leg, and chest
muscles, but more importantly directed at the development of the
brain and nerves, the main channels of life, hammering away at them
and all the vital organs day and night, while the owner, in the present
state of our knowledge about the mechanism, remains in the dark
about the form of conduct he must pursue and the precautions he
must take to save himself from injury more imminent and far more
serious than that which an athlete would suffer by a similar neglect.

But for the care taken of me by my mother in my childhood and
youth, under adverse circumstances and in the grip of poverty, and
thereafter by my wife through all the critical phases of my transformation and all the vicissitudes in my life to this day, I could never
have emerged from the terrible ordeal alive and intact. Were it not
for the colossal self-sacrifice of my wife and the anxious care lavished
by her on me every day for more than forty years after the manifestation, I would not be alive now to write these lines. Whenever I
tried to visualize how I should have acted in her position if our roles
had been reversed under similar circumstances, in spite of all my
experience of the supersensible and my claim to supersensory knowledge, I have been humbled by the thought that I would have failed
miserably to emulate her in the performance of all the tiresome yet

essential tasks which she carried out serenely and conscientiously for years.

Perhaps no one who reads this account would be as surprised as I am myself at the marvelous ingenuity of Nature and the wonder she has hidden in the frail frame of human beings, which, through the clay binding them to earth, allows their spirit to soar unfettered to giddy heights to knock for admission at the portals of Heaven itself. Like a small child for the first time venturing outdoors and finding himself on the shore of a billowy ocean, casting one look at the familiar cottage behind and another on the stupendous sight in front of him, I feel utterly lost between the two worlds in which I live—the incomprehensible and infinitely marvelous universe within and the colossal but familiar world without.

When I look within I am lifted beyond the confines of time and space, in tune with a majestic, all-conscious existence, which mocks at fear and laughs at death, compared to which seas and mountains, suns and planets, appear no more than flimsy rack riding across a blazing sky, an existence which is in all and yet absolutely removed from everything, an endless inexpressible wonder that can only be experienced and not described.

But when I look outside, I am what I was, an ordinary mortal in no way different from the millions who inhabit the earth, a common man, pressed by necessity and driven by circumstances, a little chastened and humbled—that is all.

The one really remarkable change I perceive in myself is that, not by my own effort but by what at present I can only call grace, as the result of a day-to-day observable but still incomprehensible activity of a radiant kind of vital energy, present in a dormant form in the human organism, there has developed in me a new channel of communication, a higher sense. Through this extraordinary and extremely sensitive channel an intelligence, higher than that which I personally possess, expresses itself at times in a manner as surprising to me as it might be to others, and through which again I am able, on occasions, to have a fleeting glimpse of the mighty, indescribable world to which I really belong, as a slender beam of light slanting into a dark room through a tiny hole does not belong to the room which it illuminates, but to the effulgent sun millions and millions of miles away.

I am as firmly convinced of the existence of this supersense as I am of the other five already present in every one of us. In fact on every occasion when I make use of it, I perceive a reality before which all that I treat as real appears unsubstantial and shadowy, a reality more solid than the material world reflected by the other senses, more solid than myself, surrounded by the mind and ego, more solid than all I can conceive of, including solidity itself. Apart from this extraordinary feature, I am but an ordinary human being with a body perhaps more susceptible to heat and cold and to the influence of disharmonious factors, mental and physical, than the normal one.

The truthful unembellished account of a normal life unfolded in these pages before the sudden development of the extraordinary mental and nervous condition already described is, I believe, sufficient to provide ample corroboration for the fact that initially I was no better and no worse as a human being than others, and did not possess any entirely uncommon characteristics such as are usually associated with those of vision, entitling me to special divine favor. Also that the final exceptional state of consciousness which I continue to possess now did not appear all at once, but marked the culmination of a continuous process of biological reconstruction covering no less than fifteen years before the first unmistakable sign of a new florescence.

The process is still at work in me, but even after an experience of more than forty years I am still lost in amazement at the wizardry of the mysterious energy responsible for the marvels which I witness day after day in my own mortal frame. I regard the manifestation with the same feelings of awe, adoration, and wonder with which I regarded it on the first occasion, the feelings having increased in intensity and not diminished as is generally the case with material phenomena.

Contrary to the belief which attributes spiritual growth to purely psychic causes, to extreme self-denial and renunciation, or to an extraordinary degree of religious fervor, I found that a person can rise from the normal to a higher level of consciousness by a continuous biological process, as regular as any other activity of the body, and that at no stage is it necessary or even desirable either to neglect the flesh or to deny a place to the human feelings in the heart. A higher state of consciousness, able to liberate itself from the thraldom of senses, appears to be incompatible, unless we take the biological factors into account, with a physical existence in which passions and desires and the animal needs of the body, however restricted, exist side by side.

But I can say confidently that a reasonable measure of control over appetites coupled with some knowledge of the mighty mechanism and a befitting constitution proved a surer and safer way to spiritual unfoldment than any amount of self-mortification or abnormal religious fervor can do.

I have every reason to believe that mystical experience and transcendental knowledge can come to one naturally as the flow of genius, and that for this achievement it is not necessary, save for well-directed efforts at self-ennoblement and regulation of appetites, to depart eccentrically from the normal course of human conduct.

Even the most arduous exercises of hatha yoga, practiced to the end of one's life, cannot radically alter the inherited constitution of the cerebrospinal system. The forced ascent of kundalini, even up to the *sahasrara*, cannot induce the perennial turiya state or the state of extended consciousness which is the ultimate aim of yoga. After a certain usually brief duration, kundalini returns to the *muladhara*, reverting the yogi back to normal consciousness.

This is the reason why, even in hatha yoga manuals, after initial success with the methods prescribed, practice of raja yoga is considered necessary for liberation. The *Hatha Yoga Pradipika* of Svatmarama Svamin, an esteemed treatise, specifically states that hatha yoga is a preparation for raja yoga (the total path of mental and spiritual development). The ancient masters recognized the important role played by the inherited mental capacity of a seeker in the attainment of a higher dimension of consciousness or the state of "Shiva" or "Vishnu" or "Brahman," as figuratively denoted in the traditional works on the subject.

What are popularly known as raja yoga, kriya yoga, bhakti yoga, karma yoga, or jnana yoga are comparatively easier forms of spiritual discipline aimed at bringing about the same activity of the nervous system which the more strenuous hatha yoga practices aimed to achieve by the use of force.

The Tantric and the oral tradition which form the basis for hatha yoga appear to be of remote origin, extending to the time of the Indus Valley civilization, more than 2,000 years before the birth of Christ, and probably even much earlier than that. The conservative element in human nature tries to preserve an ancient tradition in its intrinsic form as a sacred or precious legacy from the past. Considered in the light of this fact, the disciplines, practices and rituals prescribed in the Tantras and books on hatha yoga must have been oriented for seekers in a less developed state of culture, or intellectually inferior to the seekers of today. The milder practices and disciplines of the easier forms of yoga might have come into being in later times to suit mentally more advanced aspirants. In the Puranas (later scriptures of legends of gods), both types of yoga practices, the rigorous and the easier ones, are mentioned side by side.

The practices enjoined in the other forms of yoga can also fructify in the case of a limited number of seekers as much as in the practices of hatha yoga. Meditation, constant thinking about the Divine, selfless service done in the name of the Lord, prayer and worship, combined with a healthy, honest, and humane way of life have the potentialities to stir kundalini to action in those cases in which the organism is prepared for the new activity. In some exceptional cases, mere company of an illuminated soul, the transport of love with a keenly sought beloved, listening to pure music or a spiritual discourse, the contemplation of a beautiful piece of art, an image of God or the picture of an adored and highly revered prophet can also act as a trigger to raise kundalini to *brahmarandhra*, inducing a transporting visionary experience or ecstasy.

Whether the transformative process is set in motion by voluntary effort or is spontaneous, purity of thought and discipined behavior are essential to minimize resistance to the cleansing and remodeling action of the mighty power on the organism. The subject must emerge normal in every way from the great ordeal, metamorphosed but mentally sane and with unimpaired intellect and emotion to be able to evaluate and taste in full the supreme happiness of an occasional enrapturing union with the indescribable ocean of consciousness in the transcendental state, by marking the difference between the frail human element on the one hand and the immortal spirit on the other.

It is only in this way that the incomparable bliss of liberation can be realized because unconditioned existence, being beyond the pale of enjoyment or its opposite, the actual enjoyer in the ego-bound conditioned human creature is the visionary and no other.

The knowledge of kundalini cannot be contained in a nutshell. It is a colossal science. It is, in fact, the science of sciences. The growth of every form of knowledge—art, philosophy, or science—is the outcome of the evolutionary growth of the human brain. There would be absolutely no radical change in the mental capability of human beings, or radical improvement in knowledge, were the brain not an auxiliary to it. We are not able to measure this transformation because the subtle depths of the brain are beyond our reach.

The science of kundalini covers the entire spectrum of knowledge. All the facts about the universe or about ourselves, our bodies and the earth, which we have gained so far or shall gain in the future, will ultimately serve the survival of the race. The more the knowledge gained, the more will it contribute to the evolution of the brain. This indicates the colossal dimensions of the science of kundalini.

What I am stating is based on the observations of two generations of kundalini arousal—that of my father and myself. I am now observing the third generation also, that is, my children. My younger son was born after the initial awakening of the Power in me, but the system had not been adapted to the change. Even so, he is, in some respects, more sensitive than his elder sister and brother and at times displays signs of clairvoyance and has premonitory dreams. It is possible that more pronounced signs of a psychic nature would be present had I allowed my children to practice meditation from an early age, or even after adulthood. They wanted to do so and sought my guidance, but I dissuaded them from this course. I was not sure that they had the stamina or the physical strength to withstand the ordeal of a full-scale awakening. Some congenital factor in the marriage, it seems, was not favorable and so they were not well equipped to withstand the tremendous strain they would have to face.

The first unfavorable symptoms that occurred in my father during the course of the gradual awakening was a distaste for society and a desire for seclusion. This was accentuated by the death of his son. The vagaries in diet and the drastic change in the food to which he was accustomed added to this reaction. Soon he became isolated from the small family and his love dried up.

I was born when he was forty-eight years of age and I do not remember a single occasion when he held me in his arms, patted, kissed, or embraced me. I do not remember sitting in his lap or trotting alongside of him hand in hand even once during my childhood. Both my sisters stood in awe of him and never ventured to come near him if they could help it. But despite his indifference and cold behavior we loved him from our heart. He was our father and that was sufficient for us.

I have deliberately dwelt on this unhappy feature of my father's life since it is of tremendous importance not only for those interested in the arousal of kundalini or in the study of the phenomenon but also assessment of the evolutionary changes involved. It can be readily inferred that the evolution of individuals, if such a process is actually at work, must be aimed to produce a more advanced type with instincts, traits of character, and appetites which can help them to live and survive in the altered condition.

It is obvious that in order to survive as a cosmic conscious race, humanity must continue to remain in possession of all the ethical virtues and higher emotions and even add to them, as without these the harmonious continuance of society is not possible. For instance, if there is loss in the feelings of love, pity or compassion this will, after numerous generations, culminate in a race of highly intelligent, cosmic conscious but at the same time heartless specimens who sooner or later would bring about their own destruction.

Unilateral development of the intellect is not a sign of healthy evolution. It must be attended by a corresponding growth of the higher emotions and the refinement of animal instincts and appetites. It is a most complex process, of which all the parameters will not be available to human knowledge for centuries to come. To conform to the evolutionary target, the whole personality of the human race must change to create a more advanced, more harmonious, and more noble species in rapport with the sublime planes of creation that are not at present generally accessible to our senses. It is not the work of a day nor of centuries, nor perhaps of millennia, but will be performed during this and the coming ages. When the laws of evolution become better known, a superior class of human beings will be able to create a more appropriate and congenial milieu.

NINETEEN ═══════════════════════

A Complete
Metamorphosis in
Consciousness

IN ORDER TO SHOW correspondence between my experience and the
traditional ideas expressed in the Tantras and Shakti Shastras it
should be sufficient to reproduce the following passages from Arthur
Avalon's *The Serpent Power*, an authoritative translation and discussion of several Tantric texts, describing the conditions that follow
the ascent of kundalini into *sahasrara*.

> By this method of mental concentration, aided by the physical and
> other processes described, the gross is absorbed into the subtle,
> each dissolving into its immediate cause and all into Chidatma or
> the Atma which is Chit. In language borrowed from the world of
> human passion, which is itself but a gross reflection on the physical
> plane of corresponding, though more subtle, supersensual activities
> and bliss, the Shakti-Kundalini who has been seized by desire for
> Her Lord is said to make swift way to Him, and kissing the lotus
> mouth of Shiva, enjoys Him (S.N. v. 51, *post*). By the term
> Samarasya is meant the sense of enjoyment arising from the union
> (Samarasya) of male and female.
> This is the most intense form of physical delight representing on
> the worldly plane the Supreme Bliss arising from the union of Shiva
> and Shakti on the "spiritual" plane. So Daksa, the Dharma-
> shastrakara, says: "The *Brahman* is to be known by Itself alone,
> and to know It is as the bliss of knowing a virgin." Similarly, the
> Sadhaka in Laya-siddhi-yoga, thinking of himself as Shakti and the
> Paramatma as Purusha, feels himself in union (Sangama) with
> Shiva, and enjoys with him the bliss which is Sringara-rasa, the
> first of the nine Rasas, or the love sentiment and bliss. This Adirasa
> (Sringara) which is aroused by Sattva-guna, is impartite (Akhanda),

self-illuminating (Svaprakasa), bliss (Ananda) whose substance is Chit (Chinmaya). It is so intense and all-exclusive as to render the lover unconscious of all other objects of knowledge (Vedyantara-sparsa-shunyah), and the own brother of Brahma-bliss (Brahma-svadasahodara). But as the Brahma-bliss is known only to the Yogi, so, as the Alamkara-Shastra last cited observes, even the true love-bliss of the mortal-world "is known to a few knowers only" (Jneyah kaischit pramatrbhih), such as poets and others. Sexual as well as other forms of love are reflections or fragments of the Brahma-bliss.

This union of the Shakti-Kundalini with Shiva in the body of the Sadhaka is that coition (Maithuna) of the Sattvika Pancha-tattva which the Yogini-Tantra says is "the best of all unions for those who have already controlled their passions," and are thus Yati. Of this the Brihat-Srikrama (S.N. v. 51, *post*) says: "They with the eye of knowledge see the stainless Kala united with Chidananda on Nada. He is the Mahadeva, white like a pure crystal, and is the effulgent Cause (Vimba-rupa-nidana), and She is the lovely woman of beauteous limbs which are listless by reason of Her great passion." On their union nectar (Amrita) flows, which in ambrosial stream runs from the Brahma-randhra, to the *muladhara*, flooding the Kshudra-brahmanda, or microcosm, and satisfying the Devatas of its Chakras. It is then that the Sadhaka, forgetful of all in this world, is immersed in ineffable bliss. Refreshment, increased power and enjoyment, follows upon each visit to the Well of Life.

In the Chintamani-satva, attributed to Sri-Sankaracarya, it is said: "This family woman (*i.e.*, Kundalini), entering the royal road (*i.e.*, *sushumna*), taking rest at intervals in the sacred places (*i.e.*, Chakras), embraces the Supreme Husband (Para-Shiva) and makes nectar to flow (*i.e.*, from the Sahasrara)."*

As already explained in the preceding chapters, the awakening of kundalini and her ascent into *sahasrara* through the spinal canal represents, in terms of modern knowledge of the human body, a new form of activity of the cerebrospinal system, with the reproductive mechanism at one end and the cranium at the other.

---

*Arthur Avalon (Sir John Woodroffe), *The Serpent Power, Being the* Shat-Chakra-Nirupana *and* Paduka-Pancaka, 4th ed. (Madras: Ganesh, 1950), 238–240.

The start of this new activity draws upon the procreative organs for increased production of the reproductive fluids and also the spinal and other nerves for enhanced extraction of the gross substance from the body, which is converted into psychic energy. The repeated reference to the "nectar" on the spinal axis and the feeling of surpassing bliss resembling the rapture of the climax of love said to attend the union of Kundalini with Her lord Shiva in the *sahasrara*, provides clear support to the statements I am making about my own experience.

The fact that the experience is extremely short-lived in most cases and needs an interval of sustained practice to prolong it is a clear indication that biological processes are involved. In fact, the whole discipline of yoga, more so of hatha yoga, represents a series of psychosomatic exercises designed to manipulate the bodily organs and the brain, through concentration of the mind, to achieve specific psychosomatic results.

If Kundalini were actually an occult "astral force" or an incorporeal divine Power that could, by Her own miraculous potency, raise an average individual to a superhuman stature, then why should one have to spend years and years of one's life in practicing *shat-karma*, the six processes of body cleaning, postures, control of breath, mudras, *bandhas*, and exercise a strict regimen in diet and a rigid control of behavior? Why should not a simple invocation, repeated time after time, be sufficient to arouse the astral force or the Goddess from Her slumber at the base of the spine? Again, why should the ancient authorities take special pains to locate to the fraction of an inch the place between the anal aperture and the genitals where Kundalini lies asleep, coiled three and a half times, closing with Her mouth the entrance to the passage leading to *sahasrara* in the brain?

A brief glance at the ancient treatises on alchemy, astrology, hermetic sciences, medicine, and surgery, both in the West and East (including India), clearly shows what figurative and flowery language, combined with myth, superstition, and fantasy, have been used to express scientific and esoteric religious ideas that are not readily intelligible in our day.

The awakening of kundalini and its ascent to *sahasrara* is a strictly biological phenomenon, as amenable to study and investigation as any other phenomenon of nature. The main reason why it has remained so long outside the pale of scientific research is because its scientific nature has remained unknown. Whatever has been written about it by ancient or modern writers has kept it shrouded in supernaturalism, myth, and metaphor. For the average seeker, even today, kundalini is a supernatural force which can work wonders when aroused. Only, like the Philosopher's Stone of the alchemists, one should know the secret by which it can be aroused or manipulated. Sometimes I find it difficult to convince an earnest seeker that the stories he has heard are unfounded and that the arousal of kundalini is as down-to-earth an event as the birth of a child.

Pranayama (regulation of the breath), which is an indispensable adjunct of hatha yoga, proves effective in the awakening of kundalini because of the physiological factors involved. The intensely sustained effort of the will needed to hold the breath beyond the normal duration, in opposition to the usual nerve impulses and the movement of the lungs can, with repeated practice, create such an impact on the command center in the brain that the paranormal chamber is forced to open.

The students who practice intensive forms of *pranayama*, as enjoined in the hatha yoga manuals, experience this intensity. In the advanced stages, the body often perspires with the effort, and tingling sensations are felt at nerve endings all over the body.

We are not concerned here with the directions contained in some of these manuals that the sweat should be rubbed in. The utility of such a course appears doubtful and has to be established by experiment. What we are concerned with is that this tingling sensation all over the body, sometimes likened to the creeping of ants over the flesh, is an indication of the effect of a powerful effort of the will, directed to changing the normal rhythm of an organ, on the entire nervous network of the body. *Pranayama* helps in the awakening of kundalini because it stirs up the entire nervous system and forces it to the activity necessary for production of an enhanced supply of the pranic fuel to the brain.

Why should such dramatic methods be necessary if kundalini is a divine force and *nadis* only astral conduits for its activity? But even the force applied in hatha yoga practices does not work if the cerebrospinal system is not yet ripe for the self-regulating process necessary for the transformation of consciousness. The pressure exerted through pranayama and the intense state of concentration of the sadhaka might force a slight activity at the *muladhara chakra*, with erotic sensations round the genitals or even some way up the spine for a short while every day during the course of the practice.

This is what happens in some cases of hatha yoga practitioners. The sadhakas feel happy and the practice is repeated day after day because of the rapture eventually experienced. In some cases the stream of kundalini might rise higher and still higher up to the heart center. The area of the transport increases with every rise in the stream, but that is all. In a few cases, the kundalini current might rise to the *ajna chakra* in the brain. The rapture is then intensified. The light in the head and sounds in the ears become more pronounced. There might be visionary experiences during the duration of the practice and a state of intense absorption with ecstasy might supervene for a short while, ending as soon as the supply of the pranic force is spent. Arthur Avalon writes:

> Kundal(in)i does not at first stay long in Sahasrara. The length of stay depends on the strength of the Yogi's practice. There is then a natural tendency (Samskara) on the part of Kundal(in)i to return. The Yogi will use all effort at his disposal to retain Her above, for the longer this is done the nearer approach is made to the time when She can be in a permanent manner retained there. For it is to be observed that liberation is not gained by merely leading Kundal(in)i to the Sahasrara, and of course still less is it gained by stirring it up in the *muladhara* or fixing it in any of the lower

centers. Liberation is gained only when Kundalini takes up Her permanent abode in the Sahasrara, so that She only returns by the will of the *sadhaka*. It is said that after staying in Sahasrara for a time, some Yogins lead the Kundalini back to Hridaya (heart), and worship Her there. This is done by those who are unable to stay long in Sahasrara. If they take the Kundalini lower than Hridaya— i.e., worship Her in the three Chakras below Anahata they no longer, it is said, belong to the Samaya group.*

When successful, every hatha yoga practice should culminate in samadhi or mystical experience. It is not possible to draw a picture of samadhi for one who has not had the experience. For this reason it is said to be indescribable and incommunicable. It is an extremely rapturous state of mental elevation in which consciousness contemplates itself. The association with the body present in the average mind, and the world image contained in it, recede to a distance and consciousness alone dominates the scene, assuming colossal proportions which swallow up the material world. Compared to the reality of this oceanic consciousness the gigantic cosmos appears to be like variously patterned clouds sailing across the face of a sun of infinite dimensions. The descriptions left of their own experiences by the great mystics of the earth are extremely varied. There are, however, some charcteristics common to most of them. These I have discussed elsewhere in my own writings.†

There are various degrees of samadhi. In the case of individuals in whom the cerebrospinal system is not fully prepared for the new activity, samadhi can be only a poor affair compared to the resplendent visionary experience of the mature yogis. In a large number of cases, the samadhi attained is only a self-induced hypnotic trance or a swoonlike state of which little or nothing can be remembered when the yogi returns to the normal state.

Although many people claim to have achieved it, genuine samadhi is a rare phenomenon. Among the more perfect cases of samadhi are

---

*Avalon, pp. 243–244.
†Gopi Krishna, *The Secret of Yoga* (New York: Harper and Row, 1972).

ones described in the principal Upanishads or by some of the greatest mystics of different religions in various parts of the world. It is a rare condition since it represents a state of transformed consciousness that will be the heritage of the future race.

In the initial stages of awakening brought about by hatha yoga practices, the pleasureable sensation is felt around the *muladhara chakra*, rising higher and higher by small degrees with the daily exercises practiced by the sadhaka. This is a very delicate operation and care has to be taken that the nerves involved are not damaged by too frequent repetition of the process. It is for this reason that the guidance of a guru, who knows the intricacies of the new development, has always been considered as essential for the success of the effort.

The ascent of the kundalini force or, in other words, the gross pranic essence, is almost always attended by flashes of light in the brain and a peculiar blend of sounds in the ears. In the conventional cases, the minds of the sadhakas are already filled with ideas inculcated by the guru. The diagrams of the chakras, their colors, number of petals, the presiding deity, the *bija* mantras, and the letter of the Sanskrit alphabet on each petal all tend to be impressed on the mind of the sadhaka. When the ascent of the power starts, when the light is seen, sounds heard and the rapturous sensations experienced, combined with the expected images in the mind, the experience presents all the semblance of a divine manifestation. The disciple, transported with joy at this breathtaking fulfillment of the guru's promises, throws himself at his feet, vowing implicit obedience to his word and gesture forever.

Even in those cases where the ascent does not proceed beyond the first two, three, or four chakras, the phenomena witnessed and the bliss experienced provide sufficient reward for all the labor undergone and the self-denial practiced by the initiate. A celibate life, completely devoid of marital happiness, loses much of its rigor for one who succeeds in awakening the Serpent Power.

"What need have I for an external woman when I have an 'inner woman' in my own interior?" says a Tantric practitioner quoted by Arthur Avalon.

In some of the Tantras and other works on Kundalini, She is alluded to as a "widow," "washerwoman," "sweetheart," "damsel," or "virgin," or even a "harlot." To the uninitiated it appears paradoxical to find these endearing or even vulgar names applied to one who, at the same time, is regarded as a Goddess, a Divine Mother, or as the Creatrix of the universe.

It is not possible to explain this enigma except by an understanding of the somatic effects which follow the movement of kundalini through the spinal cord. Through a strange process started in the cerebrospinal system, all the alluring and transporting play of love now begins to occur in the interior of the initiate, keeping the mind enchanted with the newly discovered fount of joy in the body. The Tantras do not speak of an imaginary Goddess nor of the practices or rituals enjoined by them as mere obscenities, as those in complete ignorance of the magnitude of the physiological phenomena involved are sometimes inclined to call them. They have a firm basis in reality which a thorough scientific study of kundalini can establish.

There can be nothing further from truth than the mistaken notions current in many places that the Tantras are a repository of secret or magical methods by which the pleasures of sexual union can be greatly prolonged or enhanced. The desire for unrestricted delights of love burns in countless human hearts. Frankly speaking, Eros is the presiding deity who prescribes our dress, our behavior, our discourse, our reading material, our favorite songs and stories, our athletics, our health and beauty aids, our associations and our habits, even our mode of worship or attendance at church.

The hitherto undivulged secret of kundalini is that the human cerebrospinal system is capable of an amazing activity which is still competely unknown to modern science. The practice of meditation, carried on in the proper way regularly for a sufficient duration of time, tends to force a normally silent region in the brain to an astonishing activity which, like an electric current, galvanizes the nervous system to an action which is never experienced in the normal state. From every fiber and tissue of the body a subtle organic essence, extracted by nerve fibrils spread everywhere, is carried to the brain through the spinal canal to give rise to the ecstatic and visionary conditions associated with religious experience from earliest times.

In my own experience, the organic essence was not so clearly marked on the first occasion of arousal as on the second, several years later. But there is not the least shadow of doubt that it is this subtle organic substance which is behind the exquisite sensations of the arousal. We have not yet been able to determine how the intense rapture of the climax of love is experienced by an individual. What kind of biochemical reagent or electrical discharge is at the back of the delicious transport of the orgasm? Modern research has shown that there is a certain area in the brain which, when electrically stimulated, gives rise to the same sensation which marks the sexual climax. It is obvious that there must occur some kind of a chemical or bioelectrical activity to cause a momentary rapture that has no parallel in the other pleasures experienced by the human mind and body. It is in this extremely delightful, sense-ravishing transport of the conjugal union, and the release from pressure which it grants to the mind, that the compelling power of the reproductive urge resides.

There is little general awareness that this intense rapture of the erotic union can occur at places in the body other than the genitals and other erogenous zones. To make an assertion of this kind before an assembly of the learned is to evoke incredulity and even ridicule. The whole mystical literature of the world and many extant works in Sanskrit on kundalini, including the Tantras, provide the testimony of thousands of individuals of unquestionable honesty and truth about the reality of this phenomenon.

It is not possible to describe the intensity of orgasmic sensation that occurs in the spinal cord and the brain on the arousal of kundalini. Except for the related character of the transport experienced, there is no comparison between the climax of conjugal union and the rapture caused by the flow of the kundalini force from the base of the spine to the head. The duration of the former may be only of a few moments, followed by a sense of relief and lassitude on the part of the individual. The latter can last for several minutes, creating almost a swooning condition of the mind at the intensity of the rapture experienced. It seems to the individual as if one has been in an ocean of incomparable bliss to taste the rapture as long as one likes or as long as there is sufficient vitality in the body to cause it. On returning back to normal, there is usually no sense of lassitude or satiation. On the contrary, the experiencer feels mentally more fresh and invigorated than before.

After studying my condition for more than forty years, I now feel that even if I had studied all the literature available on kundalini at the time, I could not have solved the problems of insomnia, psychic disturbances, and the organic symptoms that I experienced immediately after the awakening. Right up to this day, I have not been able to find a detailed account of the arousal of kundalini, meticulously describing its effects on the body-mind complex and the changes that occur in them until a paranormal state of consciousness is attained. From my point of view, there is no aspect of my experience so important for study and investigation as the slow metamorphosis which my cerebrospinal system underwent to equip the brain for a new pattern of consciousness, not in evidence in the average ranks of human beings. This transformation raises problems which, so far as I know, have not been discussed in detail in any work on yoga or mysticism or any other occult or esoteric system, ancient or modern.

This slow metamorphosis in consciousness, which occurred imperceptibly from the very moment of my first experience, provides the key to the conclusion I have arrived at—that kundalini represents the upgrading mechanism behind the evolution of the human brain. What has led many scientists to believe that the human brain has reached the peak of its organic evolution is a riddle to me and to other thoughtful minds.

What evidence exists for this premature conclusion, when human evolution is still a profound mystery, no one is ready to explain. How the primate brain evolved to human dimensions during the course of past millions of years, raises a problem that no one has solved so far. The books written on the subject contain merely speculation, exciting narratives of vanished species, and suggested transitions from lower to higher forms.

The whole theory of evolution as propounded by Darwin and his successors is only a huge mass of observation and data, extending now to over a century, without any final solution. What is the basic mechanism that came into operation in the evolution of the human brain from that of the primates, and what intelligent agency coordinated the functions of the entire system to make changes in a complex organ like the human brain at each step of the ascent, and transmit the advances gained from generation to generation? Something more profound than an urge to survive is clearly involved.

Looking back at the events that followed the first kundalini awakening, it seems to me now that the intensity of concentration, exercised for many years, had slowly stimulated to activity a small area in the brain directly above the palate and below the crown of the head. The exquisite sensations I felt moving up the spine, which stopped and disappeared when my mind was diverted, was the beginning of a new activity in the cerebrospinal system which will be confirmed by science in the course of time. Two distinct entities moved up the spine side by side with the intensely pleasurable sensation which I experienced. One was a kind of radiation, orange in color in the beginning, which later on changed to silver with a slightly golden color in it. The second was an organic essence which entered the brain at the same time as the radiation.

The different stages of inner growth through which I passed during the course of my transformation have led me to conclude that there is a subtle organic compound in the body, extracted from the organs and tissues, that the nerves carry to and fro, which supplies the vehicle through which the incorporeal pranic energy acts. There is a particular reason that has led me to this conclusion. Shortly after the night of horror when I hovered between death on the one side and insanity on the other and was saved from an awful fate by what was almost a miracle, I noticed a rather disquieting change in my observation. It seemed as if every object on which I looked was coated with a thin layer of white. This did not affect the color or the shape of the object. It appeared only as if a very thin coat of white added to it. I noticed this strange alteration in the state of my vision but could not assign any reason for it. I wondered within myself, and even worried over it at times, but try as I might I could not find any satisfactory explanation for the change.

The other fact I noticed was that there had occurred an expansion in my consciousness. This position is rather difficult to explain to the average individual. But perhaps it might be possible to convey a clearer picture of it in this way. Every one of us, when sitting in a room with eyes closed, perceives a certain area of awareness round the head, extending even to the body when the atention is called towards it, which one experiences as one's own self, one's own inner being or personality. Every one of us is conscious of this area of awareness or, let us say, our mind, but is not able to perceive or to measure this area of awareness in another individual. We assume by inference that the other, too, has the same area of his inner being qualitatively and quantitatively, but we cannot actually share this because we are conscious only of our own inner personality subjectively, and we have no means at present to make it a subject for objective observation. Hence, in the present state of our knowledge, it is not possible to detect the quantitative and qualitative differences in the consciousness of two different individuals, apart from what is inferred from their respective intellectual, artistic, or aesthetic expression.

Although I never understood it at that time, my very first experience of the awakening of kundalini was actually the outcome of a widening of the cognitive center in my brain. When I returned back to my normal state of consciousness, after the expansion which I witnessed during the period of my ecstasy, I was not the same inner being as before. The area of my awareness had widened and this expansion has since become a permanent feature of my personality. During the whole period of the first memorable experience, the expansion witnessed was oceanic, and I had felt myself spreading in all directions until my consciousness exceeded the limits of the cosmic image present in my mind. When the enormous proportions I had gained in my inner being began to shrink and I came slowly back to myself, I was still basically the same individual I had been before, but a little of the expansion still remained and continued to exist day and night—a fact which I could not understand at that time.

It is clear to me that the human seed is not the product of the gonads alone. It is a compound of a subtle organic essence drawn from the body by the nerves and the secretion produced by testicles in men and ovaries in women. Modern science has not identified this subtle nervine essence which is, in reality, the concentrated fuel of life. The ancient notion that the male seed is actually produced in the head and from there descends into the genital organs has, therefore, some foundation of truth in it. The idea, expressed in the Upanishads, that semen is drawn from all parts of the body, including the vital organs, is nearer the mark. In the normal individual there occurs a constant process in the nervous system which is imperceptible to us and still undetected by science. The subtle element which imparts vitality to the seed is imported by the nerves lining the reproductive system from all organs and tissues in the body, from the head, heart, lungs, liver, stomach, intestines, spleen, kidneys, genitals, and the rest.

This organic element is extremely subtle, extracted and carried by the nerves in such a minute measure that it remains beyond detection by the individual. As far as I have been able to determine, there are special nerves connecting the reproductive system with the different organs in the body. After extraction by vast networks of nerves, the essence travels to the erotic zone to commingle with that arriving from other organs and parts of the body, ultimately to form an ingredient of the human seed. The essence from the brain in some mysterious way comes down through the spinal cord to reach the same place of confluence as the other nerve channels serving the same purpose.

The impregnated ovum, the first germ of human life, starts to divide and subdivide, adding brick after brick automatically to a blueprint of genes and chromosomes, until the marvelous structure of the human organism is complete, ushering a ready-made, tiny human being into the world. To suppose that the unintelligent atoms and molecules that constitute the impregnated seed, with any amount of chemistry and mutual interaction, could produce a marvelous organ like the brain, the eye, the ear, the nose or the mouth is to suppose the impossible. The tragedy is that science has still no instruments to detect the vibrations in the life energy or prana which is the real dynamic source behind all the phenomena of life in the universe.

Prana is present in atoms and their constituents. It is behind the energy fields into which matter is resolved at dissolution. It is the agent responsible for the unimaginably complex chemical and physical reactions in living bodies, as also in the incredibly intricate mechanisms at the back of all the complex movements of the organs and the activity of the brain. Prana is possessed of a superhuman intelligence and memory, beyond the range of our thought. It is an element of the universe infinitely subtler and more complex than the element we call matter.

The study of life bewilders and confuses us by its complexity and profound mystery. We are dumbfounded because the element we set out to explore is infinitely more intelligent and more profound than the mind that attempts to probe its mystery.

TWENTY ═══════════════════════

Creating a Mental
Climate to Remove
the Threat of War

WITHOUT PRIDE OF ACHIEVEMENT, without the least pretension to any divine office, I humbly submit, on the strength of knowledge gained, that true religion, infinitely more than what is or has been supposed to be, is in reality the expression of the evolutionary impulse in human beings, springing from an imperceptibly active though regularly functioning organic power center in the body, amenable to voluntary stimulation under favorable conditions.

Further, that the transcendental state, of which as yet only a faint though unmistakable picture is available from the descriptions furnished by visionaries, is the natural heritage of the human race; with all its feelings and desires refined and restrained to act in consonance with the needs of a higher kind of perception. Also, that the happiness and welfare of humankind depends on its adherence to the yet unknown laws of this evolutionary mechanism, known in India as kundalini, which is carrying humanity towards a glorious state of consciousness with all their capacities to act, love, and enjoy intact, enhanced rather than diminished, but functioning in response to a cultivated will, in obedience to the dictates of a properly developed conscience, and in accordance with the decrees of a correctly informed intellect fully aware of the goal in front of it.

From my own experience, extending to over forty years, I am irresistibly led to the conclusion that the human organism is evolving in the direction indicated by mystics and prophets and by men and women of genius, by the action of this wonderful mechanism, located at the base of the spine, depending for its activity mainly on the energy supplied through the reproductive organs.

Though not in its general application as the evolutionary organ in the race but in the individual sphere as the means to develop spirituality, paranormal faculties, and psychic powers, the mechanism has been known and manipulated from very ancient times. When aroused to intense activity by individuals already advanced on the path of progress and subject to numerous factors, especially favorable heredity, constitution, mode of conduct, occupation, and diet, it can lead to most remarkable and extremely valuable results, developing the organism by general stages from its native condition to a state of extraordinary mental efficiency, conducting it ultimately to the zenith of cosmic consciousness and genius combined.

It is a transformation so extraordinary that I feel at a loss to make it intelligible to my fellow human beings. When I say that "My inner self is now wrapped in a sheath of light," I wonder if it is possible for others to grasp what I mean. What I came to realize afterwards is that from the very day of the awakening my consciousness started to expand. My trials and suffering stemmed from the fact that I had no awareness of what had happened, what forces were now active in my body, and what the target of this activity was.

The process of evolution is active in the body of almost every human being. At its natural pace, the individual has no indication of it throughout life. His body functions in the normal way, in health and disease, able to sustain stresses and pressures, hardships and privations, overexertion, lack of sleep, and insufficient diet with the help of the strong reserves built into it.

A good many readers of my first book* were appalled by the suffering I underwent for years after my kundalini awakening. Some even believe that the experience of lights and sounds, prophetic dreams, and the ability to compose in inspired verse was out of proportion to the ordeal I had faced. Since no one can visualize my inner being, it is rather difficult for me to convince the world that I

* *Kundalini: The Evolutionary Energy in Man* (1967, rev. ed. 1970).

have been compensated a hundred times over. If I were offered the choice of braving the same grueling ordeal again to reach the same state of inner illumination and beatitude, I would accept it without a moment's hesitation, even if I had a kingdom to sacrifice.

I put more value on the verdict of future investigators than on that of my own contemporaries. This is an entirely unknown territory for the latter and hence some doubt is natural. The difficulties and dangers inherent in a metamorphosis of the brain, through the awakening of kundalini, resulting in a transcendental state of consciousness, will come to light when the phenomenon is subjected to investigation.

Study of the hazardous practices and disciplines of hatha yoga shows what mastery over the vital functions of the body had to be gained and what iron will had to be cultivated by those who ventured to arouse the Serpent from her sleep. The first experience of a sudden awakening of the Power is that of a raging psychic storm, as if a tornado had been let loose in the system which, if not handled with a rigorous grip on the mind, can drive one mad with its unimaginable violence.

Long years of careful preparation will always be needed in the case of those who would like to brave the hazards of arousing kundalini to activity before its proper time. The exploration of the inner world is beset with far more difficulties and dangers than the exploration of outer space. Only healthy, strong, and highly intelligent men and women who can subjugate their ambitions, desires, and emotions have the capacity to accomplish the undertaking without severe harm to themselves.

All great sages and seers of the past and all great founders of religion, whether guided intuitively by evolving life itself or led by observation, have consciously or unconsciously laid emphasis mostly on such traits of character and modes of conduct as are definitely conducive to progress. The highest products of civilization—prophets, mystics, men and women of genius—clearly indicate the direction and goal of human evolution. Studied in the light of the facts discussed in this book they will all be found to have common characteristics. The motive and guiding power behind them, in all cases without exception, is kundalini.

For the attainment of a transhuman dimension of consciousness, the evolution of morals is as much if not more necessary than the evolution of the intellect.

The brute in humankind is still very much alive. We come across these deviations in the bloody acts of criminals, in devastative wars, in oppression and in the exploitation of weak, downtrodden human beings. In the present state of society these evils appear to be irremediable and have persisted for hundreds of thousands of years. Side by side with the achievements of science, the continued existence of these evils is fraught with the greatest hazard for the race.

But in our own present state of knowledge and resourcefulness we are helpless, as we do not possess any sure defense against them. On the contrary, the achievements of technology, when used for evil, can prove to be terribly destructive, obliterating all the benefits they had conferred when employed for good. One single all-out nuclear war fought between superpowers could wipe out every trace of civilization from the earth. One nuclear device in the hands of a desperado or of a terrorist group could endanger the lives of millions of human beings. In coming ages, with further irresistible advances in technology, the safety of nations and even of the whole species will always hang by a slender thread that a single mistake or imprudent act can cut asunder in the twinkling of an eye.

I am sometimes asked the question, "How can it be possible to rear up whole crops of harmoniously evolved personalities to act as guiding lights in every department of human endeavor and thought when the phenomenon of illumination has been so rare in the past? How can there arise hundreds of thousands of successful initiates, when the exercises to be performed and the self-mastery to be gained are very difficult for an average individual to understand?"

The answer is very simple. There is no awareness at the moment of the surpassing state of glory, supernal knowledge, supreme happiness, miraculous powers, and the extraordinary talents to which spiritual discipline can lead. There is no awareness because there is hardly any fully developed example of this exuberant bloom of the mental faculties alive in the world today.

There *have* been many of them in the past, including the founders of major faiths, and there will be many more in the ages to come. Scientific experiments to be conducted on the phenomenon are sure to lead to startling discoveries. There is no treasure and no position of power on the earth even remotely comparable to the fabulous wealth and majesty of Cosmic Consciousness.

Wide awareness of the marvelous and blissful possibilities latent in spiritual striving and the encouragement provided by the positive results of scientific study will create an interest in the rank and file of the human race so that millions will be prepared to make this the goal of their life, sparing no effort to achieve it.

This would mark the beginning of a new adventure and a new direction for channeling human energy which, at the present moment, finds no satisfactory outlet in the pursuit of wealth or position, sensual satisfaction, name, or fame. Even if only a few succeed out of the first millions of seekers, the precedent established would be so phenomenal that the knowledge of this new Eldorado will spread like wildfire through the length and breadth of the world, causing an enthusiasm and a rush for this fabulous prize that has no parallel in history.

The importance attached and homage paid to political leaders, financial magnates, conquerors, and great artists will then occupy only a secondary place as compared to the adoration and reverence commanded by the surpassing products of education and spiritual discipline combined—the Christs and Buddhas of the ages to come.

Once established, this possibility of a fabulous bloom of the mental faculties latent in every human organism is sure to create a revolution in human life. What proportion this revolution will assume in the ages to come we cannot even imagine at present. Suffice it to say that prospective parents, who now readily make every sacrifice for the offspring, both in the prenatal period and after birth, striving their utmost to ensure a bright and happy future for their darlings, would now weave new fantasies and dream new dreams for them.

They would see them rising to the heights of a cosmic conscious sage, commanding the respect of multitudes. But they would also know that for the materialization of this alluring dream they, too, would have to play a decisive part to provide a favorable heredity for the precious child. Like a purifying wave from the skies, the knowledge of kundalini and the verification of the phenomenon of spiritual transformation, as a result of disciplines that accelerate the evolution of the brain, will change the direction of human life from its present hunt for ignoble objectives towards the sublime quest for the glory of the soul—the fount of immortality, peace, and surpassing happiness.

I am writing more for the future than for the present generations of humanity. Today, the overhanging threat to the survival of the race is the result of mental rust which we are not able to clean—the rust of evil custom and habit, of conservatism, chauvinism, dogma, pride, prejudice, and bias. This rust is as much in evidence in the ranks of science as in those of religion, in communists as much as in capitalists, in democracies as much as in monarchies or dictatorships. It is this mental rust which is carrying humanity to the brink of disaster, awake and alert to the danger, and yet powerless to avert it.

All our social customs are the customs of this mental rust. The brain is not able to rid itself of the poisonous decay and renovate its thinking. The reason why decadent nations take pride in glorifying the achievements of their ancestors, without feeling humiliated at the degeneration that has occurred is because, like the senile, they are not able to understand the change that has taken place.

Child marriages in India were common until 1927. It was only in that year that a bill for the abolition of child marriages was introduced in the legislative assembly. During the course of discussion on the bill it was revealed that 15,625 children of all communities had been married that year. The bill was passed in the year 1929. Before this date, child marriage was common in our community. A bride went to live with her husband at the age of eight or ten years. They were not, however, allowed to sleep together until the couple grew older in age. A day was fixed for the ceremony, when a separate room was allotted to them.

The people accepted these customs as legacies left by their ancestors that had to be honored, and for which there must have been valid reasons for their imposition. The very idea of revolt against such a palpably preposterous usage seldom entered the mind of the average individual. What we now look at with horror and incredulity appeared normal and natural to the people whose minds had been enslaved by the practice.

The same is true of other hideous customs, as for instance the practice of infanticide of Indian girl children by their parents rather than face the humiliation and the heavy expenses of dowries which the birth of a girl child involved. The parents preferred to end the menace at its birth. Another diabolical abuse still current is that of bride burning by families dissatisfied by a marriage settlement. A glance at history is sufficient to show to what unbelievable extent the human mind was held in the grip of ridiculous, fantastic, or horrible customs and practices all over the world, without waking up to their cruelty and stupidity until powerful reformative influences or a revolution brought it to its senses with a jolt.

The multitudes who now inhabit the earth, born and bred in the present social and political orders or religious beliefs accept them as normal and natural in the same way that such practices as child marriage or infanticide, which now excite our indignation and contempt, appeared normal and natural to the people in India before the practices were abolished by law.

The continuance of war, political dissension, international rivalry and competition, religious dogma, and social discord at a time when humanity has gained the power to annihilate itself in a matter of hours is no better than the continuance of habits of thought and action, customs and practices that are more preposterous, more fraught with danger and more unbecoming of the present intellectual stature of mankind than were infanticide and other evil customs of the past. We are not conscious of this anomaly because our minds are working in the same old groove and we will continue to act in the same way until we are brought to our senses by a similar jolt.

In the present era of unprecedented technological development and of high explosives powerful enough to wipe out large cities in a moment, the least vagrant tendency of the mind in the leaders, especially in those holding seats of power, is fraught with the gravest danger for the race. A single unpremeditated act or an unforeseen chain of circumstances, reacting on ethically inferior minds, however dominating intellectually, can give off the spark that might suffice to reduce whole portions of the smiling garden of humanity to mounds of virulent ash.

Consequently, so long as the basic facts about mind are not known and science does not come into possession of effective techniques to control inherent propensities, which, present in men and women holding positions of authority, can cause havoc on a global scale, mankind will continue to bide precariously on the top of a sleeping volcano liable to violent eruption at any time.

The only sure safeguard against the now constantly overhanging threat of an annihilating war is comprehensive knowledge of kundalini. I feel that it is the unseen hand of destiny which, in spite of my limitations, drives me to present a demonstrable religious truth of paramount importance that can save humanity at this crucial time, when it is drifting helplessly towards the greatest disaster it has ever suffered, all because of its utter ignorance of the laws of the mighty mechanism operating in the system of every member of the race.

The only source of strength I possess is my absolute conviction of the correctness under all circumstances of the disclosures I am making about kundalini. I feel completely sure that the main characteristics of the awakening described in this work, the results

376 LIVING WITH KUNDALINI

defined, and ultimate consequences foretold will be fully established by experiment and by corroboration from unexpected sources, partly before the end of this century and mainly in the centuries to come.

I am also certain that the disclosure of a mighty law of Nature that could well have remained shrouded in mystery for a long time yet without anyone being able even to make a guess at it is in the nature of a divine revelation. I was led to the knowledge of this momentous truth step by step by the action of a superphysical energy upon my system, shaping it by degrees to the required state of nervous efficiency, as if to be instructed in the ancient science I was destined to make known in a verifiable form suited to the tendencies of the age.

One may ask how all that I can say could have such an effect on the world as to succeed in creating the mental climate that will remove the threat of wars, usher in an era favorable to the establishment of a universal religion, a new world order, and a one-world government, with the demolition of racial and color barriers and the introduction of other much-needed reforms conducive to the unhindered progress and uninterrupted happiness of mankind.

The answer is simple, so simple perhaps that many may find it hard to reconcile its apparently ordinary character with the colossal nature of the transformation it is expected to bring about. All the changes I have mentioned will be brought about by the simple device of demonstrating empirically the alteration wrought in the human organism by a voluntarily awakened kundalini. In every successful experiment the results would be so positive as to leave absolutely no room for doubt and so astounding as to demand immediate revision of some of the most firmly established scientific theories and concepts of today, leading inevitably to the transference of the world's attention from purely materialistic objectives and projects to spiritual and psychical problems and pursuits.

The fortunate individual in whom the divine energy is benignly disposed from the beginning, possessing the psychical and biological endowments, which as far as I have been able to judge, predisposed to a favorable termination, will, after varying periods normally extending to years, show remarkable developments, both internally and externally, so startling and, judging from the prevalent notions of great thinkers, so unexpected that they are sure to strike with overwhelming effect not only the subject but also the trained scientists engaged in the observation of the phenomenon.

Inwardly the individual will bloom into a visionary, the vehicle of expression of a higher consciousness endowed with a spiritual or mental sixth sense; outwardly perhaps a religious genius, a prophet, an intellectual giant, with bewildering versatility and insight, completely altered mentally from what they were before the experiment.

In exceptional cases, and such instances will occur in the era to come when more facts become known about the mode of operation of the mighty power, the favored mortal may develop into a superman or superwoman, capable of prodigious spiritual, mental, and physical feats, a source of ever-present awe and wonder to the multitudes and of inspiration and guidance to others already firmly planted on the path but not destined to reach such heights. Most of the successful hierarchs will sooner or later find access to the eternal repository of infinite wisdom to bring, in inimitable language, inspired messages suited to the need for the enlightenment and guidance of humanity.

The idea that under the direct influence of the cosmic Life Energy the human brain is still in a state of organic evolution is a fact so important that, compared to it, all other discoveries of modern science pale into insignificance. Continued evolution of the human organism, in its turn, points unmistakably towards a conclusion which is often discredited by the orthodox evolutionists of our day. What it clearly implies is that there must exist a predetermined target or, in other words, an already existing blueprint of consciousness towards which humanity is evolving. At this stage of intelligence it would be the height of folly to assume that this evolution would be governed by accidental mutations of the genes taking eccentric directions about which we can have no knowledge at present. The steady and systematic way in which the human mind has advanced in intelligence, knowledge, and skill provides a clear rebuttal to this stand. There can be no dispute about the position that this evolution is proceeding in a certain direction about which we have little or no awareness at present.

There is every likelihood that the reality of continued evolution will be brought home to scholars of our time with the shock of a thunderbolt. It is only then that the shell of disbelief that covers our thinking will be broken, never to be rejoined again. It often needs a shock to rouse the human intellect from an accustomed erroneous way of thought.

Not until the British rulers in India made the custom of *sati* a capital crime did the orthodox pandits refrain from a practice unparalleled in its horror and inhumanity. Until the utter lunacy of our present way of thinking that continues to rely on war for the settlement of disputes, even in the nuclear age, is brought home to us by a catastrophe, the human intellect will continue to act in this dangerous way.

Sufficient sleep, proper food, moderate sexual indulgence, temperance, an active altruistic life, conformity to sublime ideals and healthy principles, noble and benevolent traits of character—these are the essentials of a life spent in concordance with the demands of evolution. Even in this age when we glance round us triumphantly at our marvelous achievements, the leaders of thought and the elders of nations seem as ignorant of these laws of the healthy evolution of every individual as physicians of the past were ignorant of the bacteria that caused plague and cholera and took a toll of millions of lives. They seem unaware of the fact that crime, insanity, violence, and war are as amenable to control when these laws are known as virulent contagious diseases have proved to be controllable in our time.

The leading personalities in every sphere of life—politics, industry, trade, technology, science, art, philosophy, religion, healing, law, defense, and the like—attain to their respective prominent positions through certain qualities that they possess. Intelligence, perseverance, dynamism, eloquence, versatility, flair for a particular avocation, industrious application, courage, resourcefulness, tact, and the like are some of the qualities they must possess to supersede or excel other competitors in the field. For these precious endowments they must always depend on the capacity of their brains. Education, training, and early environment play only a secondary role. Primarily it is the inherent potential of the brain which determines the leader or the successful contestant in the battle for life.

In every branch of human endeavor it is not always the most erudite or the most widely read who distinguish themselves. Many of the greatest names in history are those who were poorly educated or who had no education at all. The exercise of the intellect as involved in education leads only to a partial development of the human personality. The exercise of the will, involved in gaining mastery over our passions, emotions, and desires, involved in spiritual discipline is at least as much, if not more, necessary to make an individual a truly cultured citizen of the world. Judging from the present conditions, it would not be possible for the race to exist with safety or security for even another hundred years in the technological age. There is hardly any sober, far-sighted lover of humanity whose heart is not filled with misgivings about the future in the context of the chaotic trends visible at present.

It is not possible to turn back the hands of the clock of time. Our current customs, conventions, laws, values, and standards are not designed for a state of society in possession of the awesome powers which science has placed in our hands. Our present ideas of religion, philosophy, justice, right, and wrong are equally inappropriate to the demands of the present or the ages to come. Materialism on the one hand and institutional religions on the other, leading to the segregation of human beings into different self-contained compartments, are limiting the powers of perception of the human mind to a dangerous extent by their antagonism and friction and may lead to a conflagration that can swallow us all.

Materialism, with its bristling armies, ideas of superiority and spirit of rivalry with neighbors can prove even more destructive. The gulf between rich and poor, learned and illiterate, white and black, high caste and low, the tussle for equality between men and women, the competition between the advanced nations and the backward— any one of these can become the focal point of a dispute highly dangerous for the safety of the race. The time has come when humankind as a whole has to shed the now worn-out scale of thought and equip itself with new ideas and values as a measure of survival in the age to come.

Only a few successful experiments would suffice to convince the world of the validity and the natural character of the kundalini phenomenon. The results obtained would furnish the evidence necessary to find out the nature and purpose of the religious impulse in men and women, reveal the mysterious sovereign power from which prophets and sages drew their authority and inspiration, disclose the source of genius, lay bare the secret fount of art, and above all, make known the immediate goal destined by nature for humanity, which it must achieve at any cost to live in peace and plenty.

On the empirical side, the effects will be uniformity of symptoms, regularity and ordered sequence of the biological processes, clearly observable day to day for years, indicative of the action of a superior form of vital energy in the organism, resulting finally in the complete alteration of personality and development of superior mental faculties. This cannot but lead irresistibly to the conclusion that by the operation of some extraordinary biological law yet entirely unknown to science, the human organism can complete within the period of a few years the evolutionary cycle needed for its ascension to the next stage, requiring in the normal course of events enormous spans of time for completion of the process.

The paramount importance of the issues raised by this psychophysiological phenomenon, viewed in the perspective of the modern scientific trend, cannot be exaggerated. The emergence of a consciousness of the transcendental type at the end of a certain period, the inevitable result of the awakening of kundalini in all successful cases, provides incontrovertible evidence for the fact that the regenerative force at work in the body is, at the very beginning, aware of the ultimate pattern to which it has to conform by means of the remodeling biological processes set in progress.

The existence of an empirically demonstrable power in the system, not only fully aware of all the perplexing psychophysical intricacies of the organism, but also capable of reshaping it to a far higher pitch of organic and functional activity so as to bring it in harmony with the demands of a higher state of consciousness, can have only one meaning: that the evolutionary force in humanity is carrying us towards an already known, and predetermined, state of sublimity of which we have no inkling save that provided by the religious concepts of prophets and visionaries.

The awakening of kundalini is the greatest enterprise and the most wonderful achievement confronting human beings. There is absolutely no other way open to our restlessly searching intellect to pass beyond the boundaries of the otherwise meaningless physical universe.

It provides the only method available to science to establish empirically the existence of life as an immortal, all-intelligent power behind the physical phenomena on earth, and brings within its scope the possibility of planned cultivation of genius in individuals not gifted with it from birth, thereby unfolding before the mental eye of the human race avenues and channels for the acceleration of progress and enhancement of prosperity which it is impossible to visualize fully at present. But the heroic enterprise can only be undertaken by highly intelligent, serene, and sober men and women of chaste ideals and noble resolves. The experiment is to be made by them on their own precious flesh and at the present moment even at the risk of their lives and sanity.

When conducted by the right type of individual on proper lines and with due precautions, partly explained in these pages and partly explained in my other works, the experiment will surely be successful in a few cases, sufficient to demonstrate the existence of the mechanism leading to the kundalini awakening with divergent results.

The reaction created in the system may subside after a while, fizzling out like an ignited match without effecting any noteworthy alteration in the subject, after existing as a remarkable and weird biological phemonenon for months, open to observaton and capable of analysis and measurement; or it may, after varying periods, lead ultimately to permanent injury, either mental or physical, or even death.

But in the really successful cases, the transformative process generated may lead to that sublime state which carries the erring mortal to superphysical heights in joyous proximity to the everlasting, omniscient, conscious Reality, more wonderful than wonder and more secret than secrecy, which, as embodied life, manifests itself in countless forms—ugly and beautiful, good and bad, wise and foolish, living, enjoying, and suffering all around us.

The experiments, besides providing indisputable evidence for the existence of design in creation, would at the same time open to view a new and healthy direction designed by nature for the sublimation of human energy and the use of human resources, at present frittered away in frivolous pursuits, debasing amusements, and ignoble enterprises unsuited to the dignity of human beings.

The knowledge of the safest methods for awakening kundalini and their empirical application on themselves by the noblest men and women, physically and mentally equipped for it, will yield for humanity a periodic golden crop of towering spiritual and mental prodigies who, and who alone, in the atomic and post-atomic age will be able to discharge in a proper manner, consistent with the safety and security of the race, the supreme office of the true ministers of God and the rulers of humanity.

It is, of course, a great mistake to suppose that the awakening of kundalini or entry into the transcendental state of consciousness can make one infallible, all-wise, and all-knowing. Attribution of infallibility and absolute wisdom to prophets and sages has been mainly responsible for the evil side of religion. If the human race is not to stagnate, knowledge must continue to grow indefinitely. The dogma of infallibility precludes further progress in knowledge and is, therefore, inimical to the evolution of the mind.

I do not feel myself to be superior in any way to my fellow human beings. There is no idea of purity or chastity, virtue or saintliness in my mind to inflate my ego. Our whole constitution stands on frailty. We live always at the mercy of forces beyond our ken. Buddha is said to have died of dysentery. Shankaracharya died of an intestinal ailment at the age of thirty-three. Paramahamsa Ramakrishna passed away with the ravages of cancer. Disease, decay, and death claimed the body of every illuminated individual without any distinction between them and ordinary mortals. It is probable that the knowledge of medical therapy now available, if applied in their time, might have prolonged the lives of some of them who died of what are now curable or preventable diseases.

I still continue to learn from my friends and associates. There is hardly any man or woman who has not a beautiful trait of character or a small store of wisdom lying inside. It is through the inherent goodness in people that the human race is able to prosper and progress. Legions hesitate to speak an untruth, to sell dear, to adulterate, to be unjust, to deceive, to blackmail, to be mean or avaricious, not out of fear of the law but because of an inner impulse which keeps them on the side of right. The great importance of religions and their founders stems from the fact that they sowed and nurtured this righteous impulse. But the materialistic thinking of the last two centuries now poses a great threat to the human race because it tends to uproot and destroy this natural, still developing inner impulse of goodness.

Entry to transhuman consciousness adds highly to human responsibilities. We have now gained awareness of the potentialities of the intellect and the almost limitless power it can exercise, both for destructive and constructive purposes. Only a century back our ancestors had no awareness of the colossal technological achievements possible to us, with the exercise of our mental ability and skill. What undreamed-of possiblities will open before us and what stupendous forces will come under our sway with the further evolution of mind to the transhuman state, it is impossible to conceive at present. It might become possible even for the human race to extend sovereignty over all the solar system as it does now over the earth.

How can nature allow us to win this sovereign position unless we have also gained the capability to shoulder the highly increased responsibility in a befitting manner and do not abuse the almost superhuman powers gained? This is the reason why in every case of the awakening of kundalini, secret devices in the brain come into play to mold the individual towards a state of mind where the possibility of abuse of psychic power is eliminated. This is also why almost all those who possess psychic talents are never able to control the power or to exhibit them at will and choice, or even to remain fully alert and conscious when the phenomena come to pass.

This is also the reason why through all the past, in spite of the great advances made in spiritual science, as for instance in India, the secret of domination over the supermundane forces of creation was never openly revealed. And discoveries, whether in the spiritual or the material realm, were made in a series of different minds and were not vouchsafed to only one individual, such as Buddha or Christ, however high their spiritual stature might have been.

In all honesty, I cannot present an exaggerated version of what I know is necessary for the knowledge of the Serpent Power or make my narrative more attractive or sensational with concocted material or even refrain from criticism when it seems it is due in order to make my books acceptable and pleasing to readers.

The only exceptional knowledge I possess is the harvest of the extraordinary experiences I have undergone. I still keep my intellect free and benefit immensely from other books I read. In my contact with the world, in my knowledge of it, and in dealing with mundane affairs, I am no better than millions of my fellow beings and maybe at times display even less practical sense than many of them. In my contact with the transcendental world to which I slowly gained entry after the awakening, I am but a child, constantly wondering at what I perceive, trying to pick up the alphabet of a language more difficult to follow than any knowledge ever gained of the physical universe.

I have never been able to understand why pilgrims to the inner shrine should arrogate to themselves positions of power as great spiritual teachers and guides, or lay claim to exceptional piety, purity, or infallibility when in every description of the divine encounter recorded during the past thousands of years we find expressions of wonder, mystification, and incomprehensibility written large across them. The supreme experience is staggering, enrapturing, blissful, and inspiring, but at the same time inexplicable and un-graspable by the intellect. The experience is supremely illuminating because it reveals the grandeur, sublimity and the eternal nature of the soul, but beyond that—what? All that is beyond lies out of the reach of the intellect and hence cannot be translated into any language devised by the mind.

The inscrutable and ineffable nature of mystical ecstasy cannot constitute a permanent barrier to the unraveling of the Great Mystery. The evolution of the human being is a transition from darkness to light. But this transition has to occur over millions of years. At the first dim dawn of reason the new processes of thought must have appeared strange and inexplicable to the evolving primate. He must have felt bewildered when the new-born faculty began to overrule the instinctive behavior of the mind.

Entry to another dimension of consciousness, where reason is superseded, must have the same perplexing and mystifying effect on the mind. When the area of study is accurately demarcated through painstaking resarch of the phenomenon, a new alphabet, a new language, and a new symbology will develop to express and interpret the experience. A time will surely come when all the resources of science and the intellect will be mobilized to gain more and more insight into this extraordinary state in terms of the intellect.

The inquiry is not to be approached in the spirit of conquest or arrogance, with the intent to achieve victory over a force of nature which has characterized man's approach to the problems of the material world, but rather with humility, in a spirit of utter surrender to Divine Will and absolute dependence on Divine Mercy.

There is no other way save this open to men and women to arrive at the solution of an otherwise impenetrable mystery of creation, no other way open to us to find out what path has been aligned for our progress by Nature, no other way for us to know and recognize ourselves, and no other way to save us from the awful consequence of conscious or unconscious violation of the mighty laws which rule our destiny. This is the only method to bridge the gulf at present yawning between science and religion, between warring political ambitions and ideologies more deadly than the most virulent disease and more awful than all the epidemics combined, between religious faiths, races, nations, classes, and finally between human beings.

This is the immortal light, held aloft by Nature from time immemorial to guide the faltering footsteps of erring humanity across the turns and twists, ups and downs, of the winding path of evolution, the light which shone in the prophets and sages of antiquity, which continues to shine in the men and women of genius and seers of today, and will continue to shine for all eternity, illuminating the vast amphitheater of the universe for the marvelous, unending play of the eternal, almighty, queen of creation—life.

Epilogue

PANDIT GOPI KRISHNA died July 31, 1984, at the age of eighty-one, after a severe lung infection.

After he attained his inspired condition of higher consciousness, he made strenuous effort to interest scientists in studying this condition in himself as a then-living example of this rare and almost legendary phenomenon, previously known only from the writings of past saints and mystics of East and West. For a time, a government-sponsored project in India actually planned to undertake this important scientific research, but with a change in government the project was abandoned. No other scientific group evinced sufficient interest in undertaking research during the Pandit's lifetime, and so an incredibly rare opportunity was lost. This is particularly surprising in view of the warm endorsement of the Pandit's experience by such a world famous physicist and philosopher as Professor C. F. Freiherr von Weizsacker, director of the Max Planck Institute for the Life Sciences, Munich, Germany. However, friends of the Pandit have established Kundalini Research Organizations in New York, Canada, and Switzerland to collate information on the subject of kundalini, collect case histories of individuals, and promote scientific and medical research. In the United States, inquiries about the work and publications of Gopi Krishna may be addressed to The Kundalini Research Foundation, Ltd., P.O. Box 2248, Darien, CT 06820, U.S.A. In Canada, books by Gopi Krishna may be ordered from F.I.N.D. Research Trust, R.R. 5 Flesherton, Ontario N0C 1E0.

Glossary

ajna chakra The sixth chakra, sometimes referred to as the "third eye." It lies in the space between the eyebrows and is regarded as the seat of consciousness.

apana One of the five pranas. Apana flows downward and is active in the lower part of the body, governing functions such as elimination and childbirth.

asana Any of the postures or positions of hatha yoga.

ashram A hermitage or center for meditation and religious study under a teacher.

bandha Lit., "bondage," "fetter." A yogic exercise involving contraction of the throat, abdomen, or sphincter muscles, associated with the practice of pranayama.

bhakti yoga The yoga of love and devotion, in which intense love for a divine incarnation or some other embodiment of God leads to merging with the chosen ideal.

brahmarandhra Lit., "Brahma's crevice" or "cave of Brahma." The crucible of consciousness; the neural network in the brain vitalized by kundalini in mystical consciousness, symbolically portrayed as an aperture in the crown of the head.

Brahman The eternal, imperishable Absolute; the supreme nondual Reality.

chakra Lit., "wheel," "circle." One of the centers of vital energy in the human subtle body. In kundalini yoga, there are seven principal chakras that lie along the *sushumna*.

hatha yoga A yoga consisting of various bodily postures, purification exercises, and breathing practices.

ida One of the main channels (*nadi*) of subtle energy that conduct prana throughout the body. The *ida* neural network is linked with the left nostril and is known as the channel of lunar energy; it corresponds to the parasympathetic nervous system.

jiva   The embodied self that exists in the realm of duality.

jnana yoga   The yoga of knowledge, which lead to God through intellectual discrimination between the false and transitory and what is true and of lasting value.

karma   Lit., "action." The chain of cause and effect operating in human relationships and individual moral evolution.

karma yoga   The yoga of action, consisting of selfless service performed without expectation of personal reward, the aspirant dedicating the fruits of action to Universal Consciousness.

kundalini   Lit., "snake," "coiled." The evolutionary force, also known as the Serpent Power, envisioned metaphorically as a female serpent which, in a dormant or potential state, lies coiled, asleep, at the base of the spine. When awakened, it rises through and vitalizes the chakras, bringing spiritual knowledge, mystical vision, psychic powers, and, ultimately, enlightenment, if the condition of *urdhavaretas* is achieved. When gone awry, the process can lead to insanity. Kundalini is also the name of the goddess who personifies this creative energy.

mantra   A verbal formula, consisting of a syllable, word, or words, which is repeated as a prayer or meditation.

maya   The principle of cosmic illusion or ignorance, based on misinterpreting a partial aspect of Reality.

mudra   A symbolic hand gesture used ritually in religious worship or meditation.

muladhara chakra   The first, or root, chakra, located at the lowest part of the *sushumna* between the genitals and the anus. In the unawakened state, the kundalini as human potential is pictured as lying coiled in the *muladhara*.

nadi   One of the energy channels through which prana passes to all parts of the body. The major *nadis* are the *ida, pingala,* and *sushumna.*

Para-Shakti   The highest aspect of the creative energy, pictured as the Divine Mother, who stands behind the entire creation.

pingala   One of the main channels (*nadi*) of subtle energy that conduct prana throughout the body. The *pingala* neural network is linked to the right nostril and is known as the channel of solar energy; it corresponds to the sympathetic nervous system.

prana   Lit., "breath." The cosmic energy that penetrates and maintains the body and that is most overtly manifest in the breath. Hinduism identifies five different pranas: prana itself, the pure life force; *vyana,* which guides the circulation; *samana,* controlling the intake and metabolism of nutrients; *apana,* which governs elimination and is active in the lower part of the body; and *udana,* which works in the upper body and creates a bridge between the physical and the spiritual. The combusting agent that converts physical energy into radiation, as sexual energy and mental activity.

pranayama   The fourth stage of raja yoga, consisting of breathing exercises aimed at controlling the prana.

raja yoga   Lit., "royal yoga." One of the important yogas leading toward union with God; the eightfold path described by Patanjali in his *Yoga Sutras.*

sadhaka   One who practices *sadhana*; a seeker or aspirant.

sadhana   Practices that lead to the mastery of one of the yogic paths.

sadhu   A holy person, often a monk, who has renounced the world in the quest for the realization of God.

sahasrara chakra   The seventh chakra, located at the crown of the head, above the upper end of the *sushumna.* Its physical correspondence is the brain.

sannyasi   One who has renounced the world and who lives without possessions solely for the realization of God.

shakti   Lit., "power," "energy." Thr primal energy, personified as the goddess Shakti, who is the consort of Shiva and who is venerated under many names.

Shiva   The third god of the Hindu trinity, along with Brahma the Creator and Vishnu the Preserver; Shiva, the symbol of higher consciousness, is the Destroyer (of ignorance or illusion). The rising of kundalini from the root chakra to the crown chakra, the "seat of Shiva," is envisioned as the union of Shiva and his consort, Shakti.

siddha   A sage or seer.

siddhi   Supernatural powers or abilities that may appear as by-products of spiritual development.

sushumna   The main channel (*nadi*) of subtle energy, extending from the base of the spine to the brain. The awakened kundalini rises in the *sushumna*, which is in the center between *ida* and *pingala*.

urdhava-retas   Lit., "reversal of the seed." The reversal of the reproductive system and the flowing of the seminal essence or nerve energy upward through the spinal cord and into the brain. *Urdhava-retas* forms the basis of kundalini yoga and, in fact, is the ultimate aim of every form of yoga practiced for the attainment of transcendent states of consciousness.

yoga   Lit., "yoke." One of the paths to union with Cosmic Consciousness. Different types include bhakti, karma, jnana, raja, kriya, and kundalini yoga. *Yoga* signifies both the union attained (between the soul and the Oversoul) and the method or methods by which this union is achieved. The aim of yoga is to accelerate the process of evolution, a natural process already at work in the human organism, to open new areas of supersensory perception in the brain capable of manifesting a transhuman state of consciousness receptive to revelation.

Other Books by Gopi Krishna

The Awakening of Kundalini. New York: E.P. Dutton & Co., 1975.
Toronto: F.I.N.D. Research Trust/Kundalini Research Foundation,
1989.

Biblical Prophecy for the Twentieth Century. Toronto: New Age
Publishing Ltd., 1979.

The Biological Basis of Religion and Genius. New York: N.C. Press,
Inc., 1971, and Harper and Row, 1972. London: Turnstone Press,
1973.

Dawn of a New Science. Part I. New Delhi: Kundalini Research &
Publication Trust, 1978.

From the Unseen. Kashmir: Gopi Krishna, 1952. F.I.N.D. Research
Trust/New Concepts Publishing, 1985.

Kundalini: The Evolutionary Energy in Man. London: Vincent Stuart
& John M. Watkins, 1970. Boston & London: Shambhala, 1985.

Kundalini for the New Age. New York: Bantam Books, 1988.

The Present Crisis. New York: New Concepts Publishing, for the
Kundalini Research Foundation. 1981.

The Riddle of Consciousness. New York: Kundalini Research
Foundation, 1976.

The Secret of Yoga. New York: Harper and Row, 1972.

Secrets of Kundalini in Panchastavi. New Delhi: Kundalini Research &
Publication Trust, 1978.

The Shape of Events to Come. New Delhi: Kundalini Research &
Publication Trust, 1979.

*Three Perspectives on Kundalini: The Real Nature of Mystical
Experience, Reason and Revelation, Kundalini in Time and Space.*
Toronto: F.I.N.D. Research Trust/Kundalini Research Foundation,
1991.

The Way to Self-Knowledge. Toronto: F.I.N.D. Research Trust/New
Concepts Publishing, 1985. Toronto: F.I.N.D. Research Trust/
Kundalini Research Foundation, 1987.

What Is and What Is Not Higher Consciousness. New York: Julian
Press, 1974. Toronto: F.I.N.D. Research Trust/Kundalini Research
Foundation, 1988.

The Wonder of the Brain. Toronto: F.I.N.D. Research Trust/Kundalini
Research Foundation, 1987.

Yoga—A Vision of Its Future. New Delhi: Kundalini Research &
Publication Trust, 1978.

Index

absorption, 264, 289, 294, 298, 301, 358
adepts, 266; ancient, 152, 243; of India, China, or Egypt, 180
ambrosia, 132. *See also* nectar
apana, 194–95
ascetics, 125, 133
avadhuts, 73, 75
Avalon, Arthur, 354, 358, 361

Bhagavad Gita, 41, 66, 83, 116
biological: changes, 330; evolution, 275; law(s), 214–16, 227, 238, 247, 248, 252, 380; phenomenon, 357; process(es), 152, 218, 247, 256, 348–49, 380–81
bioplasma, 169
bliss, 351
brain, 169, 171–72, 176, 183–88, 194, 216–17, 271, 284, 297, 340–43; conscious center in, 210; ecstasy in, 362; effects of kundalini on, 142–51, 154–55, 198, 201–03, 206, 221, 223, 232, 234, 247–48, 262, 267; evolution of, 330, 373, 377; inherent potential, 379; intoxicated condition of, 302; light in, 2, 6, 145, 163, 360; metamorphosis of, 111, 264, 370; and nerves, 346; and nervous system, 145, 185, 208, 234, 240, 243–44, 248; new attunement of, 249, 329; nourishment of, 244–45; primate, 364; secret devices in, 384; silent region in, 22–24, 361; transcendental conditions of, 300; virulent poison in, 158–62; widening of cognitive center, 365
breathing exercises, breath, 195, 218. *See also* pranayama

Buddha, Buddhism, 334, 383, 384
burning, 150, 158, 160–63

celibacy, 121, 333, 334, 360
center in the brain, 150, 155, 171, 244–47, 267; cognitive, 230; seventh, 124, 155, 190. *See also* chakra(s)
cerebrospinal system, 21, 238, 252, 254, 349, 355, 358, 361–62, 363, 364
chakra(s), 193, 253, 255, 360; *ajna*, 358; *muladhara*, 186, 358; *sahasrara*, 349, 354, 355–57. *See also* center; heart center; lotus(es)
channel of communication, 347; with the supersensible, 182
clairvoyance, 73–76, 278–79
cognitive: apparatus, 224; faculty, 147, 149, 216, 226, 227, 263
compassion, 109, 115, 353
concentration, 2, 113, 150, 158, 171, 178, 191, 200, 201, 218, 237, 252, 254, 298, 356, 358, 364. *See also* meditation
conscious energy, 217
conscious universe, 290–92
consciousness, 3, 152, 291; cosmic, 22, 34, 132, 208, 340, 369, 372; expansion in, 262, 265, 290, 330, 365–66; extended, 156, 162, 188, 224–25, 240, 343; higher, 116, 183, 248, 334, 377; lustrous, 265, 297; metamorphosis in, 363; peripheral, 226, 234; texture of, 263; transcendental, 223, 381–82; transformed, 360; transhuman, 371, 383
contemplation, 286. *See also* meditation

395

sages, 79, 210, 370, 373, 383; of
antiquities, 386. *See also* holy men;
saints; seers
saints, 9, 154, 156, 178, 180, 190,
205, 212, 214, 269, 328, 337, 387
samadhi, 155, 171, 197, 198; as self-
induced state, 359; consciousness
contemplates itself, 358
Samaj Sudhar Samiti, 281, 305, 306,
308, 313, 317, 323, 342
Sanskrit, 194, 362; alphabet, 253,
360; verses, 288, 296
schizophrenia, 117
science, 79–80, 198, 243, 283–84,
366–67, 381; ancient, 376; bridge
to religion, 386; of kundalini, 351;
and the soul, 338–39; of yoga,
208, 211
scientific: inquiry, 164; mind, 218;
observation, 283–84; research,
357
secret(s), 180, 226, 263, 330, 357; of
domination, 384; of kundalini,
124; of nature, 152; of the soul,
339
seed, 183, 223, 244, 366; sublimated, 186
seers, 184, 197, 212, 300, 327, 370,
386. *See also* holy men; sages;
saints
self-control, 332
self-mastery, 112, 117, 371
self-mortification, 349
self-realization, 252
seminal: essence, 129, 236; energy,
130; glands, 236
Serpent Fire, 15, 62, 154, 164, 178,
186, 203, 225
Serpent Power, 18, 22–23, 123–24,
157, 158, 169, 208, 236, 276, 360,
384
sexual: climax, 362; energy and
higher consciousness, 334; indulgence, 378; organ, 155, 172; region, 237, 256; union, 266–67,
362. *See also* erotic; orgasm; reproductive

Shakti, 58, 154, 190, 191, 197–98,
210, 238, 266; Shastras, 354; union with Shiva, 267
Shankaracharya, 383
Shiva, 155, 159, 211, 350; union
with Shakti, 267
sixth sense, 210, 377
sleep, 145, 210, 233, 246, 251, 273,
296, 300, 301, 342, 378
sleeplessness, 150, 242. *See also* insomnia
solar: nerve, 162, 168; plexus, 270;
system, 384
sounds, 343, 360, 369
spinal: axis, 267; canal, 355; column, 156; cord, 148, 160, 162,
176, 186, 191, 194, 236, 253, 255;
system and nerves, 356
spine, 1, 156, 369
spiritual: development, 182, 243;
discipline, 371–72; discourse, 351;
exercise(s), 182, 208; experience,
113, 249; illumination, 109, 120;
imposter, 338; laws, 339; liberation, 303; phenomena, 215, 248;
powers, 337; practice, 143; and
psychical pursuits, 376; talents,
384; teachers, 210; transformation, 373; unfoldment, 349
spirituality, 369; growth of, 349
sublimation, 236, 382; constant, 223
suffering, 155, 173–74, 192, 214,
223, 236, 256, 262, 269, 293, 304,
369
superconscious, 165, 197, 198, 217,
289; excessive absorption in, 342;
flight, 216, 294; state, 173; vision,
188
superconsciousness, 187, 240
superhuman: agency, 174; powers,
384
superman, 31, 377
supernatural, 144, 151, 173, 181,
212, 222; agency, 215, 247; fear
of, 144, 204, 220; force, 357;
powers, 326, 337
supernormal: faculties, 154, 184;

gifts, 120, 180, 182; psychic development, 243; psychic powers, 238; realm of, 164; spiritual development, 243
superphysical, 197, 216, 329, 382; attributes, 211; energy, 376; existences, 198; medium, 200
supersense, 348; supersensual realm, 301
supersensible, 182, 267, 293; experience, 240; perception, 210; realm, 297
supersensory, 193, 216, 248; channels, 216, 218, 327; experience, 182; knowledge, 185; perception, 218; plane, 265; state of existence, 301
superstition, 180, 182, 195, 216, 256, 326, 356
Supreme Consciousness, 155
supreme: experience, 385; happiness, 351, 371–72; prize, 266
survival, 373, 380
sushumna, 32, 155, 157, 162, 168–70, 170, 201, 210, 255

Tantras, 350, 354, 361, 362
Tantric, 190, 266; lore, 189; practitioner, 361; tradition, 350; yoga, 131, 255
teachers, 210, 385; pseudo-religious, 282
temperance, 251, 378
transcendence, 210, 234
transcendent state, 218
transcendental: consciousness, 223, 370, 382; experience, 183, 293, 294; knowledge, 238, 349; reality, 294; state, 217, 351, 368; visions, 154; world, 385
transformation, 187, 212, 229, 234, 241, 256, 351, 369; in awareness, 287; cellular and organic, 231; of consciousness, 115–17; of nervous system and brain, 257; of personality, 260; power of, 234; proc-

esses of, 210; spontaneous, 212. *See also* metamorphosis
truth, 117, 165, 211, 215, 300, 329, 375, 376
turiya state, 349

uninitiated, 146, 193, 223, 255, 266
Upanishads, 14, 360, 366
urdhava-retas, 130

Vajroli mudra, 129, 130, 133
vak-siddhi, 65
Vedic: age, 121; hymns, 14; religion, 211
vision, 289, 292; extended field of, 229–31; inner, 188, 232, 330
visionaries, 213, 328, 368, 381; visionary experience, 218, 278, 351, 358, 377
vital: current, 4, 154, 330, 345; essence, 237; force, 158; fuel, 343; medium, 198, 227; radiation, 175, 274
vital energy, 149, 194, 235, 346, 377, 380; cosmic, 155, 188, 195
vitality, 366; stream of, 148

war(s), 371, 374; control of, 378; nuclear, 371; remove threat, 376; for settlement of disputes, 378; threat of annihilation, 375
will, 169, 245, 272, 332, 368, 379
willpower, 147, 159, 162, 174, 270
woman, inner, 360–61
worship, 212, 350

yoga, 83, 113, 119, 120, 142, 143–44, 155–56, 165, 182, 190, 192–94, 196, 199, 201, 205–06, 211–12, 218, 254, 350, 356, 363; ancient treatises on, 210; practice(s), 141, 208, 218–19; as a progressive science, 208; Tantric, 131, 255
yogi(s) 10, 14, 158, 178, 186, 190–91, 197–98, 224, 238, 240, 246, 252–53, 274, 338; mature, 358; pseudo-, 338

(Continued on next page)

The Shambhala Dictionary of Buddhism and Zen.

The Spiritual Teaching of Ramana Maharshi, by Ramana Maharshi. Foreword by C. G. Jung.

Tao Teh Ching, by Lao Tzu. Translated by John C. H. Wu.

The Tibetan Book of the Dead: The Great Liberation through Hearing in the Bardo. Translated with commentary by Francesca Fremantle & Chögyam Trungpa.

The Vimalakirti Nirdesa Sutra. Translated & edited by Charles Luk. Foreword by Taizan Maezumi Roshi.

Vitality, Energy, Spirit: A Taoist Sourcebook. Translated & edited by Thomas Cleary.

Wen-tzu: Understanding the Mysteries, by Lao-tzu. Translated by Thomas Cleary.

Worldly Wisdom: Confucian Teachings of the Ming Dynasty. Translated & edited by J. C. Cleary.

Zen Dawn: Early Zen Texts from Tun Huang. Translated by J. C. Cleary.

Zen Essence: The Science of Freedom. Translated & edited by Thomas Cleary.

The Zen Teachings of Master Lin-chi. Translated by Burton Watson.

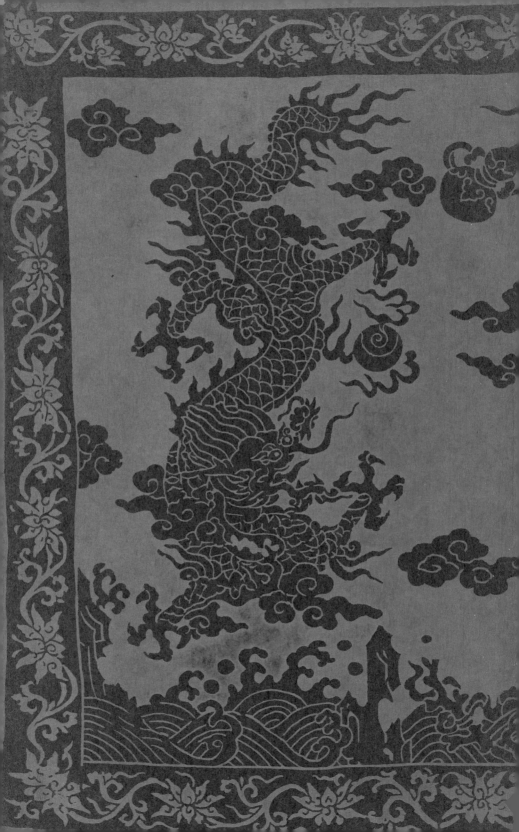